Better Health Through Natural Healing

HOW TO GET WELL WITHOUT DRUGS OR SURGERY

Dr. Ross Trattler

McGRAW-HILL BOOK COMPANY

New York   St. Louis   San Francisco   Auckland   Bogotá   Hamburg
London   Madrid   Mexico   Milan   Montreal   New Delhi   Panama
Paris   São Paulo   Singapore   Sydney   Tokyo   Toronto

This book is not intended to replace the services of a physician. Any application of the recommendations set forth in the following pages is at the reader's discretion and sole risk.

First McGraw-Hill paperback edition 1988.

1 2 3 4 5 6 7 8 9 FGRFGR 8 9 0 9 8

ISBN 0-07-065172-8

LIBRARY OF CONGRESS CATALOGING-IN-PUBLICATION DATA
Trattler, Ross.
  Better health through natural healing.
  Bibliography: p.
  Includes indexes.
  1. Naturopathy—Handbooks, manuals, etc.
2. Therapeutics, Physiological—Handbooks, manuals, etc.   I. Title.
RZ440.T73   1985   615.5'35   84-19369
ISBN 0-07-065172-8

BOOK DESIGN BY A. CHRISTOPHER SIMON

Contents

iii

Contents

Part III   APPENDIXES

Preface to the Paperback Edition

Since the release of the hardbound edition in November 1985, there have been some significant advances in our understanding of the actual biochemical mechanisms involved in the production of certain diseases. Along with this knowledge, there have also been made available several effective medications of natural origin that are not mentioned in the text of this book. I want to take this opportunity to present some of this material briefly.

A great deal of research has been done with essential fatty acids and their role in the treatment of multiple sclerosis and Charcot-Marie-Tooth (CMT) disease. Both these diseases show a progressive demyelination of nerve fibers, and in both diseases a decrease in linoleic acid in the serum and myelin has been found. A biochemical defect in the utilization of linoleic acids is strongly suspected. If this proves to be true, the supplementation of essential fatty acids further along the pathway, beyond the biochemical defect, as concentrated gamma-linolenic acid (GLA) should help prevent progression of these disorders. Although oil of evening primrose has been suggested within the text many times, higher GLA content is now available for less cost from black currant oil. The use of *both* oils is suggested as well as Max EPA and an increase in vitamin E in micellar form to help prevent breakdown of the supplemental fatty acids into substances harmful to the body. Vitamin B_{12}, beta carotene, carnitine, and taurine may also be of some benefit in these conditions.

Psoriasis is another condition found linked to abnormal fatty acid utilization. The suggestions made above should prove helpful in treating psoriasis. You may also wish to try quercetin, a naturally occurring flavinoid with anti-inflammatory activity. Clinically, I have had great success with *strict* adherence to a macrobiotic diet and the *total* exclusion of foods and substances causing an acid condition within the body. These include fruits and fruit juice, citric acid, sugar, honey, sweets of all kinds, alcohol, and tomatoes.

I also want to add a footnote on systemic Candida (yeast) infections. From clinical experience, the most important aspect of therapy is the strict adherence to a macrobiotic diet with the absolute avoidance of *anything* sweet, such as sugar, honey, fruit, fruit juice, vegetable juice, soda, ice cream, and alcohol. I have found the use of nystatin may often be avoided entirely with these dietary changes.

A modality not mentioned in the text but of great usefulness in a wide variety of musculoskeletal problems is interferential electrotherapy. These medium-frequency currents are extremely effective in cases of acute or chronic pain due to muscle spasm, strain, sprain, trigger points, joint dysfunction or trauma, and some cases of neuropathy.

Since the publication of *Better Health through Natural Healing*, I have received a great deal of correspondence that has usually been directed to the publisher. Future correspondence may be sent to me directly here in Maui at:

99 S. Market St., Suite 103
Wailuku, Hawaii 96793

My phone number at my office is (808) 244-8888. Please feel free to call or write, and I will do my best to answer any questions you may have concerning this book. For those interested in my current research, I have just completed a computer search of the medical literature throughout the world on the possible adverse effects of coffee and caffeine, antibiotics, immunizations, and dairy products. This information is available at $5 for each subject or $15 for all four by writing to me at my Maui address. Send check or money order.

I want to express my appreciation for the kind letters and presents I have received from grateful readers throughout the world and hope the paperbound edition reaches many more in need of this information.

Wishing you the *best of health,*

Dr. Ross Trattler

Introduction

This book has been written out of true need. As the years passed in my practice, I found that my memory was far from perfect. Treatments I once knew well and had used successfully sometimes evaded me at the very time they were needed most. In a busy practice, with patient following patient, a doctor is called upon to reach the essence of a problem and its cure with little time for pondering. Late in the afternoon and worn out by a hectic day, I often found myself unable to remember quickly a specifically useful prescription or other aspect of therapy, or which book it was in. The task was not easy, since I use hundreds of reference books regularly. Unfortunately, at present there is no naturopathic equivalent to *The Merck Manual* where one can quickly look up essential details of a particular illness.

After several years of work, I present this book for publication. I hope it will be of some use to both the general public and the physician interested in natural therapies. In reality, naturopathic medicine, or the science and art of natural therapeutics, can never be written down completely. Each naturopath lives and breathes his or her own philosophy and therapies differ widely. Mine is no more correct than others, but it works well for me in my practice. It is my hope and desire to make these methods easier to understand and more accessible.

How to Use This Book

Naturopathic medicine is not a subject that easily lends itself to definition. After all is said and done, naturopathy is a way of life. When practicing as a naturopathic physician, one is forced to translate a philosophical conviction in the healing power of nature, breaking it down into fractions that can easily be understood. Too often the result of this dissection is that the listener begins to feel that naturopathy is diet, or fasting, or spinal manipulation, or botanical medicine—or any of its various parts.

As you read through each chapter, always bear in mind that disease as an entity does not exist. People are at *dis-ease*, each for his or her own unique set of causes. The role of the naturopath, whatever tools he or she may use, is to educate the patient and when necessary help direct and release the inner healing power of nature.

Part I of this book examines the philosophy behind natural therapeutics and presents a brief summary and description of its most frequently used tools. Part II is the practical application of the philosophy and these therapeutic tools as they relate to the most common diseases. Each chapter begins with a brief definition and description of signs and symptoms. There then follows a list of factors possibly related to the cause of the disease. Here you will find most of the causes recognized by orthodox medicine, but, more importantly, factors as seen from a naturopathic perspective. In reviewing this list, consider how much each one may be a factor in your particular case. Next follows a general discussion drawing on the previous section, examining etiology, or causative factors, in more depth. Each discussion section should leave the reader with a clear understanding of what may cause the particular disorder.

Finally comes the treatment section, broken down into diet, physiotherapy, therapeutic agents, and botanicals. Here you will find many suggestions of therapy for each disorder. Obviously, not all of these should be employed in each case. Remember that people are unique in their requirements for cure. Therapies useful in an early stage of a health disorder may not apply later on. People vary widely in their response to therapy, and therefore individual dose prescriptions differ.

Disease is not a stagnant process. Dose prescriptions will vary as the condition changes. Also, the cause of a disease will vary from person to person, calling for different approaches to therapy.

I have tried to make each chapter as practical as possible for home use. Nothing, however, can replace the expertise and knowledge of an experienced and properly trained physician.

Dietary advice has been laid out in stages to represent progression of the disorder toward health; or, in some cases, as specific short-term regimens to be used as indicated. In the acute states of a disease it is generally best to begin with the most restricted regimen, such as a fast or mono diet (a diet containing only one substance). In some cases specific diets, such as the onion diet used for lung congestion, may be the best initial approach. As symptoms improve, one progresses to later stages until a full dietary range has been achieved, which coincides with the arrival of better health.

The choice of physiotherapy is usually very easy. In most conditions, you should do as many and as much as possible. A proper regimen should keep you too busy getting well to stay sick. This, of course, does not apply to those with diseases causing extreme weakness or debilitation, in which case you should choose less vigorous techniques.

Special attention should be given to the sections on vitamins, minerals, and botanical medicines. Many remedial agents are mentioned here, but not all are to be taken with each disease. The choice of therapeutic agents is, by their sheer number, not easy. Individuals vary so widely in their needs during the disease process that only general guidelines are possible. I have attempted to help in this process by asterisking the most frequently used therapeutic agents, and have also given specific dose prescriptions as a general guide. I suggest that you obtain expert advice on your particular needs whenever possible. In addition, I suggest reading and studying in detail a good book on vitamin and mineral therapy, such as John D. Kirschmann's *Nutrition Almanac* before you attempt self-medication.

Botanical medication is much more difficult to use wisely at home without some in-depth knowledge about individual properties of substances. I have asterisked the most-used herbs. To use herbs safely, however, I suggest researching each herb for its properties and general use prior to your use. A good beginning reference book is *The Way of Herbs* by Michael Tierra.

You will probably notice the conspicuous absence of suggestions regarding homeopathy. I feel that homeopathy can only be prescribed individually, even more so than botanicals, to derive any therapeutic results.

For serious or chronic ailments, it is always best to consult a trained physician. Should you live in an area where professional help is simply not available, and by your own choice you decide to follow the suggestions made in this book, please use common sense. Do not allow the disease process to reach a critical stage without some medical supervision.

Most diseases are curable, but not all patients. The benefit you obtain from natural therapy will depend upon the amount of effort you expend. The process of cure does not end when your symptoms disappear, but continues each day as you live more and more according to the laws of nature. Let this book function as a trained guide, giving useful suggestions to help you along the path to self-cure. The rest is up to you.

PART I

What Is
Natural Medicine?

NATUROPATHIC MEDICINE

Natural therapies have been used to treat disease since our earliest beginnings. The first known written records mention herbs and their use in healing. Every known culture has attempted to harness the healing powers in plants. Both the Old and New Testaments speak of herbs and their uses. Hydrotherapy, or the use of water in healing disease, is also very ancient. Early written records describe various uses for water therapy well before either the Roman or Christian eras. These natural therapies were on a few occasions written down, but for the most part they were passed down as oral traditions, as was the case with the American Indians.

When naturopathy as a science distinct from these loosely gathered bits of natural therapy originated, no one can say. Hippocrates is considered the father of naturopathic medicine. The Hippocratic school treated disease with diet, fasting, herbs, hydrotherapy, exercise, and spinal manipulation, prescribed from a basis of principles of healing that are now used as the foundation of naturopathy. Their most basic tenet, *vis medicatrix naturae* (only nature heals), which emphasizes the body's ability to heal itself if given a chance, is still the central theme of naturopathic philosophy.

From these origins naturopathic medicine has grown and developed. Physicians throughout the world have worked within the context of natural therapies, often specializing in one particular aspect such as fasting, hydrotherapy, herbalism, or spinal manipulation, and so developing and perfecting each natural therapeutic tool.

A great surge of development in natural therapies occurred during the last

3

century, when the orthodox medical profession drifted further and further toward the widespread use of drugs and surgery. It was not until the water cure was popularized by the work of Vincent Priessnitz, Sebastian Kneipp, and J. H. Kellogg that naturopathy once again emerged as a distinct discipline. Many schools of hydrotherapy, herbalism, and naturopathy sprang up and flourished in Europe and America. Great pioneers of naturopathy emerged at this time to help convince the skeptical public that nature, not drugs, was the path toward health. Many of these men attempted to prove their convictions by daredevil stunts, flaunting their health for all to witness. I remember reading with awe of early naturopaths swallowing vials of cholera-infected material, or fasting 40 or even 60 days, and then performing incredibly strenuous physical demonstrations to prove their unusual vigor obtained by natural means.

Many of these pioneers left written legacies of great value. Each book tells the story of powerful men of strength, conviction, and courage. Taking whatever assistance they could find from the past, they entered the labyrinth of disease only to discover not confusion, but simplicity. In an age when their colleagues of the orthodox school were finding more and more complexity in disease with the advent of the germ theory, these naturopathic physicians were discovering the very principles of health and disease.

Slowly but steadily orthodox medicine gained political power and united against the freely practicing naturopathic profession. Within a short time, most alternative medical schools were forced to close. Not only were naturopaths declared illegal and prosecuted in most states, but so were midwives and many other health professionals who were seen as either a financial or philosophical threat.

The 1970s and 1980s have been years of reemergence for naturopathic physicians. With the 1960s came a rebirth of awareness and interest in all things "natural." A new generation arose that no longer accepted the status quo blindly. All aspects of modern society were scrutinized; among these the practice of modern medicine. Thalidomide in Europe, DES-induced cancer, and other recent drug-related tragedies have led the general public more and more to ask, not "how effective is a drug," but "how safe." With each new horror story of tragedies induced by drugs thought to be harmless for years, more people are seeking a safe alternative.

Now, as in the past, naturopathic physicians are offering that alternative. The naturopathic physicians' training today encompasses both traditional and modern techniques of diagnosis and therapy. They are trained in 4-year state-accredited private naturopathic medical schools. The program includes all the basic science, diagnostic, and medical courses standard to any other medical training institution. In addition, the naturopath is trained in a wide variety of natural therapies to be used to help the body in its self-repairing efforts. The aim of naturopathy is to treat people, not disease; to remove the cause of disease, not merely its symptoms; and to cure disease, not just postpone it.

THE PHILOSOPHY OF NATUROPATHIC MEDICINE

> The natural therapeutic approach maintains that the constant effort of the body's life force is always in the direction of *self-cleansing, self-repairing and positive health*. The philosophy maintains that even acute disease is a manifestation of the body's efforts in the direction of self cure. Disease, or downgraded health, may be eliminated only by removing from the system the real cause and by raising the body's general vitality so that its natural and inherent ability to sustain health is allowed to dominate. Natural therapeutic philosophy also maintains that chronic diseases are frequently the result of mistaken efforts to cure or attempted suppression of the physiological efforts of the body to cleanse itself.

This short quote fully encompasses both the cause and treatment of nearly all disease. It begins by affirming the basic inner vitality that is life itself. The "great law of life" states that "Every living cell in an organized body is endowed with an instinct of self preservation which is sustained by an inherent force named *THE VITAL FORCE OF LIFE*."† The "great law of life" needs to be understood on many levels to be of real use. If all disease is a self-repairing effort aimed toward health, then why bother to treat disease at all, even with naturopathic therapy? Does this law not guarantee cure? Why not lie back and wait for our pneumonia, ulcer, heart disease, or diabetes to simply go away? The reason, of course, as common sense tells us, is that it probably won't.

This law means the general flow of life's energies is in the direction of positive health. If, however, this flow is hindered in any way, the final result may be less than perfect. To understand the many factors that may cause disease or hinder this life force, we must first understand what health is. Lindlahr's definition states that "Health is normal and harmonious vibration of the elements and forces composing the human entity on the physical, mental and moral (emotional) planes of being, in conformity with the constructive principle (great law of life) in nature."‡

Disease is therefore an abnormal or inharmonious vibration of the elements and forces composing the human entity in one or more planes of being.§ In the "perfectly normal" individual all aspects of life are kept in harmony. If this situation were possible to maintain, the body would live forever. The "ordinary" individual, however, is constantly being subjected to influences that upset his or her inner equilibrium. Normal changes in the physical environment, both internally and externally, are easily compensated for. The body is equipped with

†Lindlahr, Henry, *Philosophy of Natural Therapeutics*, The Lindlahr Publishing Co., Chicago, Ill., 1919.
‡Ibid.
§Ibid.

sophisticated defense mechanisms which have evolved over eons. It is designed to maintain a healthy internal environment, and can protect itself from any reasonable threat. If nothing catastrophic happens to the body other than ordinary changes, and if the life force is unhindered on all planes, the physical body would live significantly longer than the accepted three score and ten. This has been hinted at in various religious works and can be seen today in certain societies where the lifestyle is relatively harmonious.

Modern humanity, however, can no longer be considered either "normal" or "ordinary." Nearly every aspect of modern living causes disharmony in the physical, mental, and moral planes of our existence. Suddenly, in a minute fraction of our total existence on the evolutionary scale, we are being exposed to vast changes in both our internal and external environment. The physical body, designed for and requiring demanding physical exercise for its optimum functioning, now performs effortless tasks. Our diet, once composed of whole grains, nuts, raw fruits, fresh vegetables, simple proteins, and pure water, is now made up of refined, devitalized grains, highly salted nuts, frozen, canned, or poisoned fruits and vegetables, complex protein meals also poisoned by all manner of drugs and chemicals, and harmful liquids, such as coffee, tea, soda, and alcohol. Even the air is no longer pure.

As if this were not enough for the physical body to handle, many people take drugs and smoke cigarettes, pipes, cigars, and pot. We are exposed to toxic chemicals at work and at home. It is no wonder that the body reaches a point when it can no longer safely deal with these poisons.

Mental and emotional stresses have increased rapidly over the recent past. These are often of a nature that must be suppressed, such as in the employer–employee relationship, causing severe disruption of balance in the physical body.

We are equipped with various adaptive mechanisms which clear from the body a normal amount of unneeded, unwanted, or toxic substances. If, however, these safety channels are clogged, overburdened, or suppressed, the vital force can no longer slowly and safely maintain harmony, and disease results. This disease, however, is *still* the activity of the vital force to create balance. As such it is a positive *action* made to correct and remove hindrances to its proper function. Lindlahr states, "Every acute disease is the result of a healing effort of nature,"* expressing the truth that disease is an *action* made by the body as a result of a cause and effect relationship. To further understand the direction and purpose of the disease process, it is first necessary to better appreciate basic causes of disease.

Accumulation of toxic material within the body due to improper diet, poor circulation, poor eliminations, and lack of demanding exercise is a major factor in almost all disease. While it is acknowledged that other causes do exist, most

*Lindlahr, Henry, op. cit.

factors that predispose to disease result in an accumulation of poisonous substances in the body which, when the channels of elimination cannot adequately remove them, will invariably initiate a disease process. These accumulations ultimately lead to changes within the cell and eventually within the whole body.

Incorrect or unbalanced diets lead to reduced vitality, nutritional deficiency, toxemia, poor eliminations, and local tissue degeneration. Modern food processing and refining leads to an unbalanced, low-fiber, unnatural diet which drastically decreases the nutrient value of food. High-yield fertilizer usage upsets the natural balance of the soil, producing nutritionally inferior and deficient food. Pesticides and additives place a further burden on the body to detoxify unwanted and poisonous substances. Improper diet is a *major* cause of nearly all forms of disease.

Improper posture and body mechanics due to habit, poor muscle tone, accident, or injury may interfere with normal nervous activity or the circulation of blood and lymph, leading to tissue degeneration and defective function. As the normal curves of the spine are altered by weak abdominal muscles, high heels, spinal trauma, or poor body mechanics in sitting or standing, the normal relationship of internal organs and their nervous, blood, and lymph supply (and consequently their nutrition) are severely affected. These changes may lead to poor local nutrition, reduced drainage, and reduced tissue vitality. The end result is congestion, toxic accumulation, and disease.

Destructive emotions such as fear, anxiety, hate, self-pity, and resentment can affect the body by upsetting digestion, blood flow, hormone balance, and the general biochemistry of the entire body. Psychological causes of disease are increasing as society itself places greater pressures on the individual.

The administration of suppressive drugs and vaccines which inhibit the eliminative efforts of the body and place further demands on it for drug detoxification are a growing cause of disease. Many drugs, and vaccines in particular, can cause allergic reactions, chronic allergies, and other long-term health problems. The incidence of drug-induced illness is on the increase, especially in older age groups where multiple prescriptions may cause toxic interactions.

Excessive use of alcohol, coffee, and tobacco are serious health threats. These social drugs, although widely accepted and used, are major factors in many disease processes. They can severely damage the liver, lungs, pancreas, thyroid, adrenal glands, and other parts of the body or mind.

Environmental causes of disease are becoming difficult to avoid. The air, water, and soil are all becoming more susceptible to pollution as population increases and we continue to treat the earth without proper respect.

Occupational hazards may also help cause disease. Chemical contact and poor air quality are common factors in downgraded health. Some substances that have been in use for years, such as asbestos, have been found to be toxic, and are a severe health risk. Work-related stress, however, may be the greatest cause of illness among workers.

Certain inherited factors or tendencies, congenital predisposition, or abnormalities may also leave an individual more susceptible to disease or unstable conditions. Often, however, these weaknesses only become manifest when the body comes under stress from one or more of the other causes of disease above.

Parasitic, virus, or germ infection is not a primary cause of disease but rather its result. Even Pasteur, the recognized father of the germ theory, began to understand the true relationship of germs to disease late in his life when he stated "The germ is nothing, the soil is everything," meaning that a germ can only thrive in a suitable environment. The body normally is host to millions of microorganisms, some beneficial, others pathogenic. If "harmful" bacteria are allowed to multiply, then typical symptoms of disease result.

In a healthy body several factors can help keep harmful bacteria from gaining a strong foothold. The normal healthy bacterial flora in the digestive tract and vagina prevent others from proliferating, the way you or I would resist an intruder in our home. The body's secretions also act to prevent bacterial infection by their pH (their acidity or alkalinity) and their other qualities. Many mucous membranes are lined with tiny cilia, or hairs, that constantly move debris and bacteria toward the nearest exit. Glandular structures such as the tonsils are designed to screen foreign matter from the air, and internally from the circulation. Other glands perform a similar process throughout the entire lymphatic circulation, which filters the body's internal fluids. Foreign invaders that do manage to break through the body's first defenses are attacked by antibodies, consumed by white blood cells, and either digested or removed from the body.

The body is very well protected. Only when defenses are weakened can harmful bacteria gain a foothold. The factors that bring about reduced vitality are found above in the *true* causes of disease. When one or more of the causative factors predisposing to disease are present, the body is forced to act vigorously to reestablish proper equilibrium. The result is acute disease.

The body is equipped with various avenues of action to free itself of these burdens.

Fever increases the body's metabolic rate and circulation of blood and lymph, thereby speeding removal of toxins from the body, and nutrition to diseased areas. The increased circulation also acts as a carrier for the body's more complicated defenses such as white blood cells and antibodies. Fever also creates a less favorable environment for either bacteria or viruses, which generally have a very narrow temperature range for optimal growth. As fever increases, these organisms begin to die faster than they can reproduce. Hippocrates stated, "Give me fever and I will cure any disease."

Sweating carries toxins out of the system through the skin. It also helps keep the rising temperature within a range that will not endanger the long-term health of the body.

Mucous secretions also remove toxic material from the body. Cells of some mucous membranes protect against invasion by the action of the tiny cilia that move particles of foreign matter and debris toward the nearest outlet. These cilia are stimulated by external irritants, bacteria, viruses, or internal toxins.

Inflammation, swelling, and edema are actions by the body to localize a problem. Inflammation indicates a local increase in metabolic activity with increased blood and lymph supply, and an increased capillary supply to aid in transport of blood-borne defenses. Edema, or fluid accumulation, aids in diluting an undesirable, toxic, or irritating substance.

Local infection results from breakdown of vital tissues into waste matter, which then provides a suitable environment for bacterial spread until the body's forces can remove the waste material. The reduced vitality occurs first, the infection is secondary. Boils, acne, and other local infections may also be the result of an inner cleansing process.

Diarrhea and vomiting are obvious attempts by the body to rid itself of toxic substances. Local irritants may initiate this action as will systemic toxins.

Pain is a natural mechanism by which the body draws attention to a problem area. Pain indicates that the malfunction can no longer be tolerated or compensated for, and that further derangement may become injurious.

Sneezing and coughing are vigorous attempts by the body to rid the respiratory system of irritants and toxins. The coughing up of mucus can reduce the spread of infection by preventing morbid material from stagnating, and also can help prevent blockage of smaller respiratory passageways. Sneezing effectively rids the upper respiratory passages of particles and irritants.

All these acute symptoms of "disease" are in fact the result of an intelligent action by the body to reestablish equilibrium and positive health. As such they are corrective and eliminative and should not be suppressed. What is commonly called *acute disease* is really the result of nature's efforts to eliminate waste matter or poisons from the body and to repair injured tissues. If this acute condition is not allowed to run its natural course, or is treated with suppressive methods and therefore not allowed to fulfill its intended function of elimination, then eventually *chronic disease* will result. Thus, Lindlahr defines chronic disease as a

> condition of the organism in which lowered vibration (lowered vitality), due to the accumulation of waste materials and poisons with the consequent destruction of vital parts and organs, has progressed to such an extent that nature's constructive and healing forces are no longer able to act against the disease conditions by acute corrective efforts (healing crisis).*

The chronic disease condition is therefore much more permanent and often involves radical changes in the body's structures and chemistry.

*Lindlahr, Henry, op. cit.

Requirements for Health

Although the body is composed of vastly different types of structural units, each cell requires the same three factors to maintain life. These are:

- Nutrition
- Drainage
- Coordination

These factors are also essential for the health of the total organism, which depends upon the health of its individual cells.

Nutrition

The body is composed of a number of chemical elements which combine to form the basic units of protein, carbohydrates, and fats; as well as essential fatty acids, vitamins, and minerals.

- *Proteins* are built up from building blocks called *amino acids.* Eight of these are considered *essential amino acids* since they cannot be synthesized within the body and therefore must be taken in with the normal diet.

- *Carbohydrates* are essential units which must be supplied by the diet. Although complex by nature, the basic unit is glucose, which forms the major energy source for the body. Carbohydrates may be synthesized from proteins or fats within the body. In the case of proteins, this is an energy-expending pathway that yields less energy than required for the conversion and only functions when the body's dietary supply of carbohydrate is absent.

- *Fats* are used partly as structural and functional material and partly as a storage form of food. Fats may be synthesized within the body; however, food acts as the major source.

- *Essential fatty acids (EFA):* Three polyunsaturated fatty acids (linolenic, linoleic, and arachidonic) have essential fatty acid activity. In humans only linoleic and arachidonic acids are considered essential. They play important roles in fat transport and metabolism and in maintaining the function and integrity of cellular membranes. They also act as precursors to prostaglandin formation. While the body can synthesize arachidonic and linolenic acids from linoleic acid, linoleic acid itself must be ingested and cannot be synthesized in the body.

- *Vitamins and minerals* are essential to life and are used within the body's various structures as building material and are necessary for various biochemical functions. Normally these must be ingested; however, some may be synthesized within the body.

For normal maintenance of health all the above nutrients must constantly be ingested to provide the basic building blocks of life for the body's tissues to be repaired and remade, and to furnish an adequate energy supply for body action and maintenance.

Drainage

Proper drainage of the cell is necessary to get rid of toxic end products of metabolism. If these wastes are not removed, the cell's function is reduced, which can downgrade the health of tissues, organs, and ultimately the entire body, if affecting many cells.

Coordination

Coordination within single cells and also within the total organism is essential for life. Intracellular regulation is controlled by chemical means while coordination throughout the entire system is controlled by both the nervous and hormonal systems. If either of these is not functioning properly, delicate balancing mechanisms can be upset, causing downgraded local or systemic health.

In health all three of these essentials, nutrition, drainage, and coordination, are functioning and in balance, while in disease there is either disharmony or lack of performance of one or more of these essentials of life. The body's constant effort is to establish this harmony. If harmony exists, inner vitality is then able to express itself fully. Such a person appears to have an unbounded source of life and energy.

In reality very few people have completely free-flowing vitality. The total vitality available to the ordinary person equals his or her life force, minus any obstructions to this energy being expressed. Just as the quality of television reception may depend on the television receiver or antenna, so it is with the human organism. These obstructions to the life force can be any one or any combination of the basic causes of disease. In order to relieve any diseased condition, it is necessary to remove from the body any obstructive factors which interfere with its life force, allowing the body to heal itself.

We truly are what we eat and drink, what we feel, and what we think. Health can only be attained and maintained by the coordination of our body, emotions, and mind. Cures cannot come from external measures, even if they are natural therapies. True healing can only come from within with the healing power of nature freely flowing.

THE TOOLS OF NATUROPATHY

Naturopathy is a method of curing disease by releasing inner vitality and allowing the body to heal itself. The methods that the naturopath uses should be looked on only as useful tools that help release this vital healing power. In and of themselves they are not intrinsically healing. Certainly this is evident when we consider that many of the herbs used routinely in practice are potent poisons if given in the wrong doses. The beneficial effect is not due to this poison, but in the direction it urges the body to take in its self-repairing process. With hydrotherapy, healing power is in the body's action, not due to any specific medicinal power of water. The use of "natural" therapy does not of its own constitute naturopathy. Naturopathy involves the use of natural therapies according to certain established principles. This is where naturopathy as a science must be distinguished from folk medicine or any other "natural" therapy. While these techniques or tools may be employed by the naturopath, they must be used according to the basic principles of naturopathy for the end result to be naturopathic medicine.

An herb may be used to stimulate the body to action, aid in elimination, help purge the body of toxic waste, or act as a nutrient. Used in these ways the herb works *with* the healing power of nature. It may, however, be used to *suppress* the body's healing efforts, just as a drug might be used, to rid the body of its distressing symptoms with little thought for real causes or cure. In such a case the herb is *not* used according to naturopathic principles. Hydrotherapy may be used to aid in circulation, nutrition, and generally to increase vitality so that the healing efforts of nature are allowed freer action. Hydrotherapy, however, *can* be used solely to suppress pain or discomfort without concern for the final cure. The tools of naturopathy can be used in proper or improper ways.

Not all naturopaths use the same therapeutic tools. Naturopathy in its essence is a philosophy of life, not a collection of rigid, learn-by-rote prescriptions. Once the philosophy is understood, the naturopath uses whichever agents or tools his or her temperament feels most comfortable with. Some naturopaths interpret the philosophy very narrowly and use only diet, fasting, exercise, sunlight, and hydrotherapy to guide the body's healing forces toward cure. These naturopaths shun the use of herbs unless used as nutrients, and even look distrustingly on vitamin or mineral supplements. These purist or "nature cure" naturopaths are just as right as others who have added spinal manipulation, massage, physiotherapy, vitamin and mineral therapy, homeopathy, botanical medicine, acupuncture, and many other nontoxic procedures. What is important is that the procedures be used according to the basic principles of naturopathy.

BOTANICAL MEDICINE

The earliest written records of nearly all civilizations mention the use of herbs for healing. Throughout human history there has been a close relationship between people and plants. Botany and medicine have always been closely associated. The *Pentsao,* or Great Herbal of China, which dates around 3000 B.C., discusses herbal treatments in detail. Another early herbal is the Ebers Papyrus of 1500 B.C., which lists over 800 botanical prescriptions used in various disorders. Early Greek literature also has many references to the medical use of plants. Hippocrates (460–355 B.C.) was the first to list plants by their use. Several lists of pharmaceutically active plants were made throughout Greek history. The first attempt at publication of a materia medica, however, was not made until the early 1500s A.D. by Paracelsus. The first official pharmacopoeia, mostly of botanical origin, appeared in 1564. The earliest one in English was the first United States pharmacopoeia, published in 1820. Currently, over 50 percent of all new prescriptions written in the United States contain at least one ingredient either produced directly from plants, or discovered from plant sources and later synthesized.

Modern medicine draws its origins from early herbal therapies. Until the advent of "synthetic" medicine within the past 50 to 100 years, all medical doctors prescribed herbs routinely. Later research into the chemistry of plants and plant products isolated what was considered the "active principle" from plants. The active principles were prescribed as drugs whose names often still reflect their botanical origins. A commonly known example of this is *Digitalis purpurea* (foxglove). This herb had been used as a heart stimulant in folk medicine for centuries prior to the isolation of its active principle, digitoxin. Another example is the isolation in 1947 of reserpine from *Rauwolfia serpentina* (Indian snakeroot), a plant native to India and clearly described for its pharmacological uses in the *Vedas,* India's earliest written records dating from 1500 B.C.

Within the decade 1940 to 1950, hundreds of new "wonder drugs" were discovered, nearly all of botanical origin. The amazing thing about the "discovery" of these potent and clearly therapeutic drugs was not their existence, since written history was literally pregnant with specific examples testifying to the medicinal use of plants, but rather how long modern researchers took to investigate them. This nearsighted attitude has been expressed by De Ropp in *Drugs and the Mind:*

> The situation results, in part at least, from the rather contemptuous attitude which certain chemists and pharmacologists in the west have developed toward both folk remedies and drugs of plant origin. . . . They further fell into the error of supposing that because they had learned the trick of synthesizing certain substances, they were better chemists than Mother Nature who, besides creating

compounds too numerous to mention, also synthesized the aforesaid chemist and pharmacologist.*

Unfortunately, this separation of herbs from their "drug actions" was the fall from grace of the medical profession. Not only was the active principle found to be much more potent than the herb from which it was obtained, it also was usually found to be much more dangerous, with more profound toxic effects. These toxic effects were termed "side effects," but in reality were merely the normal action of the active principle in the body acting in ways other than desired by the physician. With the development of drugs came an increase in diseases caused by medication. It is now estimated that at least one-third of all diseases today are iatrogenic or the result of medication given to treat disease.

The use of botanical medicine, or preparations derived from the entire complex of the botanical plant part used, is usually safer but slower in action than orthodox drug therapy. By utilizing not only the so-called "active principle" but also the "associated factors" which naturally occur in the plant, the practitioner of botanical medicine has been spared most of the problem of drug-related diseases. The beneficial use of a botanical preparation in fact does not rest solely with the active principle, of which there may be several for a single herb, but usually in the total interaction of all its constituents.

It is, however, a common misconception that botanical medications are completely safe and nontoxic. For the most part this is true if herbs are used in their proper doses; however, any medicine can cause toxic reactions when used improperly. The use of herbs such as thyme, sage, rosemary, dill, ginger, and garlic in cooking and seasoning is an example of how widespread the safe use of herbs really is in daily life. Herbal teas now abound in most food stores and are used as pleasant-tasting drinks or to obtain mild botanical effects such as the calmative effects of chamomile, or the digestive benefits of peppermint. Even commonly used herbal teas, however, should really be reserved for medicinal use and not taken routinely. Such commonly used herbs as comfrey, goldenseal, or lobelia can cause toxic reactions. A knowledge of botanical toxicology, therefore, is essential before one tries to treat disease with herbs. Even with this warning in mind it can be fairly said that botanical medicine is usually safer and more therapeutic than the use of drugs when prescribed and monitored properly.

Herbs may be used in many ways to treat disease. If an herb is used merely to suppress symptoms without regard for cause or cure, it is little better than a nontoxic drug. If used properly, herbs act as aids in stimulating or directing the body's own healing forces, thus promoting health from within.

*De Ropp, Robert, *Drugs and the Mind*, Grove Press, 1960, p. 72.

Actions of Botanical Preparations

Botanical preparations, although often referred to as herbs, may be derived from any member of the plant kingdom, including leafy plants, weeds, trees, ferns, or lichens. The whole plant or a single part of the plant, such as its root, rhizome, bulb, stem, bark, flower, styles, stigma, fruit, seed, or resin may be used. Each part has a known action or actions; each herb stimulates the body to act in one or more directions. These actions have names which are useful as aids in prescription. Some are summarized below.

Alteratives

This herbal action elicits an alteration for the better in the course of an illness. Alteratives are often described as blood purifiers and are used to treat conditions arising from or causing toxicity. If given in proper doses over a prolonged period of time, these herbs improve the condition of the blood, accelerate elimination, improve digestion, and increase the appetite. Commonly used alteratives are:

Barberry *(Berberis vulgaris)*
Blue flag *(Iris versicolor)*
Burdock *(Arctium lappa)*
Chaparral *(Larrea tridentata)*
Coneflower *(Echinacea angustifolia)*
Figwort *(Scrophularia nodosa)*
Oregon grape root *(Berberis aquifolium)*
Plantain *(Plantago lanceolata)*
Pokeroot *(Phytolacca decandra)* (highly toxic; see p. 62)
Prickly ash *(Xanthoxylum americanum)*
Queen's root *(Stillingia sylvatica)*
Red clover *(Trifolium pratense)*
Sarsaparilla *(Smilax ornata)*
Sassafras *(Sassafras officinale)*
Tree of life *(Thuja occidentalis)*
Wild indigo *(Baptisia tinctoria)*
Yellow dock *(Rumex crispus)*

Anodynes/Analgesics

These herbs will relieve pain usually by reducing nerve excitability. These remedies are closely related to antispasmodics and sedatives. Commonly used herbs in this class are:

Catnip (Nepeta cataria)
Chamomile (Anthemis nobilis)
Dong quai (Angelica sylvestris)
Hops (Humulus lupulus)
Jamaica dogwood (Piscidia erythrina)
Mistletoe (Viscum album)
Skullcap (Scutellaria lateriflora)
Valerian (Valeriana officinalis)
White bryony (Bryonia alba)
Wild Yam (Dioscorea villosa)
Wintergreen (Gaultheria procumbens)

Anthelmintics

These include vermicides which kill intestinal worms, and vermifuges which aid in expelling worms. Most commonly used are:

Aloe (Aloe vera)
Bitterwood (Picraena excelsa)
Butternut (Juglans cinerea)
Elecampane (Inula helenium)
Garlic (Allium sativum)
Hyssop (Hyssopus officinalis)
Kousso (Brayera anthelmintica)
Male fern (Dryopteris filixmas)
Papaya (Carica papaya)
Pomegranate (Puncia granatum)
Pumpkin (Curcurbita pepo)
Santonica (Artemisia santonica)
Tansy (Tanacetum vulgare)
Worm grass (Spigelia marilandica)
Wormseed (Chenopodium anthelminticum)
Wormwood (Artemisia absinthium)

Antibiotics

These herbs inhibit the growth or kill bacteria. They include:

Bearberry (Arctostaphylos uva-ursi)
Bitter orange (Citrus aurantium)
Cajuput (Melaleuca cajuputi)
Coneflower (Echinacea angustifolia)
Eucalyptus (Eucalyptus globulus)

Garlic *(Allium sativum)*
Goldenseal *(Hydrastis canadensis)*
Horseradish *(Cochlearia armoracia)*
Mullein *(Verbascum thapsus)*
Myrrh *(Commiphora myrrha)*
Nasturtium *(Tropaeolum majus)*
Onion *(Allium cepa)*
Peruvian bark *(Cinchona ledgeriana)*
Propolis (a resinous beeswax)
Watercress *(Nasturtium officinale)*

Antiseptics

These herbs are used internally or externally to prevent breakdown of organic tissues or inhibit growth of microorganisms. Some are similar to alteratives, while others are astringents. Among these herbs are:

Barberry *(Berberis vulgaris)*
Calendula *(Calendula officinalis)*
Coneflower *(Echinacea angustifolia)*
Eucalyptus *(Eucalyptus globulus)*
Garlic *(Allium sativum)*
Goldenseal *(Hydrastis canadensis)*
Myrrh *(Commiphora myrrha)*
Pine *(Pinus spp.)*
St. John's wort *(Hypericum perforatum)*
White pond lily *(Nymphaea odorata)*

Antispasmodics

These herbs stop or prevent muscular spasm. They are used for muscle cramps, menstrual cramps, asthma, and other disorders with muscle irritability, spasm, or contraction. Commonly used herbs in this class are:

Black cohosh *(Cimicifuga racemosa)*
Blue cohosh *(Caulophyllum thalictroides)*
Chamomile *(Anthemis nobilis)*
Cramp bark or high-bush cranberry *(Viburnum opulus)*
Lady's slipper *(Cypripedium pubescens)*
Lobelia *(Lobelia inflata)*
Mistletoe *(Viscum album)*
Passion flower *(Passiflora incarnata)*
Skullcap *(Scutellaria lateriflora)*

Valerian *(Valeriana officinalis)*
Wild yam root *(Dioscorea villosa)*

Astringents

These herbs act upon the albumin of the tissue to which they are applied, causing a hardening and contraction, leaving the area more dense and firm. They prevent bacterial infection, stop discharges, diarrhea, or hemorrhages. Most astringents contain tannin as a primary ingredient. Herbs used are:

Avens *(Geum urbanum)*
Bayberry *(Myrica cerifera)*
Bistort *(Polygonum bistorta)*
Blackberry *(Rubus* spp.*)*
Calendula *(Calendula officinalis)*
Cranesbill *(Geranium maculatum)*
Myrrh *(Commiphora myrrha)*
Pinus bark *(Tsuga canadensis)*
Tormentil *(Potentilla tormentilla)*
White oak bark *(Quercus alba)*
Witch hazel *(Hamamelis virginiana)*

Carminatives (Aromatics)

These herbs, usually having an agreeable taste or aromatic odor, relieve flatulence and flatulent pain, and soothe the stomach. Many herbs fit into this category, such as:

Angelica *(Angelica archangelica)*
Anise *(Pimpinella anisum)*
Balm *(Melissa officinalis)*
Caraway *(Carum carvi)*
Cinnamon *(Cinnamomum zeylanicum)*
Cloves *(Eugenia carophyllus)*
Cumin *(Cuminum cyminum)*
Dill *(Anethum graveolens)*
Fennel *(Foeniculum dulce)*
Ginger *(Zingiber officinale)*
Peppermint *(Mentha piperita)*

Cathartics

These herbs cause copious bowel evacuation. They also usually stimulate bile secretion. Cathartics are used to expel worms after an anthelmintic herb has been used and whenever a complete bowel evacuation is desired. Their use in chronic constipation is not therapeutic and only causes further constipation as its secondary effect. Most often used are:

Black root *(Leptandra virginica)*
Butternut *(Juglans cinerea)*
Castor oil plant *(Ricinus communis)*
Jalapa *(Ipomoea jalapa)*
May-apple, or American mandrake *(Podophyllum peltatum)* (highly toxic; see p. 62)
Mountain flax *(Linum cartharticum)*
Rhubarb *(Rheum palmatum)*
Senna *(Cassia acutifolia)*

Demulcents

These herbs soothe, soften, reduce irritation, and protect the mucous membranes. Their effect may be mechanical or medicinal, depending on the herb. Among this class we find:

Chickweed *(Stellaria media)*
Coltsfoot *(Tussilago farfara)*
Comfrey *(Symphytum officinale)*
Irish moss *(Chrondrus crispus)*
Marshmallow *(Althaea officinalis)*
Slippery elm *(Ulmus fulva)*

Diaphoretics

These herbs increase perspiration and rid the body of waste material through the sweat glands. They are best given as hot infusions repeated frequently. Useful herbs in this class are:

Balm *(Melissa officinalis)*
Blue vervain *(Verbena hastata)*
Boneset *(Eupatorium perfoliatum)*
Catnip *(Nepeta cataria)*
Chamomile *(Anthemis nobilis)*
Crawley root *(Corallorhiza odontorhiza)*
Ginger root *(Zingiber officinalis)*
Peppermint *(Mentha piperita)*
Pleurisy root *(Asclepias tuberosa)*
Spearmint *(Mentha viridis)*
Yarrow *(Achillea millefolium)*

Diuretics

These herbs increase the flow of urine. Often used diuretics are:

Bearberry (*Arctostaphylos uva-ursi*)
Broom tops (*Cytisus scoparius*)
Buchu (*Barosma betulina*)
Burdock (*Arctium lappa*)
Cleavers (*Galium aparine*)
Couch grass (*Agropyrum repens*)
Hydrangea (*Hydrangea arborescens*)
Juniper (*Juniperus communis*)
Parsley (*Petroselinum sativum*)
Parsley piert (*Alchemilla arvensis*)
Pellitory-of-the-wall (*Parietaria officinalis*)
Queen of the meadow (*Eupatorium purpureum*)
Stinging nettle (*Urtica urens*)
Stone root (*Collinsonia canadensis*)
Wild carrot (*Daucus carota*)
Yarrow (*Achillea millefolium*)

Emetics

Herbs that induce vomiting include:

Ipecacuanha (*Psychotria ipecacuanha*)
Lobelia (*Lobelia inflata*)
Mustard seeds (*Brassica juncea*)

Emmenagogues

These herbs promote menstrual flow. Useful among this class are:

Arrach (*Chenopodium olidum*)
Black cohosh (*Cimicifuga racemosa*)
Blazing star root (*Chamaelirium luteum*)
Blue cohosh (*Caulophyllum thalictroides*)
Cramp bark, or high-bush cranberry (*Viburnum opulus*)
False unicorn root (*Helonias dioica*)
Life root (*Senecio aureus*)
Mugwort (*Artemisia vulgaris*)
Pennyroyal (*Hedeoma pulegioides*)
Pulsatilla (*Anemone pulsatilla*)

Rue *(Ruta graveolens)*
Southernwood *(Artemisia abrotanum)*
Squaw vine *(Mitchella repens)*
Tansy *(Tanacetum vulgare)*

Laxatives

Mild purgatives encouraging gentle bowel movements:

Cascara *(Cascara sagrada)*
Castor oil plant *(Ricinus communis)*
Chia seed *(Salvia columbariae)*
Flaxseed *(Linum usitatissimum)*
Licorice *(Glycyrrhiza glabra)*
Olive oil *(Olea europaea)*
Psyllium *(Plantago psyllium)*
Rhubarb *(Rheum palmatum)*
Senna *(Cassia acutifolia)*

Nervines/Sedatives

These herbs can calm nervous tension, nourish the nervous system, and favor sleep. Many are also antispasmodics. Useful herbs in this class are:

Betony *(Betonica officinalis)*
Catnip *(Nepeta cataria)*
Chamomile *(Anthemis nobilis)*
European vervain *(Verbena officinalis)*
Hops *(Humulus lupulus)*
Lady's slipper *(Cypripedium pubescens)*
Mistletoe *(Viscum album)*
Passion flower *(Passiflora incarnata)*
Pulsatilla *(Anemone patens)*
Skullcap *(Scutellaria lateriflora)*
Valerian *(Valeriana officinalis)*

Stimulants

Herbs that excite and arouse nervous sensibility, and stimulate vital forces to action. They increase and strengthen the pulse and restore weakened circulation. Commonly used herbs in this class are:

Cayenne *(Capsicum frutescens)*
Ginger root *(Zingiber officinale)*

Horseradish *(Cochlearia armoracia)*
Poplar *(Populus tremuloides)*
Prickly ash *(Xanthoxylum americanum)*
Snake root *(Aristolochia reticulata)*
Wintergreen *(Gaultheria procumbens)*

Stomachics

Herbs that stimulate the secretion of gastric juices include:

Avens *(Geum urbanum)*
Bitterwood *(Picraena excelsa)*
Columbo *(Frasera carolinensis)*
Sweet flag *(Acorus calamus)*

Tonics

Herbs that give vigor and strengthen the entire system or a particular set of organs or actions. Some improve general vitality while others strengthen the heart, nerves, stomach, liver, or circulation. Some examples are valerian (nerve tonic), hawthorn berries (heart tonic), and dandelion (liver tonic). Tonics must be chosen for the effect desired to obtain benefit.

These specific "properties" of botanical medication are useful in classifying herbs for easy reference, and help narrow the choice of herbs most useful with a particular condition. But these properties in themselves tell us little of the herb itself, its temperament or character. Many herbs have alterative (blood-purifying), diaphoretic (sweat-inducing), or laxative properties, but not all of these would be beneficial for everyone with a similar health complaint. Each of the herbs must slowly become known as one gets to know an old friend—each has its own personality. The relationship between botanical and practitioner is a distinctly personal one.

Since no two people with the same disease are alike and the causes of their imbalance are unique, no set herbal prescription can benefit all. Each person must be considered individually to determine the best course of botanical medicine required, if any. One must consider if the condition is acute or chronic, if the patient is weak or strong, the state of his or her internal organs, and the function of the avenues of elimination. Herbs must be chosen which aid and direct the healing powers within.

Methods of Preparation

Methods of preparing herbs depend on the part of the herb used and the manner in which it is to be taken or applied.

Infusion

This preparation is one of the most common and is similar to that used for beverage teas, except in the amount of herb used. Infusions are made from leaves, flowers, or other soft parts of the plant, where botanical properties may be extracted by water. Place ½ to 1 oz of dried or fresh herbs that have been thoroughly bruised in an enamel, porcelain, or glass container. Pour 1 pint of boiled hot water over the herbs and cover the container tightly. The herbs are allowed to steep for 10 to 20 minutes. Strain the liquid. The infusion may be taken hot, warm, or cool, depending on the herb and effect desired. The usual dose is ½ to 1 cup taken three to four times per day, or more frequently in acute disease. Occasionally honey as a sweetener is allowed although some remedies should not be sweetened. Since these herbal infusions decompose rapidly, they should be made freshly each day.

Decoction

A decoction is used to extract botanical principles that are not easily obtained by infusion, which is often the case with roots, coarse leaves, stems, or barks. Decoctions may be prepared by boiling 1 oz of herb to 1 pint of water in a covered nonmetallic container for 20 to 30 minutes. The liquid is then cooled and strained. Sometimes it is desirable to concentrate a decoction by simmering the mixture uncovered. This is not done if volatile principles are present that would be lost in steam. Softer leaves or flowers may be added in the last 2 to 3 minutes, or added after the pot has been removed from the heat and strained, as one would make an infusion, leaving the herbs to steep 10 to 20 minutes. Doses vary according to the herb—from 1 tsp to 1 cup taken three to six times per day. Decoctions, like infusions, rapidly deteriorate unless some preservative is used.

Fluid Extract

These botanical preparations are the most concentrated form of the herb, and are prepared in a variety of ways to preserve the herb's maximum effectiveness. The simplest preparation, a *green extract*, is made by thoroughly crushing the juicy parts of the herb and pressing out its juices. This is then strained. In medicinal effect, 1 oz of the fluid extract is equal to 1 oz of the pure herb. Other methods requiring special machines are used commercially. Some herbs have properties that can only be obtained by the fluid extract process. However, this is rarely done at home, with commercial preparations being the main source. Fluid extracts also deteriorate rapidly.

Tincture

An herbal tincture is a solution of the herb's active botanical principles in alcohol. Many of the principles in herbs can only be extracted in this manner, as they are not soluble in water. Often, alcohol extractions are used to provide a stable, preservable extract for principles that easily deteriorate. Nearly any herb is obtainable in its tincture form from reliable botanical pharmaceutical houses. The difference between a standard drug and a botanical tincture is that a tincture is an extract of the entire herb portion used without isolating or concentrating one single active principle. Although they may be prepared at home, only by purchasing tinctures from reliable sources can the exact percent of alcohol and strength of preparation be assured, which is essential for accurate prescriptions. Tinctures take 2 weeks to prepare at home and within this time any herbal tincture you desire can be in your mailbox. As a physician I have no time to prepare tinctures and only rarely advise them to be prepared at home, except for local herbs unobtainable elsewhere.

To make a tincture at home add 4 oz of coarsely powdered or cut herb to 1 pint of 90 proof vodka, gin, 80+ proof brandy, or, for more purity, grain alcohol. Let set for 2 weeks, shaking daily. Strain the brew and store in amber glass bottles. Tinctures may be diluted prior to storing to make a 50% alcohol dilution, depending on the percent of alcohol used. The usual dose is 25 drops in water three to four times per day. However, weaker herbs or weaker tinctures may require more. In some cases the dose may reach 1 to 2 tsp three times per day.

Syrup

Syrups are saturated solutions made with the herb and sugar, which is used as a preservative and to disguise the unpleasant taste of some medications. They are frequently employed as cough and sore throat medications. A syrup may be made in several ways. One is to add 1 oz of herb to 2 cups of water and simmer down to 1½ cups. Strain and add 1 oz honey or glycerine. Another method is to add 1 oz herbs to a mixture of water and brown sugar. Simmer until the medicine is the correct consistency and then strain. Tinctures may be added after the syrup has thickened, and require no straining. Raw syrups may be made of onion or garlic merely by slicing the bulbs thinly and covering with a small amount of honey. Cover the container, let stand overnight, mash, and strain. Dose is 1 tsp three to six times per day.

Poultice

This is a warm, moist application of crushed and bruised fresh herbs or moistened dry herbs made into a paste and applied externally directly on the surface of the body or between a thin layer of gauze. Crush and bruise the fresh herb and slightly moisten with hot water. If the dry herb is used, add a little hot water to wet it and pound the mixture to a pulp. The mixture should be just wet and not dripping. Apply directly to skin or place the mixture between gauze and strap on with tape or elastic bandage. Most poultices should be ¼ to ½ in. thick. These should be left on 3 hours or all night. An infusion or decoction may also be soaked into soft cotton and applied repeatedly or as a continuous application, like a compress. Moist heat may be applied over the poultice.

Douche

Douches are usually made from herbal infusions or decoctions; however, dilutions of apple cider vinegar or yoghurt also are used, using a douche bag or enema bag with douche applicator. The bag is hung 1½ to 2 ft above the pelvis and the medicated fluid is allowed to enter the vagina slowly and gently, under low pressure. Some douches are done by continuously flushing the area, while others are retained for 10 to 20 minutes or even longer.

Enema

Herbal enemas are used in some cases to act locally or systemically by absorption through the mucous membranes. An infusion or decoction of the herb is made, and the enema instructions under Hydrotherapy are followed.

Suppository

These are small cylinder-shaped preparations of herbs combined with cocoa butter which are inserted vaginally or rectally. Often these may be purchased from reliable botanical supply houses. However, many useful suppositories have been withdrawn from production due to lack of demand. I often have the patient make the suppository by heating cocoa butter slowly and adding powdered herbs or tinctures as required. The cocoa butter is heated only until very soft and then is reshaped into large pencil shapes, cut into 1¼-in. segments, covered with wax paper, and refrigerated until used. The usual mixture is 1 oz herb to 3 oz cocoa butter. Another method is to totally melt the cocoa butter, mix in herbs, and then pour the mixture into molds made of foil, 1¼ in. long and as deep and round as a large pencil. These are allowed to set, then covered with wax paper and refrigerated.

Ointment

Ointments are mixtures of herbs heated with cocoa butter, lanolin, and other oils or hardeners, such as beeswax. I rarely need to advise home production of ointments since they are readily available from botanical supply houses or health food stores. Details of their production at home may be found in *Herbal Medicine* by Dian Dincin Buchman. Basic ointments are made by heating dried or fresh herbs in fats or oils such as wheat germ oil, almond oil, and others desired, with lanolin, for several hours. This is strained and then reheated, adding beeswax as a hardener. The mixture is then poured into ointment jars to harden.

A good introductory book on herbalism which I suggest reading prior to using the botanical measures in this book is *The Way of Herbs* by Michael Tierra. It is simply written and will aid you in the proper choice of herbs found under each of the therapeutic sections.

DIET, FASTING, AND NUTRITIONAL THERAPY

One of the basic concepts of natural therapy may be expressed in the common phrase, "You are what you eat." Our diet has, to a large extent, determined the diseases we suffer from. Over the past 100 to 150 years our basic diet has changed drastically. We have gone from fresh, wholesome, unrefined, unsprayed food to the opposite. Our foods now are frozen, canned, or refined, and treated with toxic pesticides, preservatives, colorings, and other chemicals. Mass food production techniques have given us more food but less nutrition as the soil becomes depleted of essential nutrients and its living balance upset by fertilizers and sprays. The refining of cereal grains strips them of their fiber and germ coatings which contain the bulk of their protein, vitamins, and minerals, and leaves an unbalanced food composed primarily of starch. The consumption of refined sugar is also one of the most detrimental influences in the modern diet. Sugar consumption has increased phenomenally within the past 150 years. In 1815 the average intake of sugar was about 15 lb per year. By 1955 it had reached 120 lb per year, and is even higher now.

Consider a typical teenager's diet: refined and sweetened cereal, two fried eggs (from chickens fed hormones and confined to a cage their whole lives), and white toast with butter for breakfast; a hamburger and french fries and a Coke for lunch; boiled frozen vegetables, meat, and white rice for supper, with two other soda beverages containing 7 tsp of sugar and multiple other sweets each day. You can see how it is possible for people to eat more of less. We are literally starving ourselves nutritionally.

Not only is the *quality* of our diet extremely poor, but its quantity is often as much of a problem. The old Chinese saying that nine-tenths of the food you eat is for *your* health while the last one-tenth is for your *doctor's* is true. Whenever you eat more than the body can effectively deal with, disease is invited. This is true of the best, most nourishing foods as well as when the foods eaten are, of themselves, a health risk. A major cause of disease is accumulation of waste or toxins that cannot be silently dealt with, and overeating is one cause of this accumulation.

Another important factor in our foods' nutritional value is the manner in which it is prepared. Many foods have maximum value in their natural state, or as close to it as possible. Certainly, for most fruit or vegetables heating destroys many of their enzymes and vitamins. In the case of water-soluble vitamins, these are lost if the food is boiled and the cooking water discarded. Long-term storage or canning also results in the loss of many of the less stable vitamins. Some foods, however, require heat to be made digestible, such as whole grains, some tuberous vegetables, a few fruits, and dried beans. Some nutritionists feel that a completely raw food diet is the only natural human diet and that cooked food is a major cause of suffering and disease. Raw foods are our most natural and nutritious foods and a person following such a diet with full knowledge of necessary nutritional requirements for health will experience profound physical vigor and resistance to disease.

Such a diet may be too extreme for the general population. The body is sufficiently adaptable to be able to handle a certain amount of cooked foods quite effectively. The type of diet I usually suggest is one containing a large amount of raw vegetables, fruits, seeds and nuts, with a smaller amount of lightly cooked vegetables, beans, and whole grains. For those who wish dairy products, free-range eggs and unpasteurized, unhomogenized, goat's milk products are advised. The question of the use of raw milk products is a subject of some dispute. Raw unpasteurized milk can carry brucellosis, as well as the more common salmonella organisms. To prevent these infections and still retain the benefit of raw milk, the milk source must be continually monitored for safety. Certainly, to prevent gastroenteritis, infants younger than 6 months must not be given raw milk from any source. All fluids given to infants must be boiled or pasteurized. Goat's milk, although a better source of general nutrition for infants than cow's milk, is commonly deficient in iron, vitamin D, and folic acid, increasing the incidence of megaloblastic anemia, unless care has been given to proper supplementation of these needs. Milk, even goat's milk, is rarely advisable for adults: fermented foods such as yoghurt and kefir are best. Raw-milk goat cheese is the best cheese product when available. Those desiring fleshy foods are directed first toward fish, then free-range chicken or turkey.

The amount of red meat now consumed by the general public is a definite health risk. Many people eat meat or other animal products with each meal. If meat is to be included in the diet, it should be restricted to two to three times per week, or less. In general, it is wise to have at least two entirely lacto-vegetarian days each week.

For a proper diet to be of any use all food must be chewed slowly and thoroughly. Too many people rush their meals, putting an excess burden on their stomachs. In addition to this, the food must be eaten only when one is relaxed and under no tension. Stress completely stops the actions of the entire digestive system.

Many diseases can be directly related to improper dietary habits. The real proof, however, is seen when a disease process is reversed and cured by a simple change of diet. The prevention and cure of disease lies largely in proper diet.

Fasting and Elimination Diets

Aesculapius of ancient Greece advised "Instead of using medicine, fast." Hippocrates routinely recommended prolonged fasting. Most religions advocate periods of abstinence from food to attain physical and spiritual purity. Christ fasted 40 days in meditation. Animals and babies retain their natural instincts and refuse food when ill. Most people remain uninformed of the beneficial effects of fasting when sick and continue to advise their loved ones to "Eat and keep up your strength." Nothing worse could be done to lower vitality in illness than eating.

During fasting there is an increase in the amount of energy available for the eliminative process due to absence of large amounts of food requiring digestion and assimilation, both of which require energy. The body is able to redirect this increased energy toward elimination of the obstructions to the vital force in the form of toxic waste. Since vitality equals the life force minus any obstructions, as these are removed higher levels of vital energy are available for more rapid elimination.

The initial elimination begins as soon as the first meal is missed. Sometime during the first 3 days of the fast, usually reaching its maximum on the third day, the elimination activity is manifested by the appearance of a coated tongue, bad breath, headaches, muscular aches, and general debility. These symptoms are due to the increase in toxins in the bloodstream and passing out of the channels of elimination. The sooner these unpleasant symptoms are present, the more toxic is the system. Often we have patients complain that if they miss a meal a severe headache results. These are the people who need to fast most urgently. By the morning of the fourth day these eliminations are much less and a feeling of general well-being is often experienced, with great clarity of mind and abundant energy. This state lasts in degrees of varying intensity, interspersed with periods of lack of energy, fatigue, and difficulty in concentration as more toxins are eliminated. This period usually lasts until around the tenth day, when a *healing crisis* commonly occurs to a greater or lesser degree. During this process the body is able to eliminate a large amount of deep-seated toxins and waste matter. This manifests itself in a variety of ways from flulike symptoms, skin eruptions, or other eliminative processes. Following this crisis, the patient once again will experience a further improvement in health and vigor.

The minimum period of fasting for cleansing purposes is 3 days, while a prolonged fast may safely last 3 to 4 weeks or even longer, *under supervision.* The length of the fast must be determined by monitoring the patient's reaction and general vitality during the fasting period. It is customary to continue a fast for 3, 7, 14, 21 (or other multiples of 7) days. *All fasts of 3 days or more are best supervised by a physician.*

It is essential that the fast be terminated with extreme care, especially in more prolonged regimens. In general, the longer the period of fasting, the longer the time needed before a full diet can be resumed. This must be a gentle process of adding easily digested foods first, to gradually recondition the digestive system. A common fast-breaker for prolonged fasts is stewed apples without their skin, while fresh fruit is acceptable after a 3-day fast. Fresh goat's yoghurt is also used in some cases, especially where enemas were used during the fast. This should be continued for 1 day if the fast has been less than 1 week, or 2 to 3 days for longer regimens. This is followed by the slow introduction of other fruits for 1 day and then at least 2 days of fresh fruit and salads or steamed vegetables. Gradually over the next 1 to 2 weeks a full diet is resumed. Food must be chewed until liquefied, especially when grains are reintroduced. The food to be eaten during this building-up period must be of the best quality since the body will be building tissue from these materials. As I tell most patients, it is easy to fast, but much more difficult to break a fast properly. All the beneficial effects of fasting may be undone in a very short time by adding too much food too soon, of the wrong type or quality.

The tongue is often considered the mirror of internal health and is used as a guide to the fasting length and progress. What usually occurs is that the tongue becomes heavily coated during the first 3 days of a fast and becomes progressively clearer until the healing crisis starts, or the fast is terminated. The clearing of the tongue after the healing crisis is a good indication that the fast may be ended. If the fast is allowed to continue until the tongue is clear, and it is broken gently with wholesome food, the result will be an increase in physical well-being, vitality, and mental clarity. The body will be at peace.

The type of fast performed determines to a large extent the rate of elimination achieved. In this way it is possible to control the elimination process required by the individual patient. Fasting by definition is the elimination of solid food. The strictest fast is the *water fast*, where the patient drinks only water whenever desired. *Fresh fruit juice* or *fresh vegetable juice* fasts are also used, depending on the case and desired result. The order of fast in degree of eliminative power is:

1. Water fast
2. Citrus juice fast
3. Subacid fruit juice fast
4. Vegetable juice fast

Although the water and citrus juice fasts are more eliminative than the subacid fruit juice or vegetable juice fasts, this does not necessarily mean that they are more desirable in every situation. Some disorders need a slower, less dramatic elimination than others, and not all patients can handle citrus in excess, or could go even 1 day on only water. The various fasts are, in reality, only members of the order of elimination diets. Many regimens are employed to effect an elimination of greater or lesser strength. The following is a list in order of eliminative effect:

Citrus fruit mono diet (a diet of only one type of fruit, plus its juice)

Subacid fruit mono diet (i.e., apple mono diet)

Mixed fruit diet (only one fruit type per meal; no bananas are allowed)

Raw fruit and vegetable diet

Raw vegetable mono diet (i.e., raw carrot and raw carrot juice)

Raw fruit, raw vegetables, and some cooked vegetables

Raw and cooked fruit and vegetables plus carbohydrates

Raw and cooked fruit and vegetables with carbohydrates and vegetarian proteins

Reasons for fasting are:

During any acute disease

In any case of lowered vitality or general debility

During any healing crisis

Repeatedly in most chronic diseases

To clear the mind

The following juice or mono diets are frequently used:

- *Apple juice or mono diet:* This is a good alkaline diet for acid conditions such as gout or other inflammatory conditions.

- *Grape juice or mono diet:* This is especially useful in heart conditions or where heavy activity has to be undertaken during the elimination. Black grapes are especially called for with heart complaints. Grapes are not as eliminative as most other fruit juices or mono diets.

- *Grapefruit juice or mono diet:* This is especially useful in liver conditions, for general elimination, and with colds or mucous conditions. It is unsuitable for arthritis, ulcers, or hyperacidic states.

• *Orange fruit juice or mono diet:* Oranges are not frequently advised in too great a quantity since they tend to upset the liver. They are used primarily in mucous and lung complaints. Excess may cause inflammation and itching of the anus.

• *Lemon juice:* In dilute form lemon juice and water are highly eliminative. Most hydropathic health institutes fast their patients on cold or hot water with a slice of lemon.

• *Carrot juice or mono diet:* Especially useful in digestive problems such as colitis or ulcers. A very alkaline juice and therefore useful in all acid states.

• *Cabbage juice:* This is most effective with ulcers. It is commonly mixed with carrot juice for this purpose.

• *Onion juice and mono diet:* Excellent for any condition with excess mucus, lung complaints, sinus congestion, colds, middle ear or eustachian tube congestion, etc.

Nutritional Therapy

Most naturopaths advise specific vitamin, mineral, or other food supplements, depending on the state of the patient. A great deal of research is now being done to further understand the physiological effects of these food factors. The use of these substances as food supplements or medication has been hotly contested by most medical doctors. The average conventional physician feels that all factors necessary for health can be obtained through a normal diet and that additional supplements are a waste of money. Naturopaths, however, feel strongly that the average diet no longer supplies these needed elements in sufficient quantities for several reasons. Our foods are now grown on soils depleted by years of intensive farming, without proper understanding of organic principles of land use and ecology. Essential minerals such as zinc are already deficient in the soil of many states. Even if the food eaten looks nutritious it no longer supplies the same proportion of minerals that food 100 years ago provided. The situation becomes even worse if these already-deficient foods are canned, stored for long periods, or cooked improperly. The average person has little or no awareness of how to prevent loss of water-soluble vitamins from food, or destruction of heat-labile vitamins in cooking. The refining of foods such as we see on nearly every supermarket shelf is another obvious cause of reduced food value. The replacement of a few vitamins can in no way duplicate or make up for the wholesale destruction of our basic food groups.

Even if our food supply were the best available and we were careful to eat only organic and unprocessed foods, there still is the possibility that a certain percentage of us would be nutritionally deficient. The reason for this was first expressed by Dr. Roger Williams some years ago when he presented what is now termed the concept of "biochemical individuality." Briefly, this is the recognized fact that each person is unique in his or her biochemical makeup.* We, as members of the group *Homo sapiens*, are not exact replicas of a common ancestor, but rather evolving and genetically variable beings, with unique variations in our biochemical makeup and requirements.

Much evidence is now available to support this concept. Some 50 or more relatively rare conditions have been recognized where, due to a genetic biochemical alteration, an individual may need many times the recommended amount of a nutrient simply to maintain normal function and health. What is less well known and recognized, is that it is far more common for there to be a *partial* block in the ability of the body to utilize a nutrient. This metabolic fault may be genetic or acquired. An example of a genetic cause would be the production of abnormal enzymes that are either deficient in number or are unable to bind to their cofactors (vitamins are cofactors for enzyme functions). Without this bond many biochemical pathways are unable to be completed, resulting in what may appear to be a nutritional deficiency of a single nutrient, when in fact an average, or even above average, amount of that nutrient is consumed in the diet. To correct this situation, a very large amount of the cofactor must be supplied to "force" the enzyme reaction to occur.

The exact manner in which this excess cofactor functions is not entirely clear, but it appears that in the case where the enzyme is normal in number, but slightly abnormal in structure, the saturation of cofactor bombarding the enzyme eventually finds a site of attachment, allowing the reaction to continue. In the situation where total enzyme production is low, but the enzyme is normal in structure, the increased supply of cofactors in some way stimulates the production of more enzymes.†

In addition to a reduced number of abnormal enzymes, other factors may result in a nutritional deficiency state, even with what should be an adequate diet. Impaired absorption from the gastrointestinal tract is a common problem. This may be due to gastric or pancreatic enzyme deficiency, which in turn may be partly genetic or acquired. There may also be impaired transport of nutrients into the cells, insensitivity of the tissues to a given nutrient, or increased excretion of a nutrient. Recent studies in animals have found that severe maternal deficiency of a single nutrient such as zinc can be passed on as an excess need for

*Williams, R. J., "The Concept of Genotrophic Disease," *Lancet*, 1:287, 1950.
†Davis, Donald R., "Nutritional Needs and Biochemical Diversity," in Jeffrey Bland, *Medical Applications of Clinical Nutrition*, Keats Publishing Co., New Canaan, Conn., 1983, pp. 41–63.

that nutrient, not only in the immediate progeny, but as far as three generations later. *, †

When we consider that even by the most orthodox estimates and techniques of estimating the biochemical need of a nutrient, as expressed by the recommended daily allowances of the known essential nutrients, 1 to 2 percent of the population will need more than the RDAs of an individual nutrient to maintain proper health. When we multiply this 1 to 2 percent by the 50 or so known essential nutrients, you can see how probable it is that a given individual might be nutritionally deficient in at least one if not more of these essential health factors, if the diet supplied only the RDA recommendations.

From these and similar observations emerged the concept of orthomolecular medicine. "Orthomolecular" literally means "right molecule" and describes a form of medicine that treats disease by supplying the right amount of individual nutrients, according to the individual needs of the patient.

Also, stress places a further burden on the body, rapidly depleting the stores of many vitamins. Cigarettes, alcohol, coffee, and air pollution do the same.

Obtain and retain as many vitamins, minerals, and other nutrients from food by using organically grown foods, increase the consumption of uncooked foods, and minimize cooking of foods that are cooked. If you take great care, you can obtain all the nutrients your body needs from a "normal diet." In this case, "normal" means a properly balanced, organic, unrefined diet, and not the diet most people consume.

The aim of supplemental therapy is to supply essential elements deficient in the diet to aid in the healing process. On some occasions supplements are taken more for specific therapeutic effects. In such cases they are more like medicines and less like nutrients. An example is high doses of garlic taken to dissolve mucus or high doses of vitamins A and C to increase the effectiveness of the body's immune system.

Some naturopaths also employ glandular substances such as raw ovary concentrate, raw adrenal, raw pituitary, and others. These are used to nourish the body's glandular system and strengthen it, and not as a traditional doctor might use a hormone extract, which naturopaths feel weakens the gland.

Your body is continually undergoing a process of death and rebirth, with old cells being replaced by new. It is essential for this continual regeneration and repair that all of the necessary building blocks be made available. Diet is one of the most crucial factors in the production of health or disease.

*Prasad, Ananda A., *Nutrition Reviews*, 41:197–208, 1983.
†Beach, R., *Science*, 218:469–471, 1982.

HOMEOPATHY

Dr. Samuel Hahnemann (1755–1843) is the father of homeopathy. Hahnemann, a medical doctor and researcher in pharmacology, gave up his busy practice after becoming disillusioned with the barbaric medical practices of his day. His daughter's severe illness sent him speculating whether safer techniques might be found to treat disease. Later, when translating a text on pharmacology, Hahnemann began to question the author's description of the action of Peruvian bark (cinchona). He decided that the only way to resolve the question was to take the drug himself and observe its actions. To his great surprise, he found that the action of the drug created exactly the same symptoms that it was commonly employed to cure! From this he speculated that the first law of cure was in fact the law of similars. *Similia similibus curantur,* "Let likes be treated by likes," was an old concept dating back to the days of Hippocrates. It had, however, become bastardized into the simplistic concept that an herb, fruit, or food that "looked" like the disease was the best therapeutic agent. Thus something red might be for blood-building, an herb that looked like the heart was used for heart ailments, and so on.

Hahnemann set out to prove or disprove his initial findings by testing more drugs, both on himself and others. The result was the rediscovery of the true law of similars, the foundation of homeopathy. According to Hahnemann, a medicine will cure a patient if his or her total set of symptoms corresponds almost exactly to the symptoms produced by the same medicine when given to a healthy person:

> The curative power of medicines, therefore, depends on their symptoms, similar to the disease but superior to it in strength, so that each individual case of disease is most surely, radically, rapidly and permanently annihilated and removed only by a medicine capable of producing (in a healthy individual) in the most similar and complete manner the totality of its symptoms, which at the same time are stronger than the disease.*

This new or rediscovered science of homeopathy, or the treatment of disease with substances that produce symptoms *similar* to those of the disease, was diametrically opposed to the already established allopathic school which by definition treated disease with agents that produce effects *different* from the symptoms of the disease.

From his early conclusions regarding the true law of similars Hahnemann further proposed that the only useful diagnosis could be made by compiling a detailed list of the patient's symptoms, both physical and mental, and then finding

---

*Hahnemann, Samuel, *Organon of Medicine,* 6th ed., B. Jain Publishers, New Delhi, India, reprint 1982 (original 1921), p. 112.

the "proven" medicine that matched those symptoms exactly. He felt that the tissue changes of a clinical case of disease were merely the results of disease but not the disease itself. Emphasizing a holistic concept, he often said, "There are no diseases, only sick people." This was entirely different from the typical allopathic approach, both then and now. Too often we naturopaths and homeopaths see patients who have been to every specialist in town and through almost every conceivable laboratory test, only to be told that they have nothing wrong with them, even though they may suffer from a multitude of symptoms. This physically undiagnosable condition, however, if left untreated, may eventually settle down into a clinical syndrome so that some time later, if no treatment has been introduced, the doctor will proclaim that you have kidney disease, liver disease, or heart disease, etc. The problem, as Hahnemann explains, is that disease is a disorder of the vital life force *first*, which then is manifested in the physical (material) plane. Of this life force he says:

> The material organism, without the vital force, is capable of no sensation, no function, no self-preservation; it derives all sensation and performs all functions of life solely by means of the immaterial being (the vital force) which animates the material organism in health and disease.*

The language of this vital force is first expressed as symptoms and only much later as tissue changes.

This concept of the vital force, or the inner person being the first cause of disease, led Hahnemann to the conclusion that tissue changes in no way indicated the remedy. As Dr. James Tyler Kent explains, "Do not say the patient is sick because he has a white swelling, but that the white swelling is there because the patient is sick."†

Homeopathy specifically condemns the removal of external manifestations of disease by any external means whatsoever. If an external problem is thus removed (suppressed) the disease is driven inward, causing chronic disease. Early homeopaths warned that the final result of allopathic suppressive treatments would be a rapid increase in chronic disease in the future.

According to homeopathic philosophy it is the inner person (vital force) that is ill, so the cure must take place from within, outwards. If properly treated in this manner disease follows a set path of elimination. Homeopathic physicians believe that disease elimination proceeds from more important to less important organs, from above downwards, from within outwards, and in reverse order of its origin. Thus, according to this philosophy, since all chronic disease has its origin on the surface and then progresses deeper, as proper cure is effected, first

---

*Hahnemann, Samuel, op. cit., p. 97.
†Kent, James Tyler, *Lectures on Homeopathic Philosophy*, B. Jain Publishers, New Delhi, India, 1979, p. 60.

the inner manifestations of disease will be removed while the external manifestations will *resurface*, only later being removed as final cure results. This progression of symptoms tells the doctor that the disease is in fact once and for all being removed.

Not all conditions are treatable with homeopathic remedies. A condition such as appendicitis is better left to surgery.

The preparation of homeopathic remedies is unique. Hahnemann found that by diluting medicine to reduce its natural effect of aggravating the disease, which by definition was its therapeutic attribute, not only was the aggravation made less, but its beneficial effect was surprisingly enhanced. Later he came to realize that a vital disorder could only be corrected by a medicine similar in quality to the vital force. To attain this similarity in quality, medicines were "potentized" to be effective on the subtle forces of man. This "minimum dose" medicine is prepared by diluting one part of the original substance with nine parts of milk sugar, or in an 87% solution of alcohol, or diluted with water. This mixture is then treated in a specific way until it is uniformly dispersed. It is then known as the 1× dilution. The process is then repeated as many times as required, taking one part of the previous mixture and mixing it with nine parts as above, to create 2×, 3× and so on up to 30×, 200× and so on. The "higher" the dilution the more dilute the mixture.

This dilution process creates great difficulties for the physically minded scientist in understanding how a more dilute medicine may in fact be more therapeutic in a particular case than the more concentrated substance. The fact that these medicines are found by homeopathic physicians in practice to be even more effective in some cases than more concentrated doses supports Hahnemann's vital force concept of both the medicine and the disease itself.

According to Hahnemann,

> The dose of the Homeopathic remedy can never be sufficiently small as to be inferior to the power of the natural disease, which it can, at least, partially extinguish and cure, provided it be capable of producing only a small *increase* of symptoms immediately after it is administered.*

Actual diagnosis and treatment along homeopathic lines is extremely complex and not suited for self-administration. The patient must be interviewed in depth regarding symptoms, with each detail carefully noted. A remedy must be chosen with a complete understanding of its ability to be able to reproduce exactly the disease symptoms described. Homeopathic prescribing is not possible along "disease" categories. There is no set remedy useful for everyone with arthritis or migraines. It is in the subtle differences between each patient that the correct

*Hahnemann, Samuel, op. cit., p. 112.

remedy is chosen, and its proper dilution prescribed. The treatment process is not stagnant, with the original dose being repeated until symptoms are removed. It is in fact by a change in symptoms that the homeopath judges the prescription and alters it as required.

In this book you will find few homeopathic remedies recommended. The treatment by homeopathy must be undertaken with the guidance of someone competent in homeopathy and is not easily applied with only a little knowledge at home. For homeopathic therapy, consult a qualified naturopathic or homeopathic physician.

HYDROTHERAPY

The history of hydrotherapy dates back well before Hippocrates. Water was worshipped by primitive peoples as far as recorded history, and probably before. Many great rivers such as the Nile in Egypt and the Ganges in India have long been considered to have sacred healing powers. Many cultures, such as those of the early Egyptians, Arabians, Mohammedans, Hebrews, Greeks, Hindus, Chinese, Japanese, and American Indians used mineral waters for healing purposes. Many centuries before Hippocrates, physician-priests established temples near thermal springs or mineral waters where the sick came to bathe, be massaged, and fast in communion with their gods. Hippocrates himself gave detailed prescriptions for the use of water in the treatment of many diseases. The Romans established extensive hydrotherapy spas for both social and health purposes. The Finnish, Turkish, and Russian sweat baths are other examples of water therapy with ancient origins.

In the early middle ages the Church set up opposition to the treatment of disease with water therapy, labeling it paganism. A dark cloud was then cast on the history of hydrotherapy in the western world until the late 1600s. Water therapy continued undaunted, however, in Japan and the eastern countries even during these dark times. In 1747 John Wesley, the founder of Methodism, wrote a text on hydrotherapy entitled *An Easy and Natural Method of Curing Disease.* Hydrotherapy as a science is commonly credited to Vincent Priessnitz, a Silesian peasant. In the early nineteenth century when Priessnitz was 17 years old, he suffered a severe accident that his doctors fully expected to be fatal. Having had some experience in treating his animals with water therapy, Priessnitz applied the same measures to himself, and in a short time was completely cured. Hearing of his remarkable cure peasants from near and later far came to Priessnitz for treatment. Soon his whole time was devoted to this new "hydrotherapy." He employed douches, wet sheet packs, cold purges, sweat baths, wet compresses, sitz baths, and other treatments commonly used today.

Unfortunately, Priessnitz did not record his therapies in book form. The first modern hydrotherapy text came out of Bavaria in 1886. Father Sebastian Kneipp was from youth a rather frail, sickly sort, until hearing of the use of cold water to harden and strengthen the body. He thereupon determined to give it a try and proceeded to take daily swims, first in summer and then in the heart of the icy Bavarian winters. Soon he developed extraordinarily good health and strength. Moved by the plight of the underprivileged poor, who he felt were too often neglected and forsaken, he expanded and developed hydrotherapy, and dedicated his life's work, *My Water-Cure*, to them. His hope was to send this newly rediscovered knowledge throughout the world and be relieved of his self-appointed task as healer of the tens of thousands who sought his aid. In this task he succeeded well. In less than 10 years his English translation had already undergone fifty printings, and made its way onto many orthodox physicians' bookshelves. Water-cure establishments or "hydros" sprang up all over Germany and Europe, later spreading to the United States.

Up until this time the use of water in the treatment of disease was based mostly on empirical results; in the late 1800s Dr. J. Winternitz of Vienna developed the scientific theory that the action of water was upon the nervous system, and its effects were either direct or reflex. The extent of its influence depended upon the water's temperature, and the force with which it was applied. By 1906 Dr. H. Kellogg of the United States had written *Rational Hydrotherapy*, the first scientific text on hydrotherapy, which still serves as the basic text on the subject.

Principles and Physiology of Hydrotherapy

Even though we now possess a better understanding of how the application of water at different temperatures affects the body, the science of hydrotherapy has advanced little since the days of Kellogg. To understand how something as simple as the application of water could profoundly affect the body, we must review the mechanisms of heat regulation since it is by these basic bodily responses that hydrotherapy is able to produce its reactions. The balance between heat gain and loss is controlled primarily by the nervous system. Numerous areas in the nervous system control changes in superficial and deep circulation of blood, sweating, shivering, and general metabolic rate in response to changes in the environment and body temperatures. In the central nervous system the most important area is the hypothalamus. This thermoregulatory center regulates general body temperature, responding to nerve impulses passing from the various parts of the body, or as a result of its direct sensitivity of the surrounding blood's temperature. Another part of the brain, the medulla oblongata, controls the vasoconstricting (narrowing) tone of the blood vessels and is modified by impulses coming from the cerebral cortex and hypothalamus. The parasympathetic and sympathetic branches of the nervous system control the constriction or dilation of blood vessels throughout the body, responding to nervous and hormonal stimulation.

The degree of threat to the body's temperature equilibrium determines the extent that the nervous system is brought into play. If the stimulus is local and at a temperature slightly higher than normal, only local nerves are excited. If the thermal threat is greater, more extensive spinal reflexes are stimulated. If the heating is more prolonged, of greater temperature, or over a larger area, the hypothalamus centers in the brain are brought into play and a general reaction throughout the system is initiated. In these general reactions the body responds with superficial dilation of the blood vessels, increased blood volume, increased cardiac output, and increased pulse rate. This rapidly increases the skin's circulation and permits heat loss by conduction, convection, and radiation. Sweating then results if further heat loss is needed. The secretion of adrenalin and thyroxin is inhibited.

When the application of heat is not sufficient to raise the general body temperature and therefore does not stimulate the heat loss center in the brain, spinal vasoconstrictor centers play an essential role in heat regulation. Nervous reflexes produced by heating the skin inhibit these centers and vasodilation results. This dilation of the blood vessels occurs not only in and about the heated area, but also in other areas reflexly related. It is in this distant reflex response that most of the beneficial results of the superficial application of heat occur for the treatment of internal disorders.

The effects of cold on the body are controlled primarily by the nervous system. Heat loss is reduced by superficial vasoconstriction of blood vessels. This reduces the amount of heat transferred from the central parts of the body to the surface. Heat production is then initiated by involuntary muscular activity which may be irregular and imperceptible as individual muscle units contract out of harmony with each other, often termed "thermal muscular tone"; or it may result in the regular in-phase contractions known to all as "shivering." Thus, the body can speed up its general metabolic rate two to five times and keep the body temperature at acceptable levels. Other mechanisms helping to control body temperature are the secretion of adrenalin and thyroid hormones which increase the metabolic rate, a rise in blood pressure, an increase in heart rate, and the erection of the body's hairs ("goose flesh") to prevent heat loss.

The body responds to the application of water at different temperatures and pressure in a two-step process. The *initial* action of the body is the immediate response to a threatening external stimulus. It is strictly defensive in origin. For example, when ice-cold water is applied to the skin, the body acts to prevent heat loss by sudden vasoconstriction of the local blood supply. The opposite is true when hot water is applied to the skin, with vasodilation occurring to encourage heat loss.

If the application of either hot or cold stimuli is of short duration, a secondary reaction occurs in the body. This reaction begins just after the stimulus is removed and is usually complete within 20 minutes, and occurs due to reflex stimulation of the vasomotor and heat regulation centers. In general, the reaction is the opposite of the initial action made by the body.

The following tables summarize the body's initial actions and secondary reactions to both hot and cold stimuli if of short duration.

COLD

Action	Reaction
1. Contraction of small blood vessels of skin, with dilation of reflexly related internal vessels after a brief contraction	1. Dilation of small blood vessels of surface, with contraction of internal vessels
2. Pallor of skin	2. Redness of skin
3. Goose flesh and rough skin	3. Smooth, soft skin
4. Sensation of chilliness	4. Sensation of warmth
5. Trembling, shivering, and some pain	5. Comfort and relaxation
6. Quickened pulse	6. Slowed pulse
7. Quick, gasping respiration	7. Free, slow, deep, and easy respiration
8. Cooling of skin	8. Warmth of skin
9. Perspiration halted	9. Perspiration increased

HEAT

Action	Reaction
1. Vasodilation of surface blood vessels	1. Surface congestion due to inactive dilated blood vessels
2. Redness	2. Pallor
3. Pulse slowed at first, then quickened	3. Pulse frequent
4. Perspiration increased	4. Perspiration decreased
5. General nervous excitation	5. Nervousness and mental tiredness, drowsiness, and depression
6. Increased muscular irritability	6. Muscular weakness, atonic, sedative

The primary effect of cold is therefore excitant while the secondary reaction is invigorating, restorative, and tonic. The primary effect of heat is also excitant, while its secondary reaction is depressant, sedative, and atonic. Neutral applications are calmative.

Hydropathic Use of the Primary Effect of Heat or Cold

As a general rule the shorter the application and the more extreme the temperature, the more purely excitant will be the effect of hot or cold.

General Primary Excitant Effects

Any method of application may be used to initiate a *general primary excitant effect*. In practice, heat is usually employed for this purpose. The effect of alternate hot and cold applications of very short duration is to continually renew the excitant effect of heat. The cold source is applied only as long as is necessary to return the skin to its preheated temperature. These applications are usually 15 seconds for each temperature; however, heat may be prolonged slightly longer than cold with good effect. This technique allows an indefinite extension of the primary excitant qualities of heat without its depressant reaction. The general primary excitant effect of heat is useful in cases of severe exhaustion, collapse, fainting, shock, drowning, fright, or suffocation. *Extremes of temperature are not advised with heart conditions, advanced age, or in the very young.*

Local Primary Excitant Effects

More extensive use is made of the *local primary excitant effect*. There is no more powerful method of increasing heart activity than short very cold applications over the chest or back. This is used only as a last resort to stimulate a failing heart into increased activity in emergency situations where no other help is available. Very short cold applications almost anywhere on the body, hands, cheeks, face, or trunk are useful to arouse one from a faint. Intense cold of short duration to the umbilicus will excite and stimulate intestinal activity in nervous and motor dysfunctions of the bowels causing constipation. The uterus may be stimulated to contract by short, sudden cold applications to the breast, and is of use in delayed labor.

Hydropathic Use of the Secondary Excitant Effect

Usually, only cold applications are used for their secondary excitant effects since the secondary effect of heat is always atonic, or sedative. Heat, however, may be used in conjunction with cold to enhance the reaction, especially if the patient is sensitive to cold, or of poor vitality. Here, too, alternate hot and cold application is used, but with each temperature applied longer, anywhere from 1 to 3 minutes.

General Secondary Excitant Effects

General secondary excitant effects can produce a powerful systemic excitation where every nerve and cell is activated as well as many hormonal secretions. The intense cold application may be reinforced by percussion, as in a cold shower, giving intense excitation to the whole body. The effect may be restorative or tonic.

A single application of cold is restorative after physical or mental exhaustion. Muscular strength and mental alertness follow a short ice-cold shower or bath.

The tonic effect of cold is its most useful characteristic. It excites the entire system, increases circulation, nutrition, assimilation, and healing. Unlike coffee, which extracts energy from already depleted energy stores, leaving the body in a weakened state, cold water has only beneficial effects. The function of the brain and nervous system is stimulated and a sense of well-being follows a cold application, partly due to increased brain circulation. Ice pond plungers use this dramatic therapy to harden and strengthen their bodies for increased health and vigor.

In using the cold bath there are a few principles to keep constantly in mind. Like other great tonic agents, cold is a double-edged sword, capable of great benefit or harm. A patient I once saw in a totally devitalized and depressed state had heard of these tonic effects of cold applications and reasoned that if something was good, then twice as much must be that much better. He proceeded to take a 10-to-15-minute ice-cold bath two or three times each day. No wonder he felt devitalized. The best tonic effects are obtained by daily very cold and very *short* baths or douches, followed by massage, friction rub, and exercise.

Local Secondary Excitant Effects

Local secondary excitant effects are the most often used hydropathic effects. The application of water of varying temperatures, duration, and pressure may affect the function of any organ of the body in whatever way desired. The skin may be cleansed, toned, and purged of impurities; the circulation of blood and lymph increased; and nerve and glandular structures normalized by sweating baths or packs. Inhalations, sweat baths, and vapor baths may be used to clear congested mucous membranes and aid in expectoration. The kidneys may be stimulated by cold douches to the sternum or upper legs, or by application of a wet sheet trunk pack for 3 to 8 hours. The liver may be stimulated by cold or alternate hot and cold compresses or douches. Hot fomentations may help relieve gallbladder pain and dilate the ducts, allowing passage of stones. Gastric juices may be stimulated by cold douches over the stomach, or alternate hot and cold applications. In cases of amenorrhea prolonged hot foot baths, hot sitz baths, or enemas may be used along with ice-cold douches to the thighs for 2 to 10 seconds and daily hot and cold sitz baths. Any pelvic congestion may be relieved by alternate hot and cold sitz baths and this treatment is used for the ovaries, uterus, fallopian tubes, bladder, and prostate. Hot foot baths with ice to the back of the neck will help relieve cerebral congestion and thus remove many headaches. The hot foot bath alone is a cure for insomnia.

These and many more effects can be obtained easily with hydrotherapy.

Benefits of Hydrotherapy

The benefit that a patient will receive from hydrotherapy depends on how strong a reaction is achieved. This depends on the patient's vital reserve, which must be carefully considered before vigorous treatments are prescribed, as no two people are alike. Aesculapius' disciple Antonius Musa attained fame by curing the emperor Augustus of chronic lung congestion and catarrh by using the cold bath. As a reward for this his statue was erected on the temple of Aesculapius. But lack of discrimination in the use of hydrotherapy led to his downfall. Being called upon to treat the emperor's nephew, a rather effeminate young man, he employed the same cold bath that worked so well for the athletic soldier and emperor, with the result that the youth was so prostrated that he soon died. Father Kneipp made a similar mistake. In treating the Pope for chronic rheumatism, he advised an ice-cold bath, with the result that on the very first treatment the Pope, then a frail and aged man unaccustomed to such heroic treatment, was in such pain that he cried for hours. Had the patient been a sturdy young peasant as Kneipp was accustomed to treating, rather than a feeble Italian gentleman, the prescription might have worked.

Several factors influence the degree and speed of a positive reaction to either heat or cold. The most important of these is the general vitality of the patient. Prolonged illness, fatigue, nervous exhaustion, and anemia may reduce the body's ability to react properly. Poor reactions sometimes occur in the very young, due to incompletely developed heat regulation, and in the very aged. In general, the more the temperature of the application differs from the body's temperature, the better will be the reaction. The reaction will also be directly proportional to the size of the area exposed. Sudden applications of short duration and high intensity give a better reaction than graduated or slowly applied applications.

The actual method of application can also influence the degree of reaction. Friction or pressure will enhance a reaction. Hot drinks taken during or after a treatment, as well as general exercise, will increase certain reactions. In some cases a warm application preceding a cold one will enhance its reactive effect. However, the prolonged application of either heat or cold may cause tissue damage and inhibit the natural reaction.

Once the basic concepts of hydrotherapy are understood (and I have given only a brief and incomplete summary here), they may be used to produce any of the following effects:

Anodyne—pain reliever
Antipyretic—lowers fever
Antispasmodic—reduces cramps
Anesthetic—local
Diaphoretic—increases perspiration
Diuretic—increases urine production
Emmenagogue—stimulates menstruation
Hypnotic—induces sleep
Purgative—causes bowel evacuation
Pyrogenic—causes temperature increase
Sedative—quieting and soothing effect to nervous system
Stimulant—exciting action
Tonic—increases physical or mental vigor

Hydropathic Procedures

Following are just a few examples out of many developed by the fathers of hydrotherapy and of hydropathic applications used successfully over the years. Those procedures mentioned in this book and which are beneficial and practical for home use are discussed below.

Baths

ALTERNATE HOT AND COLD SITZ BATH

This frequently used bath may be applied with benefit in nearly any disorder of the lower abdomen or pelvic region, including menstrual disorders, diseases of the uterus, ovaries, or fallopian tubes, prostatitis, constipation, digestive disorders, and others.

Hydropathic institutions have specifically designed sitz baths, often like two water-filled armchairs, facing each other. One is filled with very hot water, the other with ice-cold water. The patient sits with his or her bottom in the hot water and feet in the cold water for 3 minutes, and then reverses, with the bottom in the ice-cold water and the feet in the hot water for 1 to 2 minutes. The patient alternates back and forth from hot to cold for three immersions in each temperature, and ends with the bottom in the cold. The patient finishes the bath by drying vigorously with a rough towel and exercising until sweating is produced.

Although these ready-made sitz baths are ideal, they are rarely available to the home patient. Simple home sitz baths may be improvised by using two large plastic tubs or galvanized washtubs. These must be large enough to accommodate the patient's bottom easily, and hold enough water to cover the person from umbilicus to midthigh. The hot water temperature should be as warm as the body can comfortably bear and the cold must be *very* cold. In most areas this means that ice needs to be added to cold tap water and allowed to melt first to lower the water's temperature.

For maximum benefit these baths must be done daily from one to four times per day, depending on the patient's condition. The effect of this bath increases the circulation of blood and lymph to the pelvic region, removes internal congestion, and improves tissue vitality and nutrition.

Cold Sitz Bath

The patient sits in a container as described previously, with cold water but no contrasting hot foot bath. The duration should be short—from 30 seconds to 1 minute. This bath is used much less frequently than the alternate hot and cold sitz bath. This bath may be very useful in enuresis, with the duration of the cold gradually increased to 3 to 5 minutes. Friction rubbing with a loofa mitt may be administered with the cold sitz, rubbing the hips, back, and thighs vigorously to increase the body's reaction. This is a powerful tonic bath and may be continued 3 to 5 minutes daily. It is useful with bed-wetting, impotence, difficulty in conception, and uterine malposition.

Hot Sitz Bath

This bath is the same as the cold sitz bath, except for the hot water, and is of longer duration—from 3 to 10 minutes. It is useful in relieving colic and spasm or pain due to menstrual cramps, low back pain, hemorrhoids, and intestinal disturbances.

Full-Immersion Bath

These baths are similar to either hot or cold sitz baths except that the effect is more generalized since the entire body is covered with water.

Cold Full Bath

The cold full bath may be used as a tonic, but is less profound in effect than the cold plunge. Repeated cold plunges may be used to cause the temperature to rise, creating an artificial fever. In practice, the cold bath is not used frequently for anything other than its tonic effect.

Hot Full Bath

This is the common bath in most households, which is in many ways very unfortunate. A full hot bath should only be taken for short intervals of 2 to 10 minutes and for definite therapeutic purposes. Very hot full-immersion baths daily create debility, poor circulation, mental lethargy, physical weakness, and depression. The Japanese *furo* is also a hot full-immersion bath and if prolonged will cause the same atonic effects. Short periods of heat need to be interspersed with ice-cold plunges to be of any use, and should end with a cold application if for general use and not specific therapeutic purposes. Hot baths may be beneficial if prolonged and taken at the time menstruation is expected in case of suppressed periods, or for dysmenorrhea as an antispasmodic. Other forms of colic benefit, as found under the heading of Hot Sitz Bath.

HOT FULL EPSOM SALTS BATH

This bath is similar to a full hot bath except that 1 to 1½ lb of Epsom salts are dissolved in the water. This bath is used for various therapeutic purposes and is very antispasmodic and cleansing. The bathwater should be as hot as the body can reasonably bear, and prolonged for 20 minutes. After the bath it is best to go to bed, cover up well, and sweat. After 3 hours or more of sweating the patient is sponged off with tepid water or given a tepid douche or bath.

NEUTRAL OR TEPID FULL-IMMERSION BATH

A tepid bath is calmative and soothing if prolonged. It may last 30 minutes to 4 hours. Acute hysteria or mental disorders are relieved by this simple bath, as is insomnia. Generally this bath is taken at 94 to 98° F. If a high fever is present no better bath may be used than this gently cooling application. To be effective for this purpose the bath must last at least 20 minutes or longer. Always remember, however, that fever is your body's friend and should not be indiscriminately or routinely reduced.

LOCAL BATH

Hot, cold, or alternate hot and cold water may be applied to any part of the body to elicit specific effects. The most frequently used is the alternate hot and cold bath. Simply obtain two containers larger than the part to be treated, and fill with hot and cold water. The method of application is simply to first immerse the part in hot, then cold water. The usual interval is 3 minutes in hot water to 1 minute in cold, although equal time in both temperatures may be used. Repeat this three times, always ending with cold water.

SWEATING BATH

The Turkish bath and Finnish sauna are essentially dry heat baths, while the Russian bath is that of moist heat. The bather sits on wooden benches until sweat is produced. Depending on the type of sauna, water is poured on hot stones to produce steam, or ice-cold water is poured periodically over the head and body, after which a masseur or partner will apply birch branches vigorously, all over the body, to increase the skin's action. The bath lasts 10 to 20 minutes and then a cold shower, cold plunge, or even a roll in the snow cools the body off and encourages a strong circulatory and nervous reaction.

This procedure is then repeated one to three times, with the individual remaining in the sauna 2 to 10 minutes after perspiration becomes noticeable. Saunas are used to increase circulation, skin function, respiration, and general vitality. They also stimulate the nervous and hormonal systems, and encourage mental relaxation and sleep. Cabinet baths are used in a similar way and allow the head to be cooled by wet compresses. This can usually be done with less severe bodily reactions.

Compresses

COLD COMPRESS

The application of cold water, using two to four layers of cotton cloth. For home use cheescloth folded to eight thicknesses, cotton diapers folded to four thicknesses, or toweling may be used. The effect depends on the temperature of the water and the length of application. Cold or ice-cold water may be used, depending on the need. Where prolonged cold applications are required, several compresses are used and alternated, one following the other with no resting interval. Intermittent cold compresses may be applied for 1 to 3 minutes, with an interval allowing a reaction to begin, followed by a reapplication of the compress. This is in essence similar in effect to alternate hot and cold water, since the value in a hydropathic application depends on a difference in temperature between the application and body. Continuous cold or ice compresses are used for pain relief or to prevent swelling in an acute injury. They also stop hemorrhages and reduce congestion in local applications—for example in sinusitis. Cold compresses often are used in conjunction with hot applications to aid further in the reaction desired. An example would be a cold compress to the back of the neck and a hot foot bath at the same time for headaches and cerebral congestion.

HOT COMPRESS (FOMENTATION)

Applied like a cold compress, using hot water and several thicknesses of cotton cloth or toweling. Thick compresses hold their heat better and are therefore usually more efficient. The compress may be covered with dry material or a towel to prevent heat loss. Where prolonged heat is needed the compress is replenished frequently, as with continuous cold compresses. Duration depends on the temperature of the compress and effect desired. Local heat is antispasmodic, pain-relieving, and sedative. It dilates the local blood vessels and draws blood into the region. Take care not to apply heat too often or too continuously, which may cause damage to tissues and effusion of blood into the area, resulting in congestion.

ALTERNATE HOT AND COLD COMPRESSES

Tonic and curative, increasing blood flow and nutrition through a local area. They are used frequently in therapy, alternating hot and cold compresses at varying intervals, depending on the effect desired. The usual frequency is 3 minutes hot and 1 to 2 minutes cold. Alternate hot and cold compresses are often used just after the first 48 hours of an injury, until healing is complete.

Packs

All packs are basically similar in design, having an inner wet cotton fabric covered by dry blanketing. They act by stimulating the body with cold for the positive reaction that later results. Among commonly used packs are the cold full-body wet sheet pack, trunk pack, abdominal pack, chest pack, and throat pack.

FULL-BODY WET SHEET (COLD) PACK

This pack has long been termed "the cold pack," which is misleading, since the end result is warmth. First, fold a sheet lengthwise and lay this across the upper end of the bed so that the top covers the lower one-third of a thin pillow, thus covering the upper one-half of the bed, except for a few inches at its upper end. Then spread a large double blanket so that it reaches from the lower edge of the pillow to well over the foot of the bed. The upper edge should leave at least 2 in. of sheeting exposed. One side of the blanket should extend at least 2 ft over the edge of the bed. Next, a thin linen sheet is soaked in ice-cold water and wrung out so that it is just wet and then spread out on the blanket so that its upper edge is an inch or two below the upper edge of the blanket. The patient lies on his back on the sheet so that the sheet extends 2 to 3 in. above the shoulders, and raises his arms above his head. The helper rapidly draws the sheet across the body and tucks it snugly underneath the side of the body. From the hips the sheet is wrapped around the leg on the same side, leaving the opposite leg uncovered. The arms are now lowered and the opposite side of the sheet is wrapped snugly over the arms and body, fully enveloping the entire body, except the head, within the sheet and in contact with it. The remaining sheet is tucked comfortably under the feet and lower legs. Next, the short end of the blanket is drawn across the body, tucked under the shoulder, side, and leg; followed by the long side, which is drawn tightly across the body and pinned. The lower end is tucked under the feet. The bottom folded sheet is then drawn across the body and tucked comfortably around the neck to prevent discomfort or irritation from the blanket.

No air draft should be present. If necessary, to produce the sensation of warmth, an extra blanket or two may be laid over the patient and tucked close to the head and shoulders. These may be removed later if needed. If the subject does not experience a sensation of warmth within 5 minutes, the pack must be removed, and after 10 minutes of brisk walking about while receiving friction massage, it may be reapplied, this time with a hot water bottle placed at the feet. In the case of nervous people or those who feel too restrained with the arms bound, they may be left out of the wet sheets, but still included in the blanket wrap.

In practice, the wet sheet pack is used with almost all acute diseases, especially conditions with fever or due to toxemia. The fever is not lowered by the pack; in fact it will be raised, but as a result of the pack if continued 3 hours or all night, the fever will have been aided in its work by increased elimination and thus be lowered due to decreased need. Wet sheet packs of short duration (3 to 5 minutes) repeated many times will lower the temperature rapidly. I rarely suggest it. Its major use is for elimination. After the pack, sponge the body well with tepid water, and dress. Do not reuse the sheet used for a prolonged pack without washing, since it contains many toxins.

TRUNK PACK

This procedure is the same as the full-body pack but is confined to the area from underneath the arms to midthigh. All that is needed in this case is a lower blanket extending from underneath the arms to midthigh. On top of this is placed a wet sheet 4 in. narrower so that when the pack is completed the blanket fully covers the sheet. Once the pack is pinned in place, the bedcovers are drawn over the entire body. This pack is somewhat more convenient than the full-body pack and easier for home use. It is used for the same purposes as the full-body pack.

CHEST PACK

This pack is similar to a short trunk pack, extending from the underarm to the umbilicus. The upper portions of the chest are included in this pack by using two pieces of sheeting cut 6-to-8-in. wide and $2\frac{1}{2}$-to-3-ft long, and two additional towels.

Lay out the blanketing so that it will extend from underneath the arms to the umbilicus. Lay the towels in an X fashion at the top of the blanket so that 6 in. or more of the lower ends of the towels overlap the upper end of the blanket. Next, place the wet sheet and two smaller sheet pieces so that they fit well inside the blanketing and towels. The patient lies down on the sheets so that his head and neck are just above the crossing of the X-placed sheets. These are drawn across the chest, followed by the body sheet. The towels then are drawn across, followed by the body blanket, and pinned. The bedcovers are then drawn over the patient. Duration of the pack depends on the patient's condition. Usually, periods range from 3 hours to all night. This is an excellent method for all chest complaints.

THROAT PACK

This pack is usually used with abdomen or trunk packs. All that is needed is a thin strip of sheet, neck size, and a suitably sized towel. The sheet is soaked in ice-cold water, wrung out, and wrapped around the throat. This is then covered by the blanket layer and pinned. This may be worn for an hour or more and is very useful in tonsillitis.

Inhalations

Steam inhalations are often recommended for lung conditions, in conjunction with various herbs. One easy method is to place the suggested herbs in boiled water as if one were making tea. Let these sit for 2 to 3 minutes in the covered container. Remove the cover and place this steaming pot on a low table and drape a large towel over the pot and the patient's head so that the vapors are directed to the nose and mouth. The patient breathes in deeply for 5 to 15 minutes. Another method is to place two chairs back to front with the steaming pot on the front chair and the patient in the one behind. A large blanket is placed over all, creating a true inhalation tent. With children, another method is to place the chairs facing each other with the pot on one chair and the parent and child on the floor of the tent. This gives a less intense inhalation, but is much less suffocating and therefore more desirable with squeamish children.

The Enema

During a cleansing fast when solid food is not taken, the bowels tend to cease functioning and their contents become more concentrated and hard. Unless this residue of waste matter is eliminated, harmful substances may be reabsorbed and reduce the effectiveness of any health regimen.

The enema should be taken only when fasting, or while on a semifast. Enemas and bowel irrigations are not recommended while on a normal or reduced diet.

Obtain an enema apparatus with a 1-to-2-quart container. The container is filled with warm (about body temperature) water or medicinal tea and placed or hung about 3 ft from the floor. Adopt the knee-chest position, or lie on your left side on a towel in the bathroom, or near a toilet. Insert the nozzle into the rectum and allow the water to run in slowly by controlling the intake valve on the hose. When the pressure becomes too strong, or you feel it is becoming difficult to retain the water, stop the water intake and take a short rest; then continue. After the water has been drained off, take out the nozzle and turn on your back. Slowly massage the abdomen from lower left up to the ribs and across the abdomen to the right, with deep circular motions. Retain the water 5 to 10 minutes and then release the fluid into the toilet.

Douches

A douche is a strong jet or spray of water directed locally or generally, like an ordinary shower. The only type of shower douche I routinely recommend for home use is the *alternate hot and cold shower*. This begins with a comfortably warm shower for 3 minutes, followed by a sudden change to cold for 1 to 2 minutes. Repeat the whole process for three cycles, ending with cold. Finish off with a brisk towel rub and some exercise.

Morning Dew Walks

An old tonic measure is to walk barefooted on the wet morning grass daily, year-round. It has the same effect as local cold foot baths and is very refreshing.

Simple though many of these hydropathic techniques may be, they are very effective aids in channeling the body's vital energies toward health.

PHYSIOTHERAPY AND MASSAGE

Naturopathic physicians use physiotherapy in their treatment of soft-tissue and connective-tissue disorders. These are used for various acute or chronic injuries. Some of the more commonly used physiotherapy devices are short-wave diathermy, microwave therapy, ultraviolet radiation, galvanism, ionto-phoresis, faradism, and ultrasound.

During my student years while observing therapy sessions at the office of a prominent naturopathic and osteopathic physician, I noticed that in his office, which he shared with other physicians, there were several physiotherapy apparatuses he never made use of the entire time I was at his treatment sessions. In an attempt to draw some information from him I asked what he thought of ultrasound and the other units in the office. His reply, "They are wonderful for a practitioner who does not have hands," was characteristic of the pure osteopath.

While acknowledging that one of an osteopath's greatest attributes is trained hands, I have found in practice that certain physiotherapy modalities can greatly accelerate the healing process when properly used in conjunction with standard osteopathic soft-tissue techniques. When weeks of agonizing frictions across fibrocystic and calcified muscle fibers would otherwise be necessary, the use of ultrasound and frictions together might cut therapy time in half. Ultrasound in particular is very useful in removing calcified spurs that would normally require surgery.

Massage, per se, another form of physiotherapy, is not usually performed by the naturopath or osteopath in a busy office practice, although many practitioners recommend massage therapy and many have a massage therapist working in their office. As described previously under Spinal Manipulation, a specific soft-tissue therapy, sometimes called the neuromuscular technique, is practiced by many osteopaths as an integral part of their therapy. Hydrotherapy, as described under that section, is another frequently used form of physiotherapy.

SPINAL MANIPULATION

Basic History and Philosophy

One of the main therapeutic techniques used by naturopaths as well as chiropractors and osteopaths is spinal manipulation. This method originated in ancient civilizations such as Egypt and Greece, many years before Christ. Hippocrates left detailed suggestions for spinal traction and manipulation. More recently a loosely knit group of lay "bonesetters" practiced widely in Europe and England in the early 1800s. Early in the 1870s a country doctor named Andrew Taylor Still from Virginia expounded the early philosophy of osteopathy. Still, disillusioned with drug therapy by the death of three of his children from spinal meningitis, sought new concepts of healing. Ultimately he became convinced that structural abnormalities affected the function and well-being of the body. In explaining this new science of "osteopathy" he evolved the "rule of the Artery." This stated that the cause of disease was reduced blood circulation due to spinal abnormalities. Still saw osteopathy as a complete science and that *all* disease could be treated by it successfully without any other measures. Still's fervor was a bit exaggerated. Not only has the basic concept of osteopathy changed significantly over the past 100 years to include a more complete understanding of the actual modus operandi of disease and osteopathic therapy, but its scope is now generally considered more limited and it does not dismiss other forms of medicine.

In 1895 an unqualified practitioner from Iowa, Daniel David Palmer, expounded his philosophy of chiropractic. Palmer had overheard his deaf janitor saying that his hearing loss had coincided with a feeling that something in his neck had "gone." Palmer examined his neck, felt an unusual lump, performed a manipulation and the janitor reportedly regained his hearing. Out of this one adjustment grew chiropractic. Palmer developed a theory very similar to Still's, stressing that anatomical faults caused functional disturbances within the body. Palmer espoused "the rule of the nerve," stating that minor spinal displacements caused nerve irritation, which eventually led to disease.

As years have passed, the basic theories and philosophies of osteopathy and chiropractic have grown closer together as medical research and knowledge of spinal disorders has improved. It is now fairly well accepted by osteopaths, chiropractors, and naturopaths that spinal "lesions" or "subluxations" cause both changes in blood and nerve supply. Major differences, however, still exist between the two philosophies, which are reflected in both their methods of diagnosis and treatment. The basic concept that structure governs function is accepted by both schools. However, subtle differences of emphasis have led to large differences in actual practice.

The chiropractic philosophy states that "subluxations" impinge on structures (nerves, blood vessels, and lymphatics) passing through the intervertebral foramen, resulting in disease, and that "adjustment" of a subluxated vertebra removes this impingement, thereby restoring to diseased parts their normal innervation (and blood supply). The two major diagnostic techniques used to determine these "subluxations" are palpation and x-ray. Most chiropractors (however, not all, and in fact fewer as time goes by) routinely expose the patient to diagnostic x-ray to diagnose a subluxation. Others rely more on palpation of bony prominences such as the transverse processes of vertebrae to diagnose a positional abnormality. In either case the emphasis is usually on "position." Once this position is determined, manipulation is applied to correct the alignment and, theoretically, relieve the problem either locally or due to referred symptoms elsewhere in the body.

Osteopathy also concerns structural and mechanical faults as they affect the physiological processes, but defines these in relation to the spine as spinal "lesions" rather than "subluxations." These lesions are ". . . impaired *mobility* in an intervertebral joint in which there may or may not be altered position relations of adjacent vertebrae."*

This concept stresses that the mobility and functional relationship of one bone to its neighbor is more important than its positional relationship. As a result of the basic concept of "mobility," osteopaths rarely employ x-rays, except to exclude pathological conditions. The key diagnostic technique used is called *mobility testing*, or *motion palpation*. With this technique each spinal segment is evaluated for proper mobility in all its planes of motion in relation to both the vertebrae above and those below. It is used for peripheral joint diagnosis, as well. Once a spinal lesion is diagnosed, osteopathic therapy is directed to this area to remove these restrictions and allow restoration of proper nervous, blood, and lymph supply, both locally and in referred areas elsewhere in the body. From the two basic philosophies, once again vast differences in actual treatment have evolved between osteopathy and chiropractic. Chiropractic, with its stress on "position," routinely and almost exclusively has used "chiropractic manipulation." This usually involves the use of short levers or direct contacts to bony prominences, with high-velocity, short-amplitude thrust to alter the position of the subluxation into alignment.

An historical distinction has been made in the past that osteopaths tend to use the principle of longer levers and indirect contact in their manipulations.

*Stoddard, Alan, *Manual of Osteopathic Practice*, Hutchinson, London, 1969, p. 36.

While this may have some historical fact, in reality actual techniques of many spinal manipulations of either chiropractors or osteopaths are the same. It is also fair to mention that there is an incredible variation, practitioner to practitioner, in both schools of healing. The main distinction, however, between a typical or traditional chiropractic and osteopathic treatment is that the osteopath routinely spends much time and energy working on the soft-tissue and connective-tissue structures prior to actual osseous manipulation. This soft-tissue manipulation is considered even more essential to complete healing than the more dramatic "clicking" and "popping" elicited from osseous manipulation. Quoting Stoddard again, we find

> It is possible to restore normal alignment and yet not restore good function. Ideally we should attempt to restore both perfection of structure and harmonious function, but of the two the function is the more important. When we manipulate the spine, we are not so much concerned with putting a bone back into place as with removing any mechanical hindrances to the restoration of normal movements in the affected joints.*

In explanation, for example, it does little permanent good to repeatedly adjust a malpositioned or malfunctioning vertebra if the reason for its hindrance in function or position is a muscle or other connective-tissue structure. As with pitching a tent, if the tent is found functionally distressed or malpositioned due to an improperly set guy line, it will do little good simply to realign the tent without first loosening or tightening the abnormal supports. Thus, in osteopathy a great deal of time is spent in normalizing the relationship of muscles, ligaments, tendons, and joint capsules to their bony partners.

Although I believe that traditional osteopathy is broader in concept than traditional chiropractic therapy, the difference between any two osteopaths or chiropractors can be immense, with some osteopaths more resembling chiropractors in practice, and vice versa.

Spinal manipulation is only one of the many modalities used by the traditional naturopath. No one method is sufficient in most cases to create real harmony within the body. It is in the intelligent use of all natural therapies, for the benefit of the patient, that the best form of medicine is to be found.

The Principles as Applied in Practice

The first principle of osteopathy is not unique to this discipline at all. Just as Hippocrates stated, "vis medicatrix naturae" (only nature heals), Still reaffirmed that the greatest law governing the human body was its self-sufficiency

---

*Stoddard, Alan, op. cit., p. 38.

and ability to heal itself if all hindrances were first removed. The second fundamental principle, as has already been stated, is that "structure governs function." The manner in which structure may affect the body was unclear during the birth of osteopathy. Still's "rule of the artery" and Palmer's "rule of the nerve" were early attempts to explain how spinal lesions or subluxations did their destructive work.

Early osteopaths and chiropractors assumed that alterations in spinal function placed direct pressure on either blood vessels or nerves, causing complete or partial blockage as they emerged from the intervertebral foramina. This has been proven untrue except in very severe trauma, or possibly in relation to lesions in the upper cervical region with their close association to vertebral arteries and veins which pass through the foramina on the transverse process. Actual dislocations, disc lesions, or pathological changes can produce such effects, but the spinal lesion or subluxation per se, which remains within the normal range of the vertebral segment, can never do so. What does occur, however, is indirect compression of other nerves or blood vessels, due to irritation, inflammation, edema, metabolic by-product accumulation, and pH changes, leading to local and referred symptoms similar to actual compression. The key, therefore, to understanding spinal lesions is the soft-tissue components of the functional unit of the spinal column.

What occurs with a typical acute spinal lesion is swelling in response to improper body mechanics, or local, visceral, or peripheral trauma. This causes congestion, edema, decreased oxygen, increased carbon dioxide, and increased pH. This may lead to indirect nerve irritation or compression, causing pain, paresthesia, hyperesthesia, numbness, hyper- or hypotonicity, reflex vasoconstriction or vasodilation, and loss of muscle power or atrophy, depending on the nerve involved and the severity and length of the compression. The cause of a spinal lesion may be improper body mechanics causing abnormal strains on the spine or periarticular structures (muscles, tendons, ligaments, articular capsules, discs, etc.), or it may be due to local, visceral, or peripheral trauma.

The role of improper body mechanics is fairly easy to understand. Abnormal pressure exerted on the vertebral segment due to altered spinal curves causes local tissue changes in muscle, ligament, bones, and discs, which may result in compression or irritation of the closely associated spinal nerves, leading to altered conduction, and changes in the tissue or organs supplied. Compression of blood vessels (directly or indirectly), and vasoconstriction or dilation due to abnormal nervous impulses, can alter blood flow to tissues and organs, resulting in congestion or reduced blood flow.

Local trauma is also easy to understand as a cause of spinal lesions. This is due to the commonly occurring strained or twisted spine, or some severe local blow or fall. The immediate results are those of the typical spinal lesion, with acute symptoms of pain, edema, heat, muscle spasm, limited motion, and possibly referred or reflex symptoms. Chronic lesions show limited mobility and increased connective tissue, but less pain. Referred or reflex symptoms may or may not be apparent, but observed or unobserved degenerative changes are taking place and vitality is being reduced in the tissues and organs supplied from that vertebral nerve center.

Peripheral or visceral causes of spinal lesions is a subject usually only understood by practitioners of spinal therapy. Abnormal stimulation in a tissue or organ may cause contraction of the spinal muscles in two or three segments on the same side of the spine at levels that correspond to its nervous supply. Later this muscle spasm spreads and may set up the very conditions of a spinal lesion with indirect nerve compression which in turn sends abnormal impulses to the organ or tissue at fault, aggravating or perpetuating the original cause. Other more direct pathways may exist such as nerve irritation with subsequent neuritis.

What all of this means in simple terms is that an injury or "spinal lesion" not only elicits local and referred pain, but may also cause an alteration in the nerve, blood, or lymph supply to distant tissues and visceral organs, resulting in a disease state. Certainly this can be understood or accepted in relation to the nervous supply being directly altered to a muscle, causing pain, twitching, spasm, or even complete atrophy. The fact that spinal lesions can also profoundly affect internal organs should not seem too remarkable when we consider that their entire functioning is dependent on nervous impulses, either directly or through vasomotor nerves affecting their blood supply. There is plenty of evidence, both clinical and experimental, that the osteopathic "spinal lesion" or chiropractic "subluxation" causes physical, chemical, and tissue changes, not only in the local area, but also in the organs and viscera that receive their innervation from the same spinal segments. It is on this proven basis that spinal therapy is used to help treat internal complaints. I can remember quite well the first time I went for chiropractic therapy and listened with horror to other patients extolling the beneficial effects of chiropractic therapy for their asthma, sexual disorders, high blood pressure, their child's bed-wetting, and a whole host of other complaints. I congratulated myself that I was not so gullible as to believe such nonsense and that at least I had come for a back complaint, the *proper* realm of chiropractic, and would go away with something better than all this hocus-pocus. It was not until 15 years later, when I was literally forced into learning about osteopathy to attain my aim of becoming a naturopath, that I finally understood how accurate such assertions were.

The naturopathic approach to the use of osteopathy or other spinal manipulation is to employ this technique as one would any other tool of naturopathy. The aim of its use is to normalize nervous, blood, and lymph supply to diseased organs, or the body as a whole. This increases local nutrition, removes congestion, and raises general vitality so that healing may progress more rapidly. For those interested in pursuing this subject, I suggest Stoddard's two books, *Manual of Osteopathic Practice*, and *Manual of Osteopathic Technique*.

POSSIBLE TOXIC EFFECTS OF SOME NUTRITIONAL AND BOTANICAL PREPARATIONS

Although some nutritional and botanical preparations can have toxic effects, the dosages required to produce such effects are usually far in excess of the normal prescriptive dose. As with nearly all substances the body is exposed to, even the seemingly most benign, excessive or prolonged use may produce undesirable, or even toxic effects. The criterion for determining how safe a nutrient, botanical medication, or even a drug is lies in how wide is the span between its pharmacologically effective dose and the dose where toxic effects are known to occur.

In general, nutritional supplement therapy and botanical medicine have a fairly wide range of safety between the normally prescribed dose and the dose at which known toxic effects can occur. In the press we periodically read of cases where a particular vitamin, mineral, or herb that may have been in use for many years has been found to cause undesirable, or even dangerous effects. Such reports can often be based on slanted research, placing a cloud of fear over an extremely useful substance.

An example of this occurred recently when the press covered widely the finding that vitamin B_6 caused sensory neuropathy and ataxia in some patients. Immediately nearly every one of my patients on vitamin B_6 therapy called with concerned questions about why I could have prescribed a medication that would paralyze them! Upon investigation of these stories, it has been found that the dose used to cause these toxic effects was from 2000 to 5000 milligrams (mg) per day of vitamin B_6 for from 40 months at the 2000-mg-per-day level to as little as 2 months at the 5000-mg dose level. The recommended dietary allowance (RDA) for vitamin B_6 is 2 mg per day. The usual therapeutic dose is between 50 and 250 mg per day. The dose required to cause these problems was 2500 times the RDA or between 8 to 100 times the doses used in therapy! It was later revealed that all the symptoms spontaneously disappeared when the subjects stopped taking such extreme doses of this vitamin.

Certainly vitamins, minerals, and botanical medications can have toxic effects, just as severe and as dangerous as drugs can if taken in excess. The point is, however, that the range of safety of most of these preparations is far wider than that of most drugs.

The following survey of possible toxic effects of vitamins and botanicals, with some dose guidelines, may prove useful for reference, as you read the individual diseases in Part II. These toxic ranges do not apply to all individuals. It is possible for an individual to be more sensitive to a particular nutrient or botanical medication, just as it is possible for a person to be *less* sensitive to it. Some individuals may have an increased need for a particular nutrient due to an abnormality of their biochemistry. *

It is fairly common that a particular enzyme deficiency may require a particular nutrient far in excess of standard doses. In these patients, a higher than average dose is in reality the correct dose for their optimum health. † Other patients, who suffer from malabsorption, may in fact only be able to absorb a small percent of the oral doses given. In these cases, large doses taken orally may allow a standard dose to be absorbed internally. In this case, most of the nutrient is excreted, with only a small fraction actually having any therapeutic effect. Dose prescriptions must be chosen individually, keeping these and other factors in mind.

Vitamin Toxicity

- Vitamin A   Standard doses are from 10,000 to 25,000 IU (international units) per day. This vitamin is highly toxic if taken in excess. Main toxic effects are a transient hydrocephalus and vomiting. Chronic vitamin A toxicity can occur at supplemental levels at or above 50,000 IU per day, if taken for prolonged periods. Toxic effects include fatigue; lethargy; bone or joint pain; headaches; insomnia; restlessness; dry, rough, or scaly skin; loss of hair; loss of appetite; enlargement of liver and spleen; edema; and other cirrhotic-like changes; abnormal bone growth; and premature closure of epiphyseal plates.

   Hypercarotenosis, or the toxic effects of large doses of carotene (vitamin A precursor found in foods such as carrots), has as its only toxic effect the yellowing of the skin. This is not known to cause any clinical symptoms and is reversible by reducing or stopping excess intake of carotene-containing foods or supplements.

- Vitamin D   Vitamin D, if ingested in excess, can cause excessive calcification of bones or elsewhere in the body (i.e., organs, especially kidney) and may encourage kidney stone formation. Elevated serum calcium levels occur at high levels of intake. Vitamin D activity is enhanced by sunlight. In most people on a normal diet or with adequate sun exposure, vitamin D use is not usually warranted. Doses of 400 to 1000 IU may be used if no other vitamin D-fortified foods are used concurrently. Due to the fact that many nutritional supplements list vitamin D as an ingredient, it is possible for toxicity to occur,

---

*Bland, Jeffrey, *Medical Applications of Clinical Nutrition*, Keats Publishing Co., New Canaan, Conn., 1983, pp. 43–45.
   †Ibid.

unless labels are read carefully. Intake of 2000 to 3000 IU per day may become toxic.

- Vitamin E   Generally considered nontoxic. High levels (1200 to 1600 IU), if taken suddenly, have been reported to temporarily raise blood pressures. This later normalizes. Vitamin E may interfere with vitamin K activity, acting as an anticoagulant in high levels. Vitamin E has also caused immune suppression at high levels. Usual doses range from 200 to 800 IU per day, with doses up to 2000 IU being used in some disorders.

- Vitamin K   Used mostly in the newborn, to prevent hemorrhagic disease due to a prothrombin deficiency in the first few days of life. Also used as an adjunct to modify anticoagulant therapy. Toxic effects include hemolytic anemia and kernicterus in infants.

- Vitamin B_1 Few toxic effects of this vitamin by mouth have been reported. Rare cases of anaphylactic shock occur from intramuscular or intravenous injection in hypersensitive individuals. Other symptoms include generalized urticaria, facial edema, wheezing, and difficulty breathing.

- Vitamin B_2 No toxic effects have been reported.

- Vitamin B_3 Due to its vasodilating action, transient tingling or flushing sensations do occur at normally used doses. Other symptoms include nausea, gastric irritation, abnormal liver function, jaundice, elevated uric acid levels, and abnormal glucose tolerance.

- Vitamin B_6 Toxicity of vitamin B_6 has been considered extremely low until recently when transient sensory neuropathy and ataxia were reported at doses from 1200 to 2000 mg per day for extended periods of time. Usual doses range from 50 to 250 mg. Vitamin B_6 is completely safe at these, or even twice these levels.

- Pantothenic acid   No toxic effects have been reported.

- Biotin   No toxic effects have been reported.

- Folic acid   High doses (15 mg daily for months) may cause sleep disturbances, nausea, irritability, abnormal distension, anorexia, flatulence, and malaise. High doses mask a vitamin B_{12} deficiency and therefore recommended doses are 400 mcg as a standard dose, 800 mcg in pregnancy. High doses may be used as long as vitamin B_{12} status is adequate and no toxic symptoms are present.

- Vitamin B_{12} No toxic effects reported.

- Vitamin C   High doses (10 g or over) have been implicated in the formation of kidney stones. This has been disputed by other sources. Rebound scurvy has been reported from subjects suddenly withdrawing from very high doses of vitamin C. Diarrhea occurs at varying doses, seemingly dependent upon the body's need for this nutrient. Scurvy in newborns whose mothers took supplements of high doses of vitamin C has been reported. This is not reported in the breastfed infant. Usual doses range from 250 mg to 30 g or more per day. Given intravenously at 30 to 50 g per day in some cases.

* Bioflavonoids   No toxic effects have been reported.

* Choline   No toxic effects have been reported. High doses cause a fishy body odor.

* Inositol   No toxic effects have been reported.

* Carnitine   Neither requirement nor toxicity known.

Botanical Toxicity

The use of herbs in the usual prescribed doses is generally quite safe. Many of the toxic effects of overdose that do occur are simply the body's action to rid itself of the substances through vomiting or diarrhea. *Some herbs, however, are extremely dangerous and have a very narrow range of safety.* Thorough knowledge of botanical medications and their possible toxic effects is essential before using these remedies. The following list of herbs and their common toxic effects is partial only, concentrating on the botanical preparations used medicinally that are most toxic, or those that have been mentioned frequently throughout this book. The toxic effects listed are not complete. For a detailed description of botanical toxicology, consult *An Introduction to the Toxicology of Common Botanical Medicinal Substances,* by Francis Brinker, pp. 1–123.

* *Aconitum napellus (aconite)   This herb is extremely toxic and has a very narrow range of safety.* Its usual therapeutic dose of tincture is 1 to 8 drops, while toxic reactions may occur at only 10 drops. Fatal dose is 5 ml of tincture. Most frequently used in homeopathic dilutions, and as such is very safe. Toxic effects include nausea, vomiting, dizziness, tingling, burning, numbness, impaired speech, blurred vision, headache, anxiety, muscular weakness, low blood pressure, weak pulse, irregular heartbeat, chest pain, shallow breathing, excess perspiration, low body temperature, and death, due to respiratory failure or ventricular fibrillation.

* *Anemone pulsatilla*   Toxic effects are abdominal pain, nausea, vomiting, burning in mouth or throat, cardiac arrhythmia, slow pulse, weakness, difficulty in breathing, paralysis, convulsions, coma.

* *Arnica montana*   Topical use of the undiluted tincture can cause local irritation or eczema-type inflammation. Usual internal therapeutic dose is 1 to 10 drops tincture. Toxic dose is 2 oz tincture. Used internally mostly in diluted

homeopathic potencies. Toxic effects (internal use): nausea, vomiting, diarrhea, muscular weakness, reduced pulse, cardiovascular collapse, convulsions, coma, and possibly death.

- *Artemisia absinthium (wormwood)* Therapeutic dose of oil is 1 to 5 drops. Toxic dose is 15 ml of oil. Toxic effects: nausea, vomiting, unpleasant dreams, impotence, lack of vitality, headache, trembling, convulsions, death. Do not use in pregnancy (emmenagogue).

- *Artemisia santonica* Fatal dose is 2 to 5 grains for children, more for adult. *This herb has a very narrow safety margin.* Toxic effects: nausea, vomiting, diarrhea, cramps, vertigo, sweating, flushing of face, dilated pupils, reduced blood pressure, slowed pulse, reduced urine flow, convulsions, death by respiratory paralysis. May cause blindness or aphasia if taken over prolonged period.

- *Atropa belladonna (belladonna)* *Very toxic.* Normally used in homeopathic dilutions only and as such is safe for use. This remedy is a component of most over-the-counter teething mixtures. Toxic effects (due to atropine poisoning): nausea, diarrhea, vomiting, dry mouth, flushing, dilated pupils, rapid pulse, increased blood pressure, incoordination, speech impairment, visual impairment, hallucinations, coma, death.

- *Bryonia alba (white bryony)* Used most frequently in homeopathic dilutions. Toxic effects (of tincture): vomiting, diarrhea, bronchial irritation, cough, gastrointestinal upset, jaundice, weak, shallow pulse, dizziness, headache, dilated pupils, temperature drop, collapse, death.

- *Cactus grandiflorus* Its major action is as a cardiac stimulant. In excess may cause increased heartbeat, arrhythmias, headaches, vertigo, angina, cardiospasm, mental symptoms, and inflammation of the heart or pericardium.

- *Chenopodium anthelminticum (wormseed)* Experiments show subcutaneous application causes cancer in rats. Other routes of entry as yet are not implicated. Other toxic effects include: nausea, vomiting, headache, tinnitus, reduced audio and visual acuity, sluggish bowels, ulcers, reduced blood pressure, paralysis, death.

- *Cinchona ledgeriana (Peruvian bark)* Contains quinine and quinidine. If used for any prolonged or excessive doses, will cause the following toxic effects: nausea, vomiting, headache, tinnitus, deafness, visual disturbances, dilated pupils, abdominal pains, mental confusion, restlessness, weakness, delirium, and psychotic changes. If taken in pregnancy it is teratogenic, causing congenital visual and auditory damage.

- *Convallaria majalis (lily-of-the-valley)* Contains many cardioactive glycosides that, if taken in excess, can cause cardiac arrhythmias, raised blood pressure, mental confusion, weakness, circulatory collapse, and death. Its toxic effects occur more rapidly than with digitalis.

- *Digitalis purpurea (foxglove)* Contains many cardioactive glycosides that, when taken in excess, can cause an increase in ventricular irritability, ventricular tachycardia, and fibrillation, leading to death. Early symptoms include nausea, vomiting, appetite loss, visual abnormalities, drowsiness, and low blood pressure.

- *Hedeoma pulegioides (pennyroyal)* May cause liver damage. Standard dose is 2 to 10 drops oil. Toxic dose 4 ml.

- *Lobelia inflata* Toxic effects are due to lobeline; however, emesis normally occurs to prevent this. Toxic effects include nausea, vomiting, weakness, loss of consciousness, coma, and death.

- *Phytolacca decandra (pokeroot)* Berries from plant are very poisonous. Tincture is made from whole plant. Toxic effects: nausea, vomiting, diarrhea, gastrointestinal cramps, weakness, convulsions, reduced blood pressure, slowed pulse, coma, death due to respiratory paralysis.

- *Podophyllum peltatum (may-apple or American mandrake)* Externally can cause severe ulceration and dermatitis. Internally may cause nausea, diarrhea, emesis and severe gastroenteritis, which may lead to death.

- *Rauwolfia serpentina (Indian snakeroot)* The toxic effects are those of reserpine. These include diarrhea, abdominal cramps, sedation, pinpoint pupils, low blood pressure, and coma.

- *Sassafras albidum (sassafras)* Tests have shown safrole, its main constituent, to cause cancer when injected under the skin in rats. This has not been observed via the normal oral route.

- *Symphytum officinale (comfrey)* Hepatocellular adenomas in rats have developed after use of comfrey leaf in diet up to 8 percent of total intake or of root at 1 percent of diet for over a year. This dose is clearly above any reasonable intake, as normally prescribed. Care needs to be taken by those who consume large amounts of comfrey in the belief that its vitamin B_{12} content is high enough to be of significant nutritional value. One would need to eat 1 to 2 lb of comfrey leaves a day to get adequate vitamin B_{12} levels, and at this level toxicity may occur.

- *Urginea scilla (squill)* Toxic effects: nausea, vomiting, diarrhea, nephritis, cardiac arrhythmia, heart block, convulsions, death.

WHEN DRUGS AND SURGERY *ARE* NECESSARY

The aim of naturopathy is to remove the cause of disease without harmful drugs or unnecessary surgery. Only when the actual causes of disease are removed can real health be present.

Many health problems can be cured with natural therapy. Abundant examples of this are given in this book. Still, there are times when the use of drugs or surgery may be necessary, even lifesaving. Obviously, mechanical injuries require a mechanical solution. If an arm or leg is fractured you need it placed in a cast, not a comfrey poultice; and it might even need to be surgically pinned. If the reason your child wets the bed is due to a congenitally abnormal genitourinary system, he or she needs reconstructive surgery and not sitz baths. If you have appendicitis you need surgery, not grape abdominal packs. Surgery, in its proper place, is the most admirable of medical achievements.

Some uses of drugs and surgery, both necessary and unnecessary, are the result of ignoring early signs and symptoms of disease. Tonsils that are greatly enlarged and severely scarred may cause enough distress to warrant removal on rare occasions, but may never reach such a state if the early symptoms of the disorder are heeded and treated properly. Appendicitis may develop into peritonitis, which is an acute surgical emergency by anyone's standards, but may never develop if the diet or the early digestive malfunctions are attended to promptly. Many surgical procedures, therefore, are necessary only because the individual has not listened to the disease's calling card until it is too late.

Drug therapy, like surgery, is also mostly preventable, in my opinion. A significant number of patients currently on high blood pressure medication for 5 years or less could be cured without drugs. However, the very life of some may totally depend on these drugs. Again, as with the case of surgery, the usual cause of this dependency was years and years of ignoring or improperly treating the first signs of high blood pressure or the diseased organ system that caused the blood pressure to rise. Insulin is lifesaving for a person with congenital or juvenile-onset diabetes, but many cases of adult-onset diabetes show early warnings that could and should have been attended to. With many chronic diseases the improper treatment of acute disease acts as the major factor in their development to the point where drugs are required.

Antibiotics fall into a separate and unique class of drugs. They are a double-edged sword, being essential in some stages of infection and at the same time detrimental in terms of human ecology. Nearly any infection anywhere in the body can develop to the point that the use of antibiotics is a wise course of action. This, however, usually occurs only if the earliest signs of infection are ignored, or if the individual's vital energy and immunological resistance are so depressed by poor diet or other factors that the body is no longer capable of self-cure rapidly enough.

The times when antibiotics are required must be carefully and seriously considered. If antibiotics are reserved for the few times in a person's life when an infection is actually life-threatening, or poses a serious threat to an organ system, their use is clearly justified. But these drugs are now employed for nearly every mild bacterial infection, and even for viral infections over which they have absolutely no effect. This reduces the future effectiveness of the antibiotic when it may really be required and favors development of antibiotic-resistant bacteria. By frequent use we are setting the stage for new plagues of antibiotic-resistant diseases.

Another disturbing fact about antibiotic overuse is that the most common aftereffect of the use of antibiotics is a bacterial or fungal infection. Antibiotics are nonspecific to a large degree within the body. Although they are developed to have a specific effect on specific bacteria, in many cases they also destroy most of the beneficial bacteria within the body that either have a physiological support function, such as those that produce vitamin B_{12} in the intestinal tract, or provide a protective service against invasion by more dangerous bacteria or fungus.

The decision to use surgery, drugs, or antibiotics must be made as the very last resort, or if no other alternative exists. No general comprehensive guidelines, however, can be made as to when this point has come. Each case must be considered individually by a physician fully aware and proficient in natural alternatives as well as more orthodox methods. The central problem with the drug and surgical approach to disease is that it generally deals with the end of the disease spectrum and concentrates on localized manifestations only. Most processes have their origin long before drugs and surgery are required. We continually push the body toward catastrophe by ignoring or suppressing acute disease beginning in early childhood. If the language of disease had been heard and treated properly at these times there would be very little need at all for drugs or surgery in our lives.

PART II

How to Use
Natural Medicine

The following chapters provide information concerning common diseases. Not all of this information applies to each person suffering from a particular disease. Each causative factor and therapeutic regimen must be considered separately, according to the individual.

By supplying this information in readily available form, my aim is to help people treat their own minor ailments in early stages. While minor disorders may safely be treated at home without supervision, any serious condition must be handled by a trained practitioner.

Use common sense. If you are dealing with a condition that is, or could become a serious health risk, consult a trained health professional you trust.

ABSCESS (see Boils)

ACNE AND SEBORRHEIC DERMATITIS

Definition

An inflammatory condition of the skin where sebaceous glands are most numerous and active: on the face, neck, chest, and back.

Symptoms

Characterized by blackheads, whiteheads, pustules, inflamed and infected nodules, sacs, and cysts. Infection occurs in the pilosebaceous follicle (hair follicle in the sebaceous gland). This may cause permanently dilated pores, obstruction of the pilosebaceous opening, and severe scarring.

Etiologic Considerations

- Puberty
  Androgenic hormones increase sebaceous gland activity
  Psychological
  Zinc deficiency

- Diet
  Excess saturated fat (especially homogenized cow's milk)
  Dairy products
  Meat
  Fried food, pastry
  Hydrogenated fats
  Excess sugar, which potentiates the effect of fats; detrimental effects on system are threefold
  Nutritional deficiency or excess need for development
  Zinc
  Lack in diet, soil depletion
  Increased need for in puberty
  Rapid growth requires excess
  Malabsorption; hydrochloric acid deficiency reduces zinc absorption
  Vitamin B_6
  Individual excess need
  Menstrually related deficiency common
  Birth control medication (progesterone)-related B_6 deficiency
  Excess sugar, refined carbohydrates, junk foods, chocolate, cocoa, caffeine (Coke, Pepsi Cola, tea, coffee), salt, alcohol (see Hypoglycemia)
  Overeating
  Improper liquids, carbonated beverages
  Lack of green vegetables

- Poor eliminations
  Bowel lesion (thinning) due to diet or stress
  Constipation
  Liver congestion or toxicity
  Overstressed kidney function
  Poor skin eliminations

- Incoordination of deep and superficial circulations
  Toxic elimination via skin associated with poor eliminations
  Spinal lesions

- Menstrual acne
  Part of premenstrual triad of fluid retention, irritability, and acne flare. Vitamin B_6 related in many cases

- Food allergy
  Food additives
  Specific food allergies, especially dairy products, wheat, yeast

- Cosmetics

- Lack of exercise

- Anemia

- Rapid growth

- Family history

- Stress

Discussion

Acne occurs most frequently in the teenage years when it affects 80 percent of all teenagers to some degree. This has been associated with an increase in sex hormone activity which causes an increase in the sebaceous gland output. This can also be seen in cases of infantile acne just after birth, due to high levels of circulating sex hormones. Acne is rarely found in eunuchs. The incidence of teenage acne is so high as to be considered "normal" in developed nations. This fails to consider that not all populations experience such high rates of acne. One such population was the Canadian Eskimos who, prior to 1950, had no incidence of acne. Later, as more modern foods, including sugar and refined carbohydrates, were introduced into their diets, acne became common.*

The main dietary offender in the modern diet is its high saturated fat content. A diet high in animal proteins, cheese, and milk causes abnormal development of the sebaceous glands, leading to acne. The modern teenage diet is a prescription for acne, with cheeseburgers, hot dogs, french fried potatoes, corn chips, potato chips, fried eggs, french toast, butter, milk shakes, milk, sugar, candy, cola, and chocolate.

Although meat (especially pork fat) and hydrogenated fats are detrimental, milk fat is often the main offender. We are the only species that feeds our young milk after weaning. The situation would probably be less serious if we gave our children mother's milk, but we give them cow's milk, with its excessive fat.

The link between diet and acne has long been recognized by both naturo-

*Wright, Jonathon, *Dr. Wright's Guide to Healing with Nutrition*, Rodale Press, Emmaus, Pa., 1984, p. 21.

pathic physicians and the lay public. Every teenager knows that chocolate may aggravate acne. Other detrimental substances in the diet are coffee, tea, alcohol, and sugar. Sugar in particular facilitates the action of saturated fatty acids, making it the number two offender.

A second major cause of acne is an incoordination of the eliminations. This may include sluggish bowel and skin function, a toxic liver, or overstressed kidneys. When the eliminating organs become imbalanced, the superficial circulation becomes filled with toxic eliminants which then clog the superficial capillaries and small lymphatic vessels which feed the sebaceous glands and cause inflammation with secondary infection. This incoordination between deep and superficial circulation may also be due to spinal lesions which upset the cerebrospinal centers located in the ganglia of the automatic nervous system which control these circulations.

Another common finding is areas of the bowels that have thinned walls allowing leakage of toxins into the system. (See Psoriasis or Allergy for more details on this condition. Refer also to Constipation as it relates to incoordination of elimination.)

The habit of hot showers or baths is another factor that upsets skin function and causes an incoordination between deep and superficial circulation. Prolonged heat causes a vasodilation or a lax condition of the superficial blood vessels, leading to poor local circulation and congestion.

Certain dietary deficiencies have been associated with acne. Of these, vitamin B_6, zinc, and essential fatty acids (EFA) are the most common. Vitamin B_6 deficiency is common in acne related to the menstrual cycle, where acne is worse prior to or during menstruation and premenstrual symptoms of irritability and water retention are severe. Zinc is a common deficiency, especially during puberty with rapid growth, which requires an excess of this mineral. Zinc is deficient in most soils and therefore most foods.

Treatment

The orthodox treatment for acne is palliative rather than curative. The patient is usually told he or she will grow out of it and may be given antibiotics topically or orally if the condition is very severe. In some cases, if the acne occurs in an older female, oral estrogens are used. These treatments are not only ineffective, they are detrimental. Most teenagers grow out of their acne, but not before some scarring. Many never grow out of it and suffer acne lesions nearly all their lives.

Antibiotics are used to combat the *secondary* infections and often must be repeated every 3 to 6 months. This has a bad effect on the entire body by destroying friendly bacteria essential to our well-being.

The skin is made from the inside out. It takes 20 to 30 days for the skin now being formed to reach the surface. It is obvious then that external treatments can do little to affect this developing skin. Acne is an internal problem, not an external one. A possible exception would be cosmetic acne due to excessive use of facial creams and lotions, which clog the pores and in some cases cause an allergic reaction. Poor hygiene will also affect the skin, but the majority of cases are caused by internal factors. True healing must come from within. This healing will take some time. Even if you begin today, the results will only start to show themselves in 20 to 30 days, usually more like 60. If any severe acne lesions are present, these will take even longer, due to the great damage that has already occurred in these areas. Perseverance and absolute adherence to the dict below are essential to get rcsults.

Diet

Our main concern is to eliminate as many saturated fats as possible. Ideally the diet should contain no saturated fat. I find it best to restrict the diet to *no saturated fat* for a reasonable length of time in the beginning, so that you can begin to see true results rapidly. If you can be motivated enough and convinced that this short-term, very strict diet will have some very long-term advantages, I advise 6 to 8 weeks of a *no-saturated-fat diet.* This includes plenty of noncitrus fruits, raw vegetable juice, salads, cooked vegetables, vegetable and seaweed soups, seeds and nuts in moderation, whole grains, and vegetarian proteins such as beans and tofu. Seaweeds are suggested for their high iodine content, as are pumpkin seeds for their zinc. All junk foods, fried foods, refined foods, and carbonated drinks or alcohol are prohibited. A short *vegetable juice fast* of 1 to 7 or more days with enemas on days 1, 2, 3, 5, and 7 is useful to speed the healing process. These should be done every 2 to 4 wecks if possible. The diet that follows allows nonfat dairy products, but by no means suggest it. If possible, dairy products should be excluded from the diet until the skin is perfectly clear. This is not always possible.

The fat content of milk is fairly complex and must be understood if proper milk products are to be added safely to the diet. The following summary should prove helpful:

Ice cream	10% to 20% butterfat
Evaporated whole milk	8% + butterfat
Whole milk	4% to 6% butterfat
Homogenized milk	4% butterfat
Evaporated low fat	4% butterfat
Low fat	2% butterfat
Nonfat, skim	.5% butterfat
Dried skim**	.1% butterfat

*Asterisked foods are included depending on stage of diet or allergy.

Evaporated skim**	.25% butterfat
True buttermilk**	.5% butterfat
Dry curd cheese**	.5% butterfat

Of these milk preparations only dried skim or evaporated skim have a low enough butterfat content to be consumed in moderation daily. Skim milk yoghurt is acceptable one to two times per week. Real buttermilk (butterfat removed) is acceptable on occasion. Dry curd cheese also is acceptable on occasion. No more than 6 oz of skim or buttermilk three times per week, 2 oz powdered skim per day, or 1 cup per day of dry curd cheese is allowed. All cottage cheeses are too high in fat, as is butter. Margarine is generally made by hydrogenating unsaturated fats and making them partly saturated. Those fats are entirely unnatural to the body and should be reduced or avoided altogether whenever possible.

Commercial peanut butters also often have hydrogenated fats. Check all labels before purchasing. In general I restrict peanut butter and encourage other nut or seed butters such as almond, sunflower, or cashew. Peanuts are not nuts anyway—they are legumes.

Commercial breads usually contain about 1 percent saturated fat and must be avoided. Either buy well-labeled whole grain breads from reliable bakers or bake your own with cold pressed vegetable oils. Commercial baked goods often contain up to 20 percent fat and should be strictly avoided.

In later stages of this diet (and in some cases very early on) poultry in moderation and fish may be added, but *never* served fried. Cold water ocean fish (i.e., cod or salmon) is suggested as the best fish source and has been found to reduce blood cholesterol levels.

Cold pressed unsaturated vegetable oils in the diet are acceptable in moderation, but never heated. It is suggested that you add 400 IU of vitamin E to a newly opened vegetable bottle to prevent rancidity and keep refrigerated. These should be used as salad dressings with lemon juice (the only citrus in the diet) or apple cider vinegar. Any herbs for taste are fine. Use plenty of onion and garlic.

ACNE DIET

The following diet may be of some use as a basic guideline. Choose from the following:

Breakfast	Noncitrus fruit
	Noncitrus fruit plus skim yoghurt*

*Asterisked foods are included depending on stage of diet or allergy.
**Milk products most commonly used in diets.

	Whole grain cereal (no sugar) with soy milk, skim milk, dried skim, or evaporated skim milk* Poached eggs and whole wheat toast*
Midmorning	Whole meal pancakes* Vegetable juice (carrot, lettuce, nettle, and watercress) Potassium broth Herb tea
Lunch	Fresh raw salad with plenty of green leafy vegetables, watercress, lettuce, cabbage, kale, chard, parsley, alfalfa sprouts, celery, onions, garlic, seaweed, sprouts, etc., with carrots and other combinations. Keep the salads varied and interesting. Salad dressing used should be based on cold pressed vegetable oil and lemon juice or apple cider vinegar. Garlic, various herbs, and honey may be used to add variety to the dressing. I suggest you obtain a good salad cookbook and experiment. Tofu or soybeans* A few nuts* Brown rice or millet*
Midafternoon	As midmorning
Supper	As lunch, *or* conservatively cooked (baked or steamed) vegetables, especially green and yellow vegetables. Carrots are also good. Use a wide variety. Tofu or soy protein, beans Fish (never fried)* Turkey or chicken (never fried)* Whole grains (especially brown rice and millet) Dry curd cheese*
Evening	As midmorning and midafternoon

Drink 6 to 8 glasses of water each day.

FOODS OF SPECIAL USEFULNESS

Green vegetables	Kelp
Carrots	Seaweeds
Onions	Fish (cold water ocean)
Garlic	Whole grains
Watercress	Sprouts

*Asterisked foods are included depending on stage of diet or allergy.

Dandelion	Vegetable juices (carrot, lettuce, nettle, and watercress)
greens	
Nettles	

In some cases wheat allergy may be a causative factor and should be avoided in all stages of the diet. Prior to therapy a radioallergosorbent test (RAST) and cytotoxic test should be done. Wheat, yeast, dairy products (even nonfat), citrus, or even eggs may be a major factor in individual cases.

Refer to Constipation if this is a problem.

Physiotherapy

- Daily Wash: Warm water wash two times per day with mild calendula or castile soap. Alternate warm, then cold applications should follow.

- Ice applications directly on lesions has helped some.

- Hot steam or hot fomentations may help lesions mature.

- Ultraviolet (UV) applications daily are very useful. *Note:* Excess UV light can cause skin cancer. Use common sense and do not overexpose the skin. The exact amount of exposure that is safe depends on individual skin type.

- Lemon juice diluted in water may be applied externally for its antiseptic and astringent effect.

- Vitamin B_6 cream locally in menstrual acne. (100 mg vitamin B_6 per gram of ointment)

- Spinal manipulation—cervical and upper middorsal, weekly.

- Sun and air baths

- Ocean bathing

- Daily skin brushing to entire body with loofa or soft bristle brush. (See Appendix I)

- Sulfur ointment (3 to 10%) topical.

- Dilute calendula tincture wash as antiseptic following maturation of lesions by hot fomentations.

Therapeutic Agents

VITAMINS AND MINERALS

Vitamin A (micellized): high doses, 50,000 to 100,000 IU per day for several months in micellized form.* Care must be taken to monitor for toxic

*Asterisks indicate the most frequently used therapeutic agents.

symptoms with these and the higher doses sometimes used. Serum vitamin A levels should be tested periodically. The frequency of test depends on dose used.

Vitamin B complex: 25 to 50 mg twice daily.* If yeast allergy is diagnosed or suspected, use a nonyeast source.

Vitamin B$_6$: 50 to 250 mg two times per day in menstrually related acne.*

Vitamin C: 250 to 1000 mg three times per day; antibiotic, antioxidant, stress reducer.*

Vitamin E: 200 to 400 IU two times per day.*

Zinc: 25 to 45 mg three times per day.* Reduce dose if bowel upset occurs. Add 1 to 3 mg copper per day at higher doses. Selenium also may need to be increased 100 mcg per day at higher zinc levels.

Trace minerals*

OTHERS

Atomodine or 636 (Cayce Products) Note: Excess iodine from Atomodine or 636 could become toxic, especially if taken with kelp in the diet. Take only under medical supervision. Some patients are sensitive to iodine and experience worsening of their acne with use.

Chlorophyll: The more the better; detoxifies intestines.

EFA (essential fatty acids): 2 to 4 capsules two to three times a day.*

EPA (eicosapentaenoic acid—cold water marine body oils): 1 to 3 capsules two to three times per day.*

Garlic: 2 capsules with meals.*

GLA, or gamma-linolenic acid (oil of evening primrose)

Glandular substances (on doctor's prescription): Raw thymus, tablets helps immune response. Raw thyroid, tablets with thyroid involvement.

Glucose tolerance factor (GTF) Yeast: To normalize blood sugar levels.

Hydrochloric acid: If previous high levels of supplements were useless or other signs of mineral malabsorption exist, and hydrochloric acid deficiency has been demonstrated with hydrochloric acid adequacy test, take with meals.

Kelp: 2 to 4 tablets two to three times per day.

*Asterisks indicate the most frequently used therapeutic agents.

Lactobacillus: 2 capsules three times per day (especially following use of antibiotics).*

Lecithin (as concentrated phosphatidylcholine): 2 capsules two to three times per day.*

Sulfur: 1 to 30 grains per day, or as homeopathic dilution. Larger doses may cause intestinal irritation and loose stools.

BOTANICALS

Aloe (*Aloe vera*): Local, topical use.

Blue flag (*Iris versicolor*): Excellent alterative; corrects imperfect lymphatic elimination; is glandular stimulant (especially thyroid)*

Barberry (*Berberis vulgaris*)

Burdock root (*Arctiumlappa*): Good alterative with skin disorders. Restores oil and sweat gland function; is antibacterial.*

Coneflower (*Echinacea angustifolia*): Alterative (blood purifier), anti-infective, bacteriostatic. Dose (tincture): 15 to 60 drops (¼ to 1 tsp) diluted in water, three to four times per day.*

Dandelion (*Taraxacum officinale*): Detoxifies liver; is a cholagogue and alterative.

Oregon grape (*Berberis aquifolium*): Alterative, activates lymphatic system. Dose (tincture): 10 to 20 drops three to four times per day.*

Red clover (*Trifolium pratense*): Alterative.

Yellow dock (*Rumex crispus*): Alterative.

Therapeutic Suggestions

Initially high doses of vitamin A in micellized form are used. This should be closely monitored for toxic reactions. As found in many other conditions, those who need a therapeutic supplement most often have a greater need than the average person, and therefore a much higher dose is often well tolerated without producing toxic manifestations. It should also be remembered that in cases of malabsorption, extremely high doses may not cause toxic reactions since only a small fraction of this dose may be assimilated. *Use any dose of vitamin A over 50,000 IU per day with medical supervision only.* Monitor higher doses with serum vitamin A test regularly.

A well-balanced B complex vitamin is also routinely suggested. Try to find one that *does not* have equal portions of all the B vitamins (i.e., 50 or 100 mg

*Asterisks indicate the most frequently used therapeutic agents.

for each—B_1, B_2, B_3, B_6, etc.), but rather one more balanced to reflect the body's true physiological needs, and not just the marketing appeal for the vitamin company. If any of the B vitamins are taken in excess they tend to deplete others in the group. Vitamin B complex is needed up to three times per day with the higher doses being reserved for those with blood sugar irregularities, or those under excessive stress. Vitamin E taken once or twice daily is also useful. Take the micellized form if poor fat absorption is suspected or known to be a problem.

Essential fatty acids are also always a regular part of the regimen. In addition to suggesting an increase in dietary sources, I recommend essential fatty acids (EFA), eicosapentaenoic acid (EPA), and cod-liver oil capsules. Lecithin in its concentrated (phosphatidylcholine) form as a fat emulsifier is also suggested three times daily.

Zinc stands out as the single most important mineral used. If doses higher than 50 mg are used per day, a copper supplement of 3 to 3 mg may be necessary. With teenagers use the lower dose. Selenium may also be needed—50 to 100 mcg per day with high zinc use.

Kelp or other iodine sources (i.e., Atomodine or 636) are often helpful in stimulating the glandular system, especially the thyroid, but may aggravate some cases.

Garlic has definite usefulness and should be prescribed routinely.

The botanical remedies of choice are coneflower (*Echinacea*), Oregon grape, and blue flag. Often, botanicals are used only in the initial stages of therapy and at intervals to encourage deeper elimination, better liver function, and tonic stimulation.

ALCOHOLISM

Definition

Habitual alcoholic consumption to the point where it interferes with the performance of daily responsibilities.

Symptoms

Late symptoms include blackouts, dizziness, slurred speech, incoordination, nervousness, irritability, tremors, heart disease, liver disease, increased cholesterol, high blood pressure, and blood sugar disorders.

Etiologic Considerations

- Hypoglycemia
- Diet
  Refined foods
  Sugar
  Vitamin and mineral deficiency
  Excess coffee
- Psychological
- Stress
- Heredity

Discussion

The commonly held view of alcoholics as psychologically sick or simply lazy and irresponsible may be incorrect. There is a growing body of evidence indicating that some cases of alcoholism may be the result of a nutritional disorder.*

For years it has been recognized that a large number (95 percent) of alcoholics suffer from hypoglycemia (low blood sugar). They also show multiple nutritional deficiencies. The usual explanation of these associated nutritional disorders is that as alcohol is consumed in preference to food (as is the case with most alcoholics) deficiency and hypoglycemia will obviously result. However, there is much evidence suggesting that many of the nutritional disorders, especially hypoglycemia, precede alcoholism.† In fact, it appears that hypoglycemia may be the *cause* of alcoholism and not its result.‡

An interesting experiment to suggest this view was performed on rats. One group of rats was fed a refined carbohydrate diet typical of most hypoglycemics. Another group was fed on unrefined carbohydrates and supplemental vitamins. The last group was fed unrefined carbohydrates and high protein, a diet commonly used to prevent or treat hypoglycemia. Each group was supplied with two drinking sources—water and alcohol. The group fed refined carbohydrates, a diet known to cause low blood sugar, slowly began to prefer the alcohol over the water until they shunned the water almost completely. The low protein

---

*Bland, Jeffrey, *Nutraerobics*, Harper & Row, San Francisco, 1983, p. 113.

†Pfeiffer, Carl, *Mental and Elemental Nutrients*, Keats Publishing Co., New Canaan, Conn., 1975, pp. 380–383.

‡Airola, Paavo, *Hypoglycemia, a Better Approach*, Health Plus Pub., Phoenix, Ariz., 1977, pp. 61–62.

group drank a little alcohol, while the third group eating unrefined carbohydrates and high protein avoided the alcohol. Another study showed that rats fed a reasonably good diet but fed sufficient sugar also began to drink alcohol. *

These studies clearly show that if hypoglycemia is allowed to develop, ideal conditions then exist for the development of alcoholism. This should not be too surprising when we consider that alcohol is probably the ultimate refined carbohydrate. Alcohol gives an even quicker blood sugar rise than sucrose. If the person is a social drinker, or has been exposed to alcohol enough for the body to recognize the very rapid blood sugar rise from alcohol, a craving even greater than sugar craving becomes established under the right conditions.

The original causes of drinking may be social, but once the body establishes an alcoholic dependency (a *physiological* need to consume alcohol to maintain blood sugar levels) the person has stepped into a vicious circle. He or she drinks to relieve standard hypoglycemic symptoms of depression, tension, irritability, tiredness, inability to think, and so on. The alcohol gives a blood sugar boost which acts as positive reinforcement, conveying relaxation, increased energy, and in general a reversal of the unpleasant hypoglycemic sensations. Over a period of time the typical alcoholic displaces what little nutritious food he or she may still consume in favor of alcohol, until the diet is even lower in protein and nutrients, further setting the stage for more hypoglycemia and therefore alcoholism.

The same progression can occur for a person who takes his or her first drinks due to true psychological problems. Long after the original psychological cause is gone, the physiological alcoholic addiction remains. Most naturopaths agree, however, that an alcoholic addiction is very rare on a proper diet. Malnutrition usually precedes alcoholism and is aggravated by it.

Treatment

Diet

Initially it is best to stabilize the person on the typical *hypoglycemic diet* to provide a stable blood sugar level. If possible, a 2-week *vegetable juice fast* is the best course of action. This normalizes the blood sugar and stops the physiological alcoholic addiction. To help break the psychological addiction and make inroads against the firmly established positive associations of drinking, Alcoholics Anonymous is a very useful program.

*The Encyclopedia of Common Diseases, Rodale Press, Inc., Emmaus, Pa., 1976, pp. 2–5.

Therapeutic Agents

VITAMINS AND MINERALS

Multivitamin, multimineral supplements:

Vitamin A: 25,000 IU two times per day.*

Vitamin B complex: 50 mg three times per day; intramuscular injections one to three times per week; nervous system nutrient, liver support.*

Vitamin B_1: B_1 deficiency is extremely common in alcoholism. The final stages of beriberi are similar to late alcoholism. Dose: 100 to 3000 mg per day.*

Vitamin B_3: 100 to 200 mg two times per day (up to 5 to 20 g given in some cases). This helps reduce alcohol craving. Increase dose slowly.*

Folic acid: 800 mcg per day.

Vitamin B_6: 50 to 100 mg two times per day.*

Vitamin B_{12}: 250 to 1000 mcg per day.

N,N-Dimethylglycine (DMG): 50 to 100 mg per day.

Vitamin C: 1000 to 5000 IU three to six times per day (or more); detoxifies; antistress agent. 20 to 30 g per day intravenously to reduce withdrawal symptoms.*

Vitamin D: 400 to 1000 IU or plenty of sunshine.

Vitamin E: 400 IU two times per day.*

Calcium: 800 to 1500 mg per day. Antispasmodic, sedative.

Magnesium: 400 to 800 mg per day.

Zinc: 25 to 50 mg one to two times per day.

Chromium: 200 mcg per day.*

Selenium: 200 mcg per day. Helps protect against alcohol-induced liver damage.*

OTHERS

Brewer's yeast—1 tsp three times per day.*

Glutamine (a nonessential amino acid): 2 to 4 g per day. Provides brain cells with an energy source, reduces alcoholic craving, and decreases harmful poisoning effects of alcohol. Glutamine has glucogenic properties.*

*Asterisks indicate the most frequently used therapeutic agents.

GLA, or gamma-linolenic acid: Alcohol is an enzyme blocking factor in the metabolism of essential fatty acids. EPA, or eicosapentaenoic acid, may also be useful.

Pancreatic enzymes: Blood glucose level stabilization; digestive enzyme support.

Raw adrenal tablets: Antistress, adrenal support.

Raw liver tablets

BOTANICALS

Angelica (*Angelica archangelica*) induces distaste for alcohol.

Chelendonium majus

May-apple, or American Mandrake (*Podophylum peltatum*) (highly toxic; see p. 62)

USEFUL PRESCRIPTIONS

Oil of eucalyptus: 1 drop

Oil of turpentine: ½ drop

Compound tincture of benzoin: ½ drop

Place in 00 capsule. Dose: one, two times per day. Reportedly makes person nauseous if alcohol is taken.

Therapeutic Suggestions

The B complex group is extremely important in therapy. Isolated B vitamins may be needed in very large doses. Vitamins B_1, B_3 and usually B_{12}, DMG (N, N-di, methylglycine) and folic acid are supplemented at high doses in conjunction with a good balanced B complex. It often is useful to begin therapy with intramuscular injections of B complex as well. Vitamin C should be taken to bowel tolerance for best results, especially in the early stages, to help break the cycle of alcohol dependence. It may even be used 20 to 30 g on an IV drip once daily in the initial detoxification regimen.

The malnutrition that usually accompanies alcoholism usually requires extra magnesium, calcium, zinc, essential fatty acids, fat-soluble vitamins (A, D, and E), and a broad-spectrum multivitamin, multimineral supplement.

Glucose regulatory factors such as chromium as found in chromium-enriched brewer's yeast are essential. 1 to 2 tsp three times per day are suggested. *Spirulina* as a glucose regulator may also be useful at 1 to 3 tsp per day. L-Glutamine, of all the therapeutic agents, is the most specific and must be used regularly over the whole course of therapy.

Considering the long list of supplements required with this disorder, I often omit botanicals and rely entirely on dietary changes and nutritional supplements. Botanicals may be required where severe liver impairment has resulted from prolonged alcohol use.

ALLERGIES

Definition

The body's adverse reactions of any variety to otherwise normal stimuli.

Symptoms

Allergies can do just about anything to almost any part of the body. Common symptoms are runny nose, watery eyes, ear infections, sinusitis, rhinitis, tonsillitis, asthma, headaches, gastrointestinal complaints, nausea, vomiting, cramps, colitis, flatulence, constipation, edema, menstrual disorders, palpitations, hypoglycemia, obesity, emotional disturbances, learning disability, mental deficiency, schizophrenia, hyperactivity, skin rashes, eczema, psoriasis, hives, ulcers, neuritis, arthritis, phlebitis, epilepsy, and others.

Etiologic Considerations

- Adrenal exhaustion
    Alcohol
    Coffee, tea
    Drugs
    Hypoglycemia
    Stress

- Stress
    Adrenal exhaustion
    Vitamin deficiency (B complex and C)
    Hypoglycemia

- Diet
    Hypoglycemia
    Sugar
    Refined carbohydrates
    Deficiency: Vitamin B complex
        Vitamin B_6
        Excess pantothenic acid need

Vitamin C
Veganism
Repeated exposure to specific foods

- Improper weaning

- Milk, egg, or wheat intolerance, plus others

- Digestive enzyme deficiency: Incompletely digested foods are irritant, toxic, allergenic

- Acid diet or junk-food diet

- Acidosis: Due to pancreatic enzyme deficiency and allergic reaction itself

- Green vegetable deficiency

- Food additives, pesticides, preservatives, colorings, etc.

- Heavy metal poisoning

- Aluminum cooking utensils

- Chlorinated water

- Fried foods

- Poor eliminations

- Liver disorders

- Inhalant sensitivity (i.e., dust, mold, pollen, grasses, animal hair, etc.)

- Drugs
Vaccines
Drug reactions (i.e., antibiotics and others)

- Heredity
Immune deficiencies (i.e., gamma A-globulin, or IgA)
Defective enzyme structure
Poor pancreatic function

- Increased permeability of intestines to large protein molecules due to a thinning of the bowel walls

- Chemicals: Severe exposure

- Radiation

- Psychosomatic

- Spinal lesions, especially in neck and upper thoracic region

- Severe viral infection (i.e., mononucleosis, flu, hepatitis), causing immune system disturbance

- *Candida albicans* intestinal infection

- Free radical oxidative damage
- Antioxidant insufficiency

Discussion

What we usually are dealing with in cases of allergy is a hyperallergic system, not a system with an allergy or two. This can easily be seen in the typical allergy patient who finds himself or herself first allergic to one thing, only later to develop more allergies as time goes by. I have seen patients who claimed food allergies to nearly everything except potato chips and Coca-Cola! Another interesting fact is that allergies may be inconsistent, being worse on some days and almost absent on others. This reflects variations in the individual's reaction, due to factors other than mere exposure.

The difference in many cases between a normal reaction and an abnormal reaction to otherwise normal elements in the environment is weak and overstressed adrenal glands. This is not the only cause as we shall see later, but certainly is a major factor. Overstressed adrenals may be due to an improper diet of sugar and refined carbohydrates, alcohol, or coffee, all of which put an excess burden on these glands. Hypoglycemia, a result of such a diet, is closely associated with most cases of allergies. Prolonged psychological stress also stimulates and depletes the adrenal glands. This creates a vicious cycle of stress, adrenal exhaustion, and allergy, which in turn usually creates some degree of stress, and so on.

A very common history reported by many allergy patients clearly shows this allergy–stress relationship. As a child many symptoms of allergy were present. These disappeared sometime in the teens or earlier. For years the patient was symptom-free, until the onset of a severely stressful incident or period of life such as a divorce (or marriage), death of a loved one, stressful job, difficult child, or other similar situation. Shortly after this, *severe* allergic symptoms return.

Another common cause of allergies, especially in the form of chronic skin rashes, is the use of vaccines and other drugs. A common history obtained from those with chronic eczema or psoriasis is single or repeated vaccinations followed closely by the onset of allergy. This is probably due to a similar mechanism of thymus gland destruction as found with massive chemical exposure of severe viral disease such as mononucleosis, hepatitis, or influenza. Certain cells, called T-regulatory cells, are produced by the thymus gland and help suppress formation of excess antibodies (and thus reduce allergic reactions). These cells are easily destroyed by many vaccines, some drugs, massive chemical exposure, severe viral infections, and radiation. The thymus plays a pivotal role with most allergies. Antibiotics are notorious for allergic skin reactions that can be most difficult to resolve. In some cases, however, the roots of allergy are not so easily traced, but a history of repeated vaccinations of drugs is always suspect. Once a foreign protein is introduced into the bloodstream some degree of allergic reaction, depending on individual variables, is probable.

Certain foods may act as the primary cause of allergies. These cause different reactions in the body than the common inhalants and other topical allergens. The body may, due to inherited tendencies, have for example a gluten intolerance causing malabsorption of any grain that contains this protein. The intestines become irritated and lose their normal villi necessary for proper absorption. This thinning of the bowel's walls allows toxic substances to be absorbed into the bloodstream, which may cause allergic symptoms far from the original disorder to complicate the local intestinal complaint. Thus we see how a single digestive incompatibility may lead to multiple allergic symptoms.

Milk intolerance is also a very common problem. Some individuals lack the enzyme to digest milk sugar from birth, while others lose this enzyme (lactase) later in life. Up to 85 percent of Orientals are deficient in lactase by adult life, while up to 85 percent of the Caucasian population retain adequate levels for normal digestion. If lactase levels are too low or absent, milk cannot be digested and it ferments, causing diarrhea, constipation, gas, abdominal pain, and many other systemic allergic reactions. The protein in milk may also cause problems.

Part of the problem with these two main food groups, wheat and milk, stems from improper weaning. The infant's intestine is much more permeable than the adult's. Large proteins or protein fragments can be absorbed directly into the blood. If protein-containing foods such as milk, wheat, or eggs are introduced into the diet too early, these protein components can set the stage for life-long allergy. Breast milk seems to protect against this foreign protein absorption into the blood by sealing the intestinal mucosa and making it less permeable. Most children are either not breastfed, or are breastfed for too short a period and then weaned to pasteurized, homogenized, antibiotic-ridden, pesticide-containing cow's milk. If breastfeeding were continued for a minimum of 9 to 12 months and the child then weaned to raw goat's milk, which is closer in constitution to mother's milk, fewer allergies (and allergists!) would exist.*

Wheat also is added to the average infant's diet much too early. Digestive enzymes necessary for proper starch digestion are not even present until 4 to 6 months. I usually advise adding wheat cereal grains as one of the last, not first elements of the diet, somewhere around the first birthday. This most definitely includes breads and crackers, no matter how wholesome. I find that the children with the most colds and allergies generally eat the most starches. Children who are breastfed eat less starches and get plenty of fruit and vegetables, and are generally very healthy during their first year of life.

Eggs are the third major food allergen and should not be given until the child is about 8 to 12 months old, and then no more than one poached egg should be consumed every other day, to prevent allergies in the early years.

*Annals of Allergy, 51: 296–299, 1983.

The general procedure of weaning is also a major cause of undetected allergy. Many parents indiscriminately add foods to their young infant's diet without carefully observing for any adverse reactions. I personally have seen 3-month-old infants with chronic eczema, whose parents already routinely fed the child "a normal diet" which for them was fried sausage, fried eggs, fried potatoes, hamburgers, potato chips, candy, and Coca-Cola! It is essential that the first foods given to an infant be as close to their natural state as possible, either raw or conservatively steamed, in a small amount only, and separate from any other foods. This should be done for a period of 2 to 3 days at one meal, to observe for a rash or any other adverse reaction. If no reaction occurs, increasing amounts may be given and then may be combined with other tested and compatible foods.

Sometimes an allergic reaction will be noticed to otherwise healthful foods such as broccoli or cabbage. In these cases discontinue these foods for 6 to 8 weeks and try again. If the child repeatedly reacts, he or she may indeed have a specific food intolerance. More likely than not, however, the second or third try will be met with success. Specific food allergies are very rare when foods are introduced properly.

I emphasize the necessity for proper weaning since it is far easier to pinpoint a reaction earlier, than later on when a full diet has been introduced. In some cases it then becomes impossible to detect the offending food without reweaning the infant—a painful process for both infant and mother.

Liver congestion and toxemia due to improper diet may also be a factor in allergies. If this is coupled with digestive enzyme deficiency or other causes of incomplete digestion, the allergic reaction is enhanced. Undigested foods usually stimulate an increase in histamine which may initiate an allergic reaction by the cells. The liver normally detoxifies histamine, but a damaged or toxic liver may do so inefficiently, causing the histamine to build up in the system, initiating a reaction. Antihistamines used as allergy medication may further cause liver damage, reducing the body's ability to detoxify histamine.

Another factor of increasing importance in the last 50 years is the widespread use of chemicals, pesticides, and other additives to the food supply. Evolution naturally adapts us to our environment; however, the pace of this exposure to foreign substances has been so rapid that evolution has been unable to keep pace. A dramatic increase in various allergic reactions has been the result.

Fairly recently *Candida albicans* (yeast) infection of the digestive system has been implicated in some stubborn cases of allergies. The yeast proliferates and irritates the intestinal mucosa, causing it to become inflamed and more permeable, allowing foreign proteins to enter into the blood. A history of antibiotic use or the birth control pill is suggestive.*

---

*"Truss Co. Metabolic Abnormalities in Patients with Chronic Candidiasis—The Acetaldehyde Hypothesis," *J. Orthomolecular Psychiatry*, 13(2): 66–93, 1984.

Treatment

The object of naturopathic therapy in this case is to strengthen the entire system, especially the overburdened adrenal glands. If specific allergens exist, they may need to be avoided where possible, to allow the system time to repair itself and establish equilibrium. If an isolated food that causes a reaction can be discovered, it will need to be eliminated. Often, however, after prolonged therapy, these may once again be added to the diet, at least in moderation.

Allergy Diagnosis

Several methods exist to diagnose individual allergies. Unfortunately none of these is sufficient on its own to distinguish all allergies. In fact all of them put together still are not sufficient to identify all allergies. However, at least they can give us a good idea of the allergens mediated by the allergy systems we now know about.

THE RADIOALLERGOSORBENT TEST (RAST TEST)

This test is a method to identify specific antibodies in the blood to certain foods or other substances. The problem with the RAST test is that a person must already have a good idea of what his or her allergies may be. Since each specific test costs around $15, it can get fairly expensive pretty quickly to have substances tested at random. Usually, common foods are tested such as wheat, milk, eggs, yeast, and citrus; however, any food can be the problem. We also test for any favorite foods, since these frequently used items are the most likely to be the problem. Most good laboratories do RAST testing. The RAST test is very selective and will only show up as positive IgE-mediated allergies. Many false negative reactions therefore occur. The foods tested must have been eaten in the three days prior to the test for best results.

THE CYTOTOXIC ALLERGY TEST

This test exposes the white blood cells to a fraction of the suspected food or substance to observe for a specific reaction. This test is more convenient than the RAST test since a battery of thirty-eight to forty tests of common foods are routinely tested for at a cost of $80 to $90. Any other specific foods, inhalants, food dyes, or chemicals may be tested for by request. Cytotoxic tests are less routinely available than the RAST, but can usually be found at large medical centers. Many false positives, however, occur with this test, and there is some question about its reliability. It is subject to error in interpretation.

Unfortunately, results from the RAST and cytotoxic tests rarely ever are the same. Thus, a positive reaction to wheat on the cytotoxic test may end up negative on the RAST. This does not mean that one test is more or less valid, but that we are dealing with two out of several systems of allergic response. Most allergists feel that several as yet undiscovered systems exist, which hopefully will soon be discovered.

THE PULSE TEST

This test, originated by Dr. Arthur Coca, may be attempted in full as outlined in his book, *The Pulse Test*, or the modified approach may be used to test for single allergens. This is a very good technique in conjunction with the two previous diagnostic tests and may help to confirm both. The basic concept of the pulse test is that foods that cause an allergic reaction also cause the pulse to rise suddenly.

ELIMINATION DIETS AND FASTS

One approach is to eliminate suspected foods for 5 to 7 days to see if symptoms are removed. This only rarely is successful since most people respond to several unsuspected foods. The better approach is to fast for 5 days and then add foods individually to the diet to test for reaction via the pulse test or by eating only one food item for several days to test for negative reactions. Many reactions take 5 days to settle down and 3 to 5 days to begin again, so you can see this can be a very difficult procedure. It is, however, the best procedure to diagnose food allergy accurately.

Food rotation diets are extremely useful in reducing the allergy load, allowing a supplement program to have maximum effect. Grains, proteins, and other suspected foods are arranged in the diet so that their consumption is not repeated more frequently than every 4 to 5 days.

The typical skin patch test is of some use.

Once an attempt to isolate specific allergens is complete, these items are removed from the diet. The next stage of therapy involves the actual process of healing the body. As previously mentioned, the allergic reaction, and along with this the specific allergens, are usually only the symptoms of a deep-seated disorder. Our next step is to soothe the hyperallergic system.

Diet

Periods of vegetable juice fasting in any acute phase of an allergic reaction are very useful. Such fasts are also essential to eliminate toxins and establish equilibrium within the body. The fast may be anywhere from 3 to 21 days with supervision. Use organically grown vegetables only. Carrot is usually the base ingredient with other vegetables added for variety.

Raw food vegetarian diets are beneficial for varying periods of time, alternated with either the vegetable juice fast or the full hypoglycemia diet (minus any allergic foods). Low blood sugar is a consistent causative or coexistent factor in most allergic patients. (See Hypoglycemia for more details on this aspect of allergic reactions.) All foods or juices should be obtained unsprayed from reliable organically grown sources. Many times a "food allergy" is in reality a chemical, pesticide, or color additive allergy.

In severe cases it is often necessary to follow vegetable juice or better yet water fasting with the introduction of single food meals on a rotation basis. Unsuspected foods are introduced into the diet with the patient eating only one food type per meal and not consuming the same food again for at least 4 days. The body is thus able to rest from repeated allergic reactions and heal itself using the nutrients found under Therapeutic Agents. Once the body has become less reactive, combination meals of the tested foods are introduced and the diet is continually expanded. Any food that causes an allergic reaction is eliminated until later in the healing process, until ultimately the individual is free of all or most allergic reactions.

Physiotherapy

• Meditation two times per day.
• Relaxation exercises two times per day.
• Spinal manipulation one to two times per week.

Therapeutic Agents

VITAMINS AND MINERALS

Vitamin A: 10,000 to 75,000 IU per day or more for short terms in acute cases. Use any dose of vitamin A over 50,000 IU per day with medical supervision only.*

Vitamin B complex: 25 to 50 mg three times per day (essential in adrenal function).*

Vitamin B$_3$: 1 to 3 g or more per day.

Vitamin B$_6$: 100 to 250 mg or more in acute cases, three times per day (essential in adrenal function).*

Pantothenic acid: 100 to 500 mg two times per day (antihistamine, essential in cortisone production).*

Vitamin C: 500 to 1000 mg three times per day, or up to bowel tolerance (essential to adrenal function; antioxidant, antiallergy, detoxifies histamine).*

Bioflavonoids: 500 to 3000 mg per day.

Vitamin E: 200 to 400 IU one to two times per day (antioxidant).*

Calcium: 400 to 800 mg per day.*

Magnesium: 200 to 400 mg per day.*

*Asterisks indicate the most frequently used therapeutic agents.

Calcium, magnesium, and potassium (as bicarbonate buffers).

Manganese: 2 to 5 mg two to three times per week.

Selenium: 20 mcg per day (anti-inflammatory with chemical allergies and allergic toxemia).

Zinc: 15 to 45 mg three times daily (immune support).*

OTHERS

Amino acids: To improve digestive enzyme production, for weight control, for cerebral allergy.*

Bee pollen (locally produced is best).

Biotin: With Candida infestation: 200 mcg three times per day.

Castor oil: 5 drops in the morning on empty stomach.

Comb honey: Chew ½ tsp two times per day; especially therapeutic if local comb honey is used.*

Pancreatic enzymes: 1 to 2 tablets. Take with meals.

Evening primrose oil: Especially with eczema or other skin disorders.

Garlic: 2 capsules three times per day.

Hydrochloric acid: If hydrochloric acid deficiency has been proven, take 5 to 60 grains with meals.

Kelp: 2 to 4 tablets three times per day.*

Lactobacillus: To correct Candida overgrowth.*

Max EPA (eicosapentaenoic acid): May be useful in hypersensitivity reactions such as asthma, allergic rhinitis, or the panallergic patient.

Raw adrenal tablets: 1 to 2 tablets three times per day.*

Raw thymus tablets: Immune system support. 2 to 6 tablets two to three times per day.*

BOTANICALS

Prescribed according to individual symptoms and general needs.

Therapeutic Suggestions

Due to the extremely diverse nature of the allergic response, the nutritional supplement program must be individually tailored, depending on the organ or tissue groups affected. More vitamin A will be required, for example, with an allergic manifestation affecting the lungs' mucous membranes or skin. Extremely high doses may be required when malabsorption of fats is present in steatorrhea.

*Asterisks indicate the most frequently used therapeutic agents.

Use micellized form in these cases. Any level taken over 50,000 IU per day should be monitored closely with blood test. Use any dose of vitamin A over 50,000 IU per day with medical supervision only. The B complex group is particularly essential in reversing an allergic tendency. High levels of B_6, B_{12}, and pantothenic acid are almost always required with an additional balanced B complex. In some cases these may need to be given by intramuscular injection in the initial stages.

Vitamin C at bowel tolerance doses are also essential. In cases of severe reactions, it may be given intravenously in doses of 5 to 20 g with 500 to 1000 mg calcium (as calcium gluconate) and 250 to 500 mg magnesium (as magnesium sulfate).

Vitamin E is an excellent antioxidant and should be a regular part of any program.

Zinc acts as an autoimmunity factor, working with vitamins A and E.

Selenium is of particular usefulness with any chemical allergies or sensitivities, especially if given with kelp.

Where pancreatic digestive deficiency exists, pancreatic digestive enzymes and free amino acid powder supplements are useful to reduce the absorption of undigested antigenic proteins and also to increase the amino acid pool necessary for protein synthesis, to help encourage proper immune and digestive enzyme function. Raw thymus taken three or four times daily in the early stages of therapy helps boost immune function. In cases of intestinal *Candida albicans* overgrowth causing multiple allergy symptoms, *Lactobacillus* and biotin therapy is sometimes very effective. Other cases require nystatin for up to 3 to 6 months to rid the system of this yeast. Proper internal ecology is then restored through proper diet and the avoidance of birth control pills and antibiotic therapy when possible.

ANEMIA

Definition

Anemia literally means "without blood," and is a deficiency of red blood cells, or the presence of abnormal red blood cells due either to reduced production, abnormal production, excess destruction, or blood loss.

Symptoms

Pallor, tiredness, dizziness, headaches, depression, slow healing, loss of sex drive, bruising, nervousness, shortness of breath, and palpitation.

Etiologic Considerations

- Iron deficiency (hypochromic)
  Malabsorption
  Post hemorrhagic: Heavy menstruation, ulcers, hemorrhoids, fissure, etc.
  Sideroblastic (failure to utilize iron)

- Vitamin B_{12} or folic acid deficiency (Megaloblastic)
  Nutritional
      Vegans (no animal products); lack of vitamin B_{12}
      Lack of green vegetables; lack of folic acid
      Addisonian, pernicious
      Drugs, insecticides (may destroy bone marrow)
      Gastrointestinal
          Stomach removal
          Hydrochloric acid deficiency
      Intrinsic factor deficiency
      Colitis, malabsorption, food allergy, etc.

- Vitamin C deficiency
  Scurvy; vitamin C deficiency withdrawal in newborns from mothers on
  high vitamin C doses

- Vitamin E deficiency

- Vitamin B_6 deficiency

- Thyroid disorders
  Myxedema anemia

- Heredity (hemolytic, sickle cell, thalassemia or autoimmune anemia)

- Infancy
  Iron deficiency after 6 months
  Vitamin E deficiency in pregnancy and early life
  Iron deficiency (on cow's milk diet)
  Vitamin C deficiency

- Puberty
  Rapid growth of muscle (myoglobin) leading to iron deficiency

- Bone marrow disease

- Abnormal bacterial flora
  Blind loop syndrome
  Improper diet leading to change in bacterial flora

- Zinc-induced copper deficiency anemia

- Excess onion/garlic use

- Alcoholism
- Marathoner's Anemia
- Infectious diseases
  Malaria and others
- Autoimmune diseases
  Rheumatoid arthritis
  Lupus and others
- Old age
  Poor absorption
  Poor dentures leading to lack of green vegetable consumption
- Reduced exposure to sun
- Intestinal parasites
- Cellular obstruction to nutrients causing poor utilization
- Lead toxicity

Discussion

Anemia is a symptom caused by a very wide variety of conditions, as seen by the long list of etiologic considerations. The most significant and common forms of anemia are those related to diet. It is to these that I wish to confine this discussion.

Most people equate anemia with *iron deficiency*. This is encouraged by commercials for products such as Geritol, which extol the virtues of this product, offering it almost as a cure-all for any condition that produces tiredness. While iron deficiency anemia is fairly common for women in the childbearing years due to frequent loss of iron-containing hemoglobin in the menstrual flow, it is less likely to be the cause of anemia in the elderly who are the prime target for these advertisements.

In fact, due to years of consuming excess iron in supplement form, many elderly persons actually develop severe iron *excesses*. Extreme iron overdose can cause the dangerous condition known as siderosis, resulting in damage to the liver, pancreas, and heart, and cause a form of arthritis.

Iron deficiency should be first tested for prior to medication. It is to be suspected in infancy, puberty, pregnancy, females with heavy periods, and any other condition causing sudden or chronic blood loss, such as a chronic bleeding ulcer. Iron absorption is reduced by the consumption of coffee, tea, edetic acid (EDTA), or excess soy protein.

Vitamin B_{12} deficiency anemia is becoming an increasing concern. Pernicious anemia, a rare condition, is due to intrinsic factor deficiency, essential for vitamin B_{12} absorption. This must be corrected by vitamin B_{12} injections. Another form of B_{12} deficiency caused by restricted diet, however, is less rare. Vegans, those who abstain from all animal protein and animal products, including eggs and dairy products, may find themselves creating a vitamin B_{12} deficiency with its insidious effects. Vitamin B_{12} deficiency takes 6 to 10 years to become apparent, but once manifest the damage is permanent. It produces a nerve destruction similar to multiple sclerosis, with sensations of pins and needles, sore muscles, neuritis, stiff spine, difficulty in walking, and paralysis.

Vitamin B_{12} is found almost exclusively in animal products, with the exception of traces in comfrey, kelp, sunflower seeds, raw wheat germ, and grapes. Even in these the vitamin B_{12} is often the result of fermentation such as that found on grapes. Any fermented foods also contain significant amounts of vitamin B_{12}, and it is with these sources that the informed vegan supplements his or her diet. The amount available in vegetable sources, however, is minute. One would need to eat 1 to 2 lb of comfrey per day to get adequate vitamin B_{12}, at which levels toxicity from comfrey overdose would occur. Brewer's yeast as naturally found is deficient in vitamin B_{12}, and if this is to be used as a reliable source, B_{12} must have been added and will be so marked on the package. Seed yoghurts, unboiled miso, seaweed, kelp, sunflower seeds, and grapes should be eaten frequently.

Arguments are heard that vitamin B_{12} may be made by the bacteria of the small intestine and that these precautions are unnecessary. There are several considerations that must be kept in mind. It is true that a healthy bacterial flora will synthesize vitamin B_{12} in some people, and it is also true that a vegan diet, being high in vegetables and fiber foods, will generally favor a healthy floral colony. It has been suggested by some researchers, however, that not all vegans develop this vitamin B_{12} synthesizing ability. The reasons for this are not entirely clear. I personally feel that the problem stems from the drastic and sudden way in which many vegans have changed their diet. In many cases, for their entire lives and for the entire lives of each of their ancestors, the food eaten had some animal origin. Through the process of natural evolution, the capability to synthesize the body's own B_{12} was irrelevant as a survival factor, therefore was not favored genetic material. A further complication is that the folic acid found very prominently in the raw green vegetables so prevalent in a vegan's diet, will mask the effects of vitamin B_{12} deficiency until very late, when the damage is already extreme.

Whatever the cause, the fact is that no person can be absolutely certain that his or her own vitamin B_{12} production is active or adequate enough to prevent vitamin B_{12} deficiency anemia without the precaution of eating vitamin B_{12} source foods. If individuals wish to restrict their diets for whatever reason, be it religious, humanitarian, or health, they must become more and more aware of what special attention the body may need to prevent deficiency. I suggest all vegans take a B_{12} supplement daily.

Folic acid deficiency is most commonly caused by a diet deficient in raw green vegetables and foods, which contains insufficient vitamin C to aid absorption. Vitamin C is also a factor in the absorption of essential minerals, including iron and vitamin B_{12}, and helps conserve vitamin E.

Vitamin E is essential in blood building. Deficiency of this vitamin is often a factor in pregnancy; babies born of vitamin E-deficient mothers, and who are given prolonged feedings of cow's milk, can become deficient in vitamin E and iron.

For those on very high zinc supplementation, copper stores may be depleted since the zinc and copper ratio is interrelated. Copper is an essential ingredient in an enzyme necessary for lead to be oxidized into a form capable of being incorporated into the hemoglobin molecule. Thus a zinc excess may produce a copper deficiency leading to the production of an iron nonresponsive anemia correctable by copper supplementation.

One final but little-mentioned aspect of anemia is cellular obstruction. All the nutrients in the world are useless if they never reach the cells. This is the reason, contrary to established ideas, why many naturopaths routinely *fast* some anemic patients. Instead of hemoglobin levels falling even further during a fast, they are found to rise markedly, thus improving the condition. The reason for this is that the fast stimulates the blood-forming tissues to function more effectively. *Obviously, this must be done in selected cases where cellular obstruction is the primary cause and not, for instance, in a true case of vitamin B_{12} or iron deficiency.*

Treatment

Diet

FOODS RICH IN IRON

Meat, liver from organically raised cattle, fish, egg yolks, blackstrap molasses, dark green vegetables (i.e., lettuce, spinach, alfalfa, asparagus, cabbage, broccoli, parsley, celery, kale, cucumbers, leeks, and watercress), dried fruit (i.e., apricots, raisins, figs, dates, peaches, prunes, and pears), cherries, berries, bananas, grapes, apples, beets, carrots, yams, legumes, whole grains, rice, wheat, black cherry juice, grape juice, plus many others

FOODS RICH IN VITAMIN B_{12}

Meat, fish, eggs, dairy products, comfrey, bitter almonds, and the seeds in stone fruits* (vitamin B_{12} is synthesized from vitamin B_{17} in this case) such as

*Please note: Seeds in stone fruits contain cyanide compounds that can be toxic and even be fatal if taken in excess. Never eat more than 6 to 8 apricot, prune, or peach pits or more than 10 to 12 apple seeds per day, and only under medical supervision.

apple seeds, apricots, prunes, etc., fermented foods such as yoghurt, seed yoghurt, grapes and miso, wheat, sunflower seeds, seaweed, brewer's yeast with vitamin B_{12} added, and *Spirulina*

FOODS RICH IN FOLIC ACID

Dark green vegetables, liver, yeast, lentils, beans, grains, and *Spirulina*

GENERAL ANTI-ANEMIA FOODS

- *Vegetarian food sources:* Green vegetables, especially alfalfa, cabbage, chard, watercress, kale, parsley, spinach, comfrey, dandelion leaves, green onions, lettuce, cucumbers, leeks, nettles, beetroot tops, turnip greens, asparagus, *Spirulina*

- *Other vegetables:* Onions, beets, carrots, legumes (lentils, black beans, etc.), yams, potatoes with skin

- *Fruits:* Dried apricots, figs, raisins, dates, grapes, bananas, plums, oranges, grapefruits

- *Nuts:* Almonds, hazelnuts, sunflower seeds, sesame seeds

- *Other special vegetarian sources:* Wheat germ, whole grains, blackstrap molasses, brewer's yeast, miso, kernels of stone fruits* (i.e., apricots, prunes, etc.), apple seeds, seed yoghurts

- *Lacto-vegetarian food sources:* Yoghurt, milk, kefir, eggs, cheese, cottage cheese

- *Herbal teas:* Dandelion leaf, comfrey, yellow dock, raspberry, fenugreek

- *Nonvegetarian food sources:* Liver, muscle meats, organ meats, eggs (especially egg yolk), fish

ANTI-ANEMIA DIET

The following diet may be useful as a guideline:

On Rising	1 tbs blackstrap molasses in hot water, orange juice, or grapefruit juice
Breakfast	1. Yoghurt, fruit, almonds, sunflower seeds, hazelnuts, wheat germ, and honey
	2. Stewed dried fruits, plain or with yoghurt and wheat germ
	3. Museli (granola) or oatmeal and milk
	4. Eggs (not fried) and whole wheat toast

*Please see previous note concerning stone fruit kernel toxicity.

Midmorning	Dandelion leaf tea, comfrey leaf tea, parsley tea, yellow dock tea, raspberry tea, fenugreek tea, or any combination of the above
Lunch	1. A raw salad, primarily green, including any of the following: alfalfa sprouts, lettuce, cabbage, spinach, watercress, green onions, cucumber, parsley, beetroot tops, asparagus, kale, chard, other green vegetables, carrots, beets, and sunflower seeds
	2. Baked yam or potato in jacket if desired, *or*
	3. Cottage cheese or other cheese
Midafternoon	Same as midmorning
Supper	Choose from the following:
	1. Conservatively cooked vegetables, whole grain and fish liver, organ meat, or muscle meat
	2. Miso soup with vegetables, seaweed and/or fish
	3. Egg or cheese vegetarian savory

Physiotherapy

• Sun and sea baths
• Outdoor exercise

Fasting

Beet juice
Red grape juice

Therapeutic Agents

VITAMINS AND MINERALS

Vitamin B complex: 50 mg three times per day*

Vitamin B_6

Vitamin B_{12}: 25 mcg to 1 mg daily*

Folic acid: 400 mcg to 5 mg per day (especially needed in anemia of pregnancy)*

Vitamin C: 500 to 1000 mg three to four times daily. (Enhances hemoglobin

---

*Asterisks indicate the most frequently used therapeutic agents.

production and folic acid usage and increases iron and vitamin B_{12} absorption; conserves vitamin E)*

Vitamin B_{12} and folic acid intramuscularly: 1 mg one time per week*

Vitamin E: 800 to 1200 IU per day*

Calcium: 800 mg per day*

Iron chelate or ferrous gluconate: 20 to 50 mg per day when iron deficiency has been diagnosed*

Copper: 3 to 5 mg per day or 1 mg per every 10 to 15 mg of zinc taken*

Trace minerals

Zinc orotate: Sickle cell disorder

OTHERS

Apple cider vinegar: Acts like vitamin C as a reducing agent to increase absorption of iron

Blackstrap molasses: Source of iron*

Brewer's yeast: 1 tsp three times per day (source of B complex)*

Chlorophyll

Pancreatic enzymes: 1 to 2 tablets with meals in cases of poor assimilation

Hydrochloric acid: Where hydrochloric acid deficiency has been diagnosed, take with meals

Intrinsic factor (raw stomach tablets)*

Lactobacillus

Organic raw liver tablets: 2 to 4 tablets three times per day*

Protein supplements

Spirulina: 2 to 3 tsp per day

Wheat germ

Therapeutic Suggestions

Complete blood tests are essential to help differentiate the type of anemia and therefore the nutritional supplements required. In addition to the routine hemoglobin and the complete blood count, serum iron, B_{12}, folic acid, iron-binding capacity, serum ferritin and free erythrocyte protoporphyrin levels are

*Asterisks indicate the most frequently used therapeutic agents.

needed. The nutritional supplement program can then be selected with accuracy. Zinc-to-copper ratio levels in hair may be useful.

ANGINA PECTORIS (see Heart Disease)

ARTERIOSCLEROSIS (see Heart Disease)

ARTHRITIS: Osteoarthritis (OA) and Rheumatoid Arthritis (RA)

Definitions

Osteoarthritis (OA):   Local or generalized degeneration of the articular cartilage and the formation of bony "lips and spurs" (osteophytes) at the edges of joints. An exaggeration of the normal aging process.

Rheumatoid Arthritis (RA):   An inflammatory disease involving the synovial membranes and the periarticular structures. Localized bone atrophy and rarification of the involved bone is common, with associated muscle atrophy.

Symptoms

Osteoarthritis: Onset is gradual, with progressive pain and joint enlargement. No constitutional symptoms are present. May involve single or multiple joints, but does not migrate from joint to joint.

Rheumatoid Arthritis: Onset is abrupt or insidious. Synovial membrane thickens and joint swells with redness and tenderness. Symmetrical joint involvement is common. May migrate from joint to joint. Constitutional symptoms present. Joint deformity with contracture. Subcutaneous nodules commonly found.

Etiologic Considerations

• Poor eliminations and inadequate assimilations
    Poor digestion
      Hyperacidity
      Hypoacidity
      Enzyme deficiency
    Sluggish bowels
    Poor skin, kidney, gallbladder, and liver activity
    Poor circulation (blood, lymph)

Toxemia
Spinal imbalances causing reflex conditions as above, leading to accumulated toxins which cause an inflammatory reaction.

- Chemical imbalances and dietary deficiency
  Diet: Excess meat and soda drinks (phosphorus/calcium ratio upset)
       Excess refined carbohydrates, sweets
       Raw vegetable deficiency
       Excess acid-forming foods
       Excess coffee
       Excess phytic acid (bread) binding calcium
       Excess salt
       Multiple vitamin and mineral deficiencies, i.e., copper deficiency—RA
  Excess copper blood levels (copper pipes, low iron) may increase copper levels in joints; lack of zinc and manganese increases copper levels.
  Excess vitamin D
  Lack of sulfur
  Excess irritants (coffee, tea, salt, spices, alcohol)
  Food allergy
       Gluten intolerance
       Intolerance to foods in nightshade family (tomatoes, potatoes, etc.)
       Isolated food allergy
- Glandular imbalances
  Low thyroid
       Iodine deficiency
  Adrenal
       Stress
       Refined diet
       Corticosteroids
  Low pituitary
  Low liver plus toxicity
  Low sex hormones
- Psychological factors
  Long-held resentments
  Worry
  Envy
  Fear
  Anxiety, depression, deep shock
- Autoimmunity (RA)
  Rheumatoid factor found in blood of at least 50 percent of patients with RA
  Postimmunization Arthralsia (German measles)

- Excess wear and tear (OA)
    Joint trauma
        Excess weight-bearing (obesity)
        Overuse
- Lack of exercise
- Menopause
- Protozoal infection
    Some cases of rheumatoid arthritis have benefited by antiprotozoal medication.
- Sexual excess
- Anemia associated
- Chronic infections
    Tonsils
    Gallbladder
- Tonsillectomy
- Chronic fatigue
- Muscular tension, fibrositis
- Water allergy (locally irritant water supply)

Discussion

Of all the diseases that affect humanity, arthritis, in its multitude of forms, is one of the most debilitating and widespread. Orthodox treatments have proven unsatisfactory and completely unable to cure these disorders. The reason is simple. Due to the complex etiology and constitutional nature of most forms of arthritis, only individualized therapy has any hope of removing the cause. There is no one quick and easy cure, no magic pill, and no miracle diets suited for all. With arthritis, as with most degenerative diseases, there are as many different approaches as there are patients, and each one is unique. Only when each of the causative factors are recognized and corrected can true healing take place. It *always* involves lifestyle changes and almost *never* is the improvement rapid.

This implies that the only type of arthritis patient who can ever hope for real improvement must have a real desire for health and the persistence and patience to obtain it at all cost. The rewards, however, are worth the effort. The dream of a body free of pain can only be fully understood by one who lives day and night with severe arthritis.

As to the orthodox approach to arthritis, I have never met or heard of a single arthritic patient who received drug therapy who did not become progressively worse. Although aspirin, which is advised in most cases of painful osteoarthritis or rheumatoid arthritis, does help relieve the immediate pain, it certainly is no cure.

In addition to its other side effects, as well as reactivating or causing ulcers, aspirin lowers vitamin C levels (essential in the health of connective tissue, useful as a detoxifying agent, and needed for proper adrenal function), damages connective tissue, causes an increase in uric acid levels (a cause of gouty arthritis), depletes the adrenal glands, and in toxic doses will cause salicylism, leading to paralysis of the respiratory center as well as central vasomotor paralysis. If taken over a prolonged period of time, aspirin can mimic other diseases such as Ménière's syndrome and cause severe respiratory distress and mental confusion. Most health authorities now agree that if the present FDA regulations existed when aspirin was first produced, it would now be a prescription drug only.

Self-induced aspirin toxicity is very common. Although no physician would ever prescribe aspirin in doses that could become toxic, the fact is that patients often take more of this medication than suggested. This is particularly the case with some elderly patients who suffer from poor memory and cannot honestly remember if they took their pain medication three or thirteen times in a day. For many with pain, anything that gives some relief three times a day might be better six or ten times a day. One last word on aspirin. As one doctor put it, "Do you really think you have arthritis because of an aspirin deficiency?"

Cortisone is another prescribed drug for arthritis, especially rheumatoid arthritis. Compared to this drug aspirin is an essential vitamin! I personally consider cortisone one of the most deceptive and dangerous drugs ever produced. Its well-known anti-inflammatory effects hide its insidious side effects. Cortisone depresses the immunological system so dramatically that even minor infections can become life-threatening. It directly depresses the function of the adrenal gland, the gland that is so often the cause of the disorder in the first place. Cortisone causes calcium depletion, resulting in osteoporosis, another major cause of arthritis. It also aggravates peptic ulcers and in overdose will induce Cushing's syndrome with its symptoms of obesity, muscle wasting and weakness, poor wound healing, bruising, high blood pressure, diabetes, psychiatric disturbance, with balding, excess body hair, and menstrual disorders in the female. In short, cortisone is a very dangerous drug and its use should be reserved for life-threatening diseases only. The common medical opinions that "diet has nothing to do with arthritis" and that "you will have to live with it" are simply not acceptable nor are they true. Only when the individualized concept of disease causation is understood will the true cause and cure of arthritis at long last be recognized.

Treatment

Diet

Therapy must begin by identifying which of the etiologic factors interact to cause the abnormality. While no two arthritic patients are alike, it is usually not very difficult to pinpoint the major problem areas. Diet, as with many other degenerative or autoimmune disorders, stands out as the major detrimental influence. Many sufferers of both osteoarthritis or rheumatoid arthritis have dietary patterns that are clearly a problem.

Heavy meat consumption is a common finding. Meat contains anywhere from twenty to fifty times more phosphorus than calcium. This stimulates the parathyroid glands, responsible for the mobilization of calcium from bones. This extra calcium is then deposited around the joints, explaining the common finding in arthritis of less dense bones with calcium buildup around the articulations. This one factor alone may be the reason why vegetarians have less of an incidence of osteoarthritis than meat eaters. A good vegetarian diet will have a much better phosphorus-to-calcium ratio. Another source of excess phosphorus in the diet is soft drinks. It may have seemed odd to some that a condition such as osteoarthritis characterized by calcium deposits would be benefited by calcium and magnesium supplements, but the average diet clearly shows us why.

Another aspect of concern in the average diet is an excess of refined carbohydrates and sweets. Not only are these foods robbed of many of their naturally occurring vitamins and minerals, the relative ratios of many minerals are completely altered. As we have seen in many other conditions in this book, not only are the absolute values of vitamins and minerals important to human health, but also their ratios and interactions. Vitamin E, magnesium, vitamin B complex, and essential fibers are removed by the refining of whole grains. These are all very important in the prevention and cure of many degenerative conditions, arthritis included.

Refined carbohydrates, especially sugar, contribute to a generalized acid condition of the body, especially when accompanied by a diet low in fresh vegetables. Fresh vegetables are a protective factor against arthritic changes, whereas processed vegetables can actually aggravate the condition. Once again we find that essential mineral balances are upset in the processing. One example is the sodium and potassium ratio. Fresh vegetables usually have a higher potassium-to-sodium ratio than when canned. The amount of salt in the diet has increased dramatically over the past 50 years. Coffee is another common problem. In fact, so many facets of the average arthritic's diet are negative health factors that all of them cannot be mentioned here. A complete individual dietary appraisal is necessary to eliminate any possible health risks. The question of food allergy must also be investigated, especially in rheumatoid arthritis. *

It must be remembered that arthritis is a degenerative and possibly an auto-immune disease taking years to develop. Subtle dietary changes are rarely successful in reversing the problem. More heroic therapy is required. The following dietary manipulations will gradually help establish equilibrium, if applied diligently and coupled with a good nutritional supplement program.

RAW VEGETABLE JUICE FASTING

This is the fastest method of attaining results with RA. OA will also respond to this regimen. The fasting period depends on the patient and the condition, and may range from 7 to 21 days or longer, under close supervision. The following liquids are especially useful:

- Carrot and celery juice
- Potassium broth
- Chlorophyll drink
- Alfalfa mint or seed tea
- Watercress, celery, and parsley juice

RAW NONCITRUS VEGETARIAN DIET

This initial diet may follow the fasting period and should last 2 to 4 weeks or longer. The bulk of the diet is raw green vegetables, with no animal proteins whatsoever. All stimulants such as coffee, tea, alcohol, nicotine, or sweets are forbidden.

Food allergy tests (cytotoxic, RAST, pulse tests) should be performed prior to dietary treatments, to disclose any hidden food sensitivity.

The following foods have been found beneficial in the majority of arthritic patients with both RA and OA:

Green vegetables	Carrots
Seaweeds	*Spirulina*
Watercress	Avocado
Parsley	Bananas
Celery	Pecans
Okra	Potassium broth

*Hicklin, J.A., McGwen, L.M., Morgan, J.E. "The Effect of Diet in Rheumatoid Arthritis," *Clinical Allergy*, 10:463, 1980.

Kale   Wheat grass juice
Alfalfa sprouts   Whey
Kelp   Cod liver oil drinks
Soy milk   Apple cider vinegar and honey
Soy   Papaya
Soy products   Dandelion coffee
Distilled water   Seeds
Millet   Garlic, onions
Brown rice   Wheat germ
Egg yolks   Figs plus molasses
Raw goats' yoghurt   Cherries (gout)

The following should be strictly avoided:

Citrus   Fried foods
Dairy products   Drinks with meals
   (goat products OK in some cases)   Foods of the nightshade family:
Wheat   Tomatoes
Meat   Eggplants
Refined carbohydrates, sugar, etc. Potatoes
Alcohol   Peppers
Salt   Tobacco

These foods, members of the Solanaceae family, are related to deadly nightshade (belladonna), thus their common grouping as "nightshade" foods. Some people show a strong reaction to this food group. As with other severe food sensitivities, even minute doses in the diet can be a problem for these hypersensitive people. Care must be taken to avoid hidden nightshades found in prepared foods. For example, potato flour thickeners are used in a wide variety of products, including surprising ones such as some yoghurts. Capsicum also shows up hidden in foods such as pink-colored cheeses or herbal teas. Tomatoes are used in a large variety of prepared foods. Only strict avoidance will be of benefit to those truly sensitive to this food group.

Physiotherapy

DAILY MASSAGE
1. Peanut oil: 2 oz
   Olive oil: 2 oz
   Lanolin: 1 tsp

or:

2. Peanut oil

or:

3. Olive oil: 2 oz
   Peanut oil: 2 oz
   Oil of pine needles: ½ oz
   Oil of sassafras root: ½ oz
   Liquefied lanolin: 1 oz

HYDROTHERAPY

1. Hot and cold showers (alternate): to stimulate general circulation and act as a general tonic

2. Hot and cold compresses (alternate): local use

3. Hot compress (pain relief)

4. Hot Epsom salts baths or local bath or compress (see Appendix I)

5. Cabinet bath with or without Atomodine fumes

6. Sauna baths

7. Paraffin bath: local: 4 parts paraffin, 1 part mineral oil. Heat to 125° to 130° F, or let cool until thin film forms. Dip part repeatedly until ¼ in. thick, or paint on larger areas.

ELIMINATIONS

Correct eliminations using as many of the following as possible:

Castor oil packs (see Appendix I)
Anticonstipation foods
Epsom salts baths (see Appendix I)
Hot and cold showers
Skin brush and salt rub (see Appendix I)
Sea bathing
Sun bathing
Trunk packs
Mineral spring baths
Hot sand baths
Seaweed baths
Sulfur baths (sulfur hot springs)
Sweat baths
Wet grass walks

OTHERS
 Ultrasound
 Cabbage leaf poultices, in acute cases
 Comfrey leaf poultice
 Joint mobilization
 Infrared heat
 Flowers of sulfur in socks daily
 Counterirritant therapy

Therapeutic Agents

VITAMINS AND MINERALS

 Vitamin A: 25,000 to 100,000 IU per day.* *Use any dose of vitamin A over 50,000 IU per day with medical supervision only.*

 Vitamin B complex: 50 mg two to three times daily.*

 Pantothenic acid: 250 to 500 mg two to three times per day.

 Niacinamide: 200 to 1000 mg two to four times per day. Increases joint mobility by up to 85 percent if taken daily for 3 to 4 weeks. It is used for osteoarthritis and some rheumatoid arthritis. If nausea occurs at these doses this may be a toxic reaction and the dose should be reduced by one-half or stopped completely.*

 Vitamin B$_6$: 100 to 250 mg two to three times per day. Especially indicated for females on birth control pills and those with Carpal tunnel syndrome and nonarticular rheumatism.

 Vitamin B$_{12}$: 1000 mcg intramuscular injection one time per week, or in some cases daily for 7 to 14 days. Useful with heel spurs and other osteoarthritic joint disorders. Use 1 ml per day until pain subsides.*

 Vitamin C: 1000 to 2000 mg three to four times daily, or larger doses, up to bowel tolerance. Increases natural cortisone production; anti-inflammatory; aids adrenals. Large doses may aggravate some cases, so take care to evaluate its effect separately from other medications. Try ascorbate, if this is a problem.*

 Vitamin E: 400 IU, one to two times per day; antioxidant; anti-inflammatory.*

 Calcium: 800 to 1000 mg per day.*

 Calcium pantothenate: 2 g per day in RA.

*Asterisks indicate the most frequently used therapeutic agents.

Magnesium: 400 to 800 mg per day.*

Manganese: Superoxide dismutase activation.

Essential fatty acids: 2 to 4 capsules three times per day.*

Copper: High doses used with medical supervision only.*

Copper aspirinate (for RA): Anti-inflammatory and SOD (Superoxide dismutase) activation.*

Selenium: 50 to 200 mcg per day works in synergy with vitamin E. Selenium has also been found useful in cases of Osgood-Schlatter disease of the knees. Standard dose is 250 mcg of sodium selenite per day, along with 800 IU vitamin E per day for 1 month, later reducing to 400 IU per day; vitamin C: 3 to 6 g per day; B complex 25 to 50 mg one to two times per day; zinc: 15 to 25 mg two to three times per day; calcium: 800 to 1000 mg per day; magnesium: 400 to 500 mg per day, and a diet high in raw vegetables.

Trace minerals

Tryptophan: Some arthritics respond to 1 and 1½ g per day.

Zinc: 25 to 50 mg one to two times per day, SOD activation. Especially indicated in psoriatic arthritis.

OTHERS

Alfalfa tablets (6 to 10), plus tea, three times daily.

Atomodine or 636 (Cayce products)

Apple cider vinegar

Bee pollen

Bone meal

Brewer's yeast: 1 tsp two to three times per day.

Bromelain enzyme: 2 to 4 tablets three to four times per day. Decreases soft tissue swelling, inflammation and pain. Induces formation of prostaglandin E.*

Cod-liver oil capsules: 3 to 4 capsules three times daily.

D.L. Phenylalanine: Analgesic; 300 mg three times per day.*

Green liped muscle tablets: May help some people with RA.

Hydrochloric acid: If hydrochloric acid deficiency has been proven, take with meals. Hypochlorhydria is very common in rheumatoid arthritis patients.

*Asterisks indicate the most frequently used therapeutic agents.

Kelp: 2 to 4 tablets three times per day.*

Lecithin (as concentrated phosphatidyln choline): 1 to 2 capsules three times per day.*

Molasses plus eggs: Sulfur source.

Pancreatic enzymes*

Raw adrenal tablets: Antistress.*

Raw thymus tablets: Immune system support.*

SOD (Superoxide dismutase): While this substance is a very powerful natural antioxidant, its absorption and utility given *orally* is questionable. In *injectible* form it has proven useful in RA, gout, and other inflammatory joint disorders. It has been used as such in veterinary medicine for years. The affected joint is injected once weekly; enhancing zinc, copper, and manganese orally stimulates the body's production of native SOD. Even with questions over its effectiveness orally, I have still found that *reliable* superoxide dismutase oral tablets have proven effective in some cases. I have found the superoxide dismutase made by Biotics Research Corporation to be a reliable source.*

Wheat germ concentrate

BOTANICALS

Autumn crocus (*Colchicum autumnale*): Gout (contains colchicine).

Bee sting (*Apis mellifera*): Homeopathic dilutions used for inflammation and edema (as if by a bee sting).

Bryony (*Bryonia alba*): Low homeopathic dilutions for pain aggravated by movement.

Burdock (*Arctium lappa*): Alterative.

Celery (*Apium graveolens*): Stalk eaten in abundance; seeds used as medicine.

Devil's claw (*Harpagophtum procumbens*): Anti-inflammatory, analgesic action similar to phenylbutazone. Reduces uric acid levels.

Poison ivy (*Rhus toxicodendron*): Homeopathic dilutions used for rheumatic pain and inflammation improved by motion.

St. James-wort (*Senecio jacobaea*): Use as topical lotion.

White willow (*Salix alba*)

Wintergreen oil (*Gaultheria procumbens*): Used as topical 10 to 20% solution. Antirheumatic, local irritant; contains methyl salicylate.

Yucca

*Asterisks indicate the most frequently used therapeutic agents.

Therapeutic Suggestions

Essential medications include vitamin A, vitamin B complex, niacin, pantothenic acid, vitamin B_{12} intramuscularly, vitamin C in bowel tolerance doses, vitamin E, calcium, magnesium, essential fatty acids, bromelain, cod-liver oil, lecithin, kelp, and thymus (RA). Copper aspirinate for RA is worth a trial. Pancreatic enzymes also may be useful. Enhancing the status of zinc, copper, and manganese may stimulate the body's own production of SOD (anti-inflammatory).

Although this list is long, many other medicinal agents may be required to reach maximum results. Each patient's prescription and dose must be individually determined in light of the case history and results obtained.

ASTHMA, BRONCHIAL

Definition

Recurrent paroxysms of difficult breathing and wheezing due to air flow obstruction following constriction of the bronchi and bronchioles, and increased mucous secretion.

Symptoms

Difficult breathing, sense of choking, wheezing, coughing, difficulty in exhalation, causing use of accessory muscles of respiration. (The use of intercostal muscles and the pectoralis minor requires the patient to brace the shoulders by sitting upright and grasping the side of bed or chair.) Eventually causes "barrel chest" formation. Expectoration usually ends spasm; attack worse lying down.

Etiologic Considerations

- Diet
    Excess carbohydrates, sweets
    Excess dairy products
    Difficult-to-digest foods
    Overeating
- Allergy
    Wheat
    Milk
    Inhalants
    Other

- Food Additive Sensitivity
    Sodium metabisulfite
    Tartrazine
    Acetylsalicylic acid
    Sulfur dioxide
    Sodium benzoate and others
- Hypoglycemia
    Associated with many allergies and adrenal gland malfunction.
- Poor eliminations
    Constipation
- Toxicity
- Spinal
    Cervical
    Thoracic
- Birth Trauma
- Lesions
    In larynx and/or bronchi due to previous acute infections.
- Suppressive treatment
    Improper therapy for previous colds, bronchitis, and other disease.
- Glandular imbalance
    Adrenal
- Poor circulation
- Emotional
    Insecure, fear, overprotective mother.
- Hydrochloric acid deficiency

Discussion

Asthma is a deep-seated disorder with a complex etiology. The majority of cases, however, fall into a general "asthma syndrome." These people are hypoglycemic, have spinal lesions due to injury or birth trauma, were weaned too early and excessively onto wheat and dairy products, and received suppressive treatments to previous acute disease.

Hypoglycemia has been associated with many allergies and asthma. This may have been caused by consuming an excess of refined carbohydrates (sugar, refined cereals, etc.) or due to stress-related adrenal malfunction. The adrenal glands are usually the key to the glandular imbalances found with asthma (see Hypoglycemia).

Spinal lesions are found in nearly all cases of asthma. These may be acquired due to injury or accident, or may be due to a difficult delivery in childbirth. This is considered by some to be the most severe trauma most of us will suffer in our lives. These lesions may be found anywhere from the lower cervical (C4) to midthoracic vertebrae (T9).

Most asthmatics were weaned before the first birthday onto an abundance of wheat and dairy products. These two dietary elements are the most commonly found food allergens. Even when strict food allergy is not the cause, excess wheat and dairy products both alter the body's acid/alkaline balance and increase the production of mucus. They also predispose to frequent colds and other respiratory complaints.

A history of chronic colds and bronchitis is usually reported by asthma sufferers prior to their disorder. These may have been caused by improper diet as above, or have been due to spinal lesions or toxicity. The effort of the body in these acute diseases is to encourage elimination. If this is constantly suppressed by drug action, chronic disease such as asthma results.

Emotional insecurity has been a recognized factor in many cases of asthma. Systemic candidiasis may also be a factor.

Treatment

Diet

The best dietary therapy is an allergy-free vegetarian diet with few carbohydrates and no dairy products. Specific food allergy tests are useful to help eliminate possible irritants and allergens. These are then avoided and specific homeopathic preparations employed to desensitize the individual to these substances. The same may also be done with inhalants or contact allergens. Foods to avoid in the diet, irrespective of specific allergy are:

• Sweets
• Refined foods
• Excess carbohydrates
• Additives
• Alcohol, tea, or other nonfood irritants
• Very hot or very cold foods

Most cases also require absolute avoidance of dairy products and wheat for at least 2 months, if not longer. In some cases goat's yoghurt may then be introduced as well as free-range eggs later in the treatment regimen.

Periods of fruit juice or vegetable juice fasting or at least an all-fruit diet (see Appendix I) are necessary to help restore balance. Children may find it difficult to fast, but very easy to go on a 3-to-5-day all-fruit diet. The specific mucus-cleansing diet (see Appendix I) regimen with onions and citrus is useful in nearly all cases, and should be employed during any acute episodes.

Alternatively, the modified carrot mono diet is sometimes found more appealing and almost as effective in the severe acute case. On this diet the patient drinks an abundance of carrot juice and eats raw carrots if desired between meals, with a large plate of three-fourths cooked carrots to one-fourth cooked onions at mealtimes. After this, stage 2 of the diet below should form the basis for the general diet for the first 2 months. As improvement is seen by the use of frequent fasting, mucus-cleansing diets, and an allergy-free vegetarian diet, along with physiotherapy, spinal manipulation, exercise, nutritional supplements, and botanical remedies, the diet may be slowly and carefully expanded. If hypoglycemia is a factor, protein levels may need to be increased (see Hypoglycemia).

I have seen young children in the midst of severe asthma attacks lasting weeks that were unrelieved by any of the drugs currently on the market, respond within 24 to 48 hours and be symptom-free in less than 1 week on this regimen.

The following is a sample diet that has proved very useful in these cases.

ASTHMA DIET REGIMEN

Begin treatment with one of the following diets, depending on your doctor's advice.

STAGE 1

• Liquid Diet (3–7 days) No solid food is to be taken.

On Rising	Herb teas such as chamomile, alfalfa, mint, linden flower, etc., or a glass of fresh fruit juice from fully ripened (and if possible) unsprayed and organic grapefruit, grapes, papaya, oranges, apples, guavas, or any other fresh fruit
Breakfast	Potassium broth (hot vegetable broth, see Appendix I)
Midmorning	Any herb tea, fruit juice, or fresh vegetable juice
Lunch	Potassium broth (hot vegetable broth)
Midafternoon	Any herb tea, fresh fruit or vegetable juice (no tomato juice)
Supper	Potassium broth (hot vegetable broth)

An enema should be taken on days 1, 2, 3, 5, 7.

• All-Fruit Diet (3–7–10 days)

On Rising	Herb tea or grapefruit juice
Breakfast	Any fresh fruit (unsprayed and organic)
Midmorning	Herb tea or fruit juice
Lunch	Any fresh fruit
Midafternoon	Herb tea or fruit juice
Supper	Any fresh fruit

(*Note:* One type of fruit per meal. *No* bananas.)

• Carrot Mono Diet (modified)

On Rising	Carrot juice
Breakfast	Carrots
Midmorning	Carrot juice
Lunch	Large plate of boiled or steamed carrots and onions
Midafternoon	As midmorning
Supper	As lunch
Evening	Carrot juice

• Mucus-Cleansing Diet (3–7–10 days)

Breakfast	Citrus fruit (especially grapefruit)
Midmorning	Herb tea, fresh fruit juice, or fresh vegetable juice (carrot)
Lunch	A large plate of boiled or steamed onions; a little vegetarian margarine may be used to flavor, but no salt. An orange for dessert if desired
Midafternoon	Potassium broth, or as midmorning
Supper	Same as lunch
Evening	Potassium broth, or as midmorning

Take 2 garlic capsules with lunch and supper.

STAGE 2

Breakfast	1. Any fresh fruit, raw or stewed, *or* 2. Stewed or baked apple with soaked or simmered raisins.

Lunch

1. A large, varied raw salad composed of vegetables that grow mostly aboveground, in the ratio 3 to 1 below (e.g., lettuce, cabbage, celery, watercress, cucumber), plus carrots. Also have a large plate of boiled or steamed onions topped with vegetarian margarine or nut cream. A few walnuts, almonds, or hazelnuts may be added to the salad.
2. Tofu may be added to meal.

Evening

1. Same as lunch, or
2. A vegetarian protein meal (excluding eggs and cheese) plus steamed or baked vegetables. Fresh or stewed fruit if desired as dessert.

Later in regimen

3. Lean meat, fish, or poultry (not fried) with vegetables.

When thirsty, choose from fruit juice, vegetable juice, potassium broth, or herb teas.

Take 2 garlic capsules with meals. Always include raw onions in the salad meals.

Please refer to Allergies for an alternative approach.

Physiotherapy

EXERCISES

- Blow up balloons.

- Blow out candles.

- Stand before open window with hands behind head. Pull elbows in front and have them touch. As inhalation begins, arms are flexed outward and backward. Exhale as they return forward. Breathe slowly and deeply with full exhalation.

- Diaphragm breathing: On back, begin slow progression of abdominal diaphragm breathing to lower costals, then to upper chest. Counterpressure on upper ribs may help localize the breathing effort to diaphragm and lower costal area. Exhale normally.

- Sitting with back supported, right arm across chest, bend to right inhaling, to left exhaling, with hand helping. Then switch hands and reverse.

- Sitting, with hands on ribs, inhale and then exhale while leaning forward with pressure exerted on ribs by hands. Progress to hands above head on inhalation, bending forward until chest reaches the knees on exhalation. This may also be done in puffs and pushes rather than continuous exhalation (after only one inhalation). This is a very useful exercise in loosening mucus.

- During an attack blow through a straw into water and then inhale fresh air, or if available, oxygen.
- Relaxation exercises.
- Outdoor singing.

(Note: In these exercises it is the *exhalation* that is to be stressed, not deep inhalation. The diaphragmatic breathing is to teach the proper progression of breathing. No excessive deep inhalation breaths are required.)

OTHERS

Neuromuscular: Deep muscle massage between ribs, along spine, and along diaphragm.

Spinal manipulation: Cervical and thoracic manipulation weekly for 6 to 8 weeks. Rest and repeat cycle as needed.

Outdoor exercises: Swimming is one of the best activities for asthmatics.

Massage: Between shoulder blades (acute cases).

HYDROTHERAPY

Chronic	Hot Epsom salts baths two times per week (see Appendix I)
	Alternate hot/cold showers daily
	Chest packs nightly
Acute	Hot chest compresses plus hot foot bath
	Hot foot bath with mustard and lobelia plus ice to back of head
	Hot fomentations with olbas oil
	Warm bath for 45 minutes with relaxation and diaphragmatic breathing

Therapeutic Agents

VITAMINS AND MINERALS

Vitamin A: 10,000 IU two to four times per day in acute cases for children; 25,000 IU two to four times per day in acute cases for adults. Mucous membrane integrity, immune system support. *Use any dose of vitamin A over 50,000 IU per day with medical supervision only.**

Vitamin B complex: 25 mg three times per day for children, 50 mg three times per day for adults.*

Vitamin B$_6$ (antihistamine): 100 to 250 mg two or three times per day.*

*Asterisks indicate the most frequently used therapeutic agents.

Vitamin B_{12}: Some cases benefit from 1 to 3 mg intramuscularly daily for 1 month, then reduce dose to three times per week until stabilized. Maintain dose at level needed to control.*

Vitamin C (antihistamine): Stimulates natural Adrenalin production; antioxidant. 1000 mg three to eight times per day or to bowel tolerance.*

Vitamin E: 400 to 1200 IU per day.*

Calcium: 400 to 1000 mg per day. In acute cases, take more at frequent intervals.*

Magnesium: 200 to 500 mg per day.

Manganese: 5 mg two times per week.

Zinc: 15 to 25 mg two to three times per day for immune support.

OTHERS

Apple cider vinegar: To aid calcium absorption.

Atomodine or 636 (Cayce product): With doctor's prescription.*

Bee pollen: As preventive for inhalant allergies.*

Chlorophyll

Garlic capsules: 2 with meals.*

Hydrochloric acid: Take 5 to 60 g with meals if hydrochloric acid deficiency has been demonstrated.

Kelp: 1 to 2 tablets two to three times daily.*

Raw adrenal: 1 tablet two to three times per day, or every 15 minutes in acute cases; antistress, antiallergic nutrient.*

Raw thymus: 1 to 2 tablets three to six times per day; immune support.*

Raw comb honey*

Raw honey/onion syrup (see Appendix I)*

Trace minerals

(Note: Refer also to chapter on Allergy.)

BOTANICALS

Asthma weed (*Euphorbia pilulifera*): Useful in most asthmas. Dose of tincture: 25 drops in a small amount of water two to four times per day.*

Coltsfoot (*Tussilago farfara*): Demulcent, mild expectorant.*

*Asterisks indicate the most frequently used therapeutic agents.

Garlic syrup (*Allium sativum*): Expectorant, mucus solvent. Dice garlic and cover with 1 tsp honey. Allow to sit 4 to 8 hours, then mash and strain. Dose: ¼ to ½ tsp two to four times per day or more frequently in acute episodes. Hot garlic tea is also useful.*

Licorice (*Glycyrrhiza glabra*): Expectorant, demulcent.

Lobelia (*Lobelia inflata*): Antispasmodic, bronchodilator, expectorant, emetic, mucolytic agent. Use in severe cases. Dose: 10 to 15 drops tincture, three to four times per day, or in acute attack a once only dose of 30 to 45 drops. Larger doses become emetic and possibly toxic.*

Ma-huang (*Ephedra*): Bronchodilator; contains ephedrine. Useful in emergencies for extreme difficulty of breathing.*

Mullein (*Verbascum thapsus*): Can be used as tea, or the leaves may be smoked for asthma relief.

Skunk cabbage (*Symplocarpus foetidus*): Expectorant, mild sedative, antispasmodic. Dose of tincture: 15 to 60 drops.*

USEFUL PRESCRIPTIONS

Kloss antispasmodic:*
    Tinctures of:
        Lobelia, 1 part
        Skullcap, 1 part
        Skunk cabbage, 1 part
        Gum myrrh, 1 part
        Black cohosh, 1 part
        Cayenne, ½ part

Take 10 to 15 drops two to three times per day. In acute cases, a one-time dose of 1 tsp.

Therapeutic Suggestions

Due to the chronic nature of this complaint, many supplements are required. As with other disorders of the respiratory system, high doses of vitamin A are required. Those with fat absorption problems should use the micellized forms. In acute phases vitamin A may be taken four or even six times daily. Care, however, must be taken to monitor for vitamin A toxicity when it is used at high doses for any prolonged period of time.

Vitamin B6 helps as an antihistamine when taken in conjunction with a balanced B complex. Vitamin C is always prescribed at as high a dose as the bowels will tolerate. Other medications routinely prescribed are vitamin E,

*Asterisks indicate the most frequently used therapeutic agents.

calcium, magnesium, and zinc. Calcium is prescribed as often as every half hour in acute attacks. Iodine-containing medications such as kelp, Atomodine, or 636 are often found useful, but never taken coincidentally, to avoid iodine excess. Kelp is more frequently prescribed, but often a series with Atomodine will be a more effective glandular stimulant.

Doses must be individually prescribed with iodine, but a typical course will be 1 drop per day for 3 days; 1 drop two times per day for 3 days; 1 drop three times per day for 3 days, and then followed with at least 1 week of no iodine medication prior to a second course at the same or a lower dose.

Garlic capsules, although fairly antisocial, are very useful as mucus solvents. Raw adrenal tablets should always be on hand in case of acute reactions. Take 1 to 2 tablets up to every half hour for a few hours, along with the calcium supplement. Raw thymus should be given several times to enhance immune function.

The most useful botanicals are asthma weed, lobelia, and ma-huang.

ATHEROSCLEROSIS (see Heart Disease)

ATHLETE'S FOOT (Tinea Pedis)

Definition and Symptoms

A fungus infection of the foot caused by *Trichophyton rubrum*, *T. mentagrophytes*, and *epidermophyton floccosum*. These fungi invade the outer layers of the skin, especially between the third and fourth interdigital spaces. The lesions are macerated areas with scaling borders. The area between the toes may become dry, scaly, itchy, cracked, bleeding, and very tender. Various bacteria may also settle in this area, causing a weeping, malodorous type of athlete's foot that can be very painful.

Etiologic Considerations

• Warmth, moisture, and maceration, i.e., from exercise

• Tight shoes

• Moist socks

• Perspiration

Discussion

These fungal infections are very common among athletes who may have their feet exposed to warmth and moisture over prolonged periods of time. The toes commonly affected are the third, fourth, and fifth. These interdigital spaces are so close that perspiration does not evaporate readily, providing an ideal medium for fungus growth on the dead layers of skin. Secondary bacterial infections may occur that will not respond to antifungal treatments.

Treatment

Prevention is the best form of treatment. Always take care to dry between toes after showers, and change socks after exercise or sweating. Wear less constricting shoes when not exercising, or go without shoes if possible, for prolonged periods daily. Keep feet exposed to fresh air as much as possible. If you have a tendency to athlete's foot, it may be useful to apply powder between the toes to assure a dry, moisture-free surface. If you remove the environment for fungus development, it cannot take hold. Some people, however, have a reduced resistance to fungus infections of all kinds, and a detailed investigation of their diet and lifestyle patterns may help reveal the cause of this reduced immunity.

Physiotherapy

The following therapeutic aids have been useful in eradicating athlete's foot:

- Wash feet and between toes with dilute or straight vinegar three to four times per day.

- Sero Aseptic or Herbal Septic (Seroyal, NF Factors): Apply after vinegar wash in mild cases.

- Mutton tallow applications

- Boric acid soak: 1 tbs per quart of water. Soak feet 10 to 20 minutes three times per day.

- Castor oil, 1 part; Peruvian balsam, 1 part; Tea tree oil, 1 part; apply four to six times daily. May also be useful for secondary bacterial infection.

- Ultraviolet light exposure and fresh air

- Vitamin E (topical use)

Therapeutic Agents

VITAMINS AND MINERALS

Vitamin A: 25,000 to 100,000 IU per day. *Use any dose of vitamin A over 50,000 IU per day with medical supervision only.*

Zinc: 25 mg two to three times a day.

BALDNESS (Alopecia)

Definition

Partial or complete loss of hair on the scalp.

Symptoms

Thinning of hair over entire scalp; total loss of hair uniformly or male pattern loss.

Etiologic Considerations

- Glandular imbalance
    Thyroid (hypothyroid)
    Pituitary
    Adrenal
- Poor local circulation
- Seborrhea; excess secretions
- Excess male hormone
- Thickening of galea aponeurotica (male pattern, hormonal)
- Dandruff
- Single or multiple nutritional deficiencies
    Vitamin B complex
    Biotin
    Inositol
    Para-aminobenzoic acid (PABA)
    Vitamin B_6
    Folic acid
- Pregnancy
- Birth control pill (B_6 loss)

- Stress
- Overwork
- Improper hair treatment
    Shampoo—strong alkalies or acids
    Hair dyes
    Hair dryers
- Severe fevers
- Heavy metal poisoning
- Refined diet
- Anemia
- Alcohol; nicotine
- Some drugs or other toxicities

Discussion

Hair health depends on the amount and quality of its circulation. If the blood and lymph supply to any given hair follicle is cut off, it will die. What occurs in baldness is exactly this process. Whatever the causative factors, the end result is a reduction of the circulation and hair follicle death. This may be the result of hormonal factors, as in male pattern baldness. In this instance the galea aponeurotica membrane in the scalp becomes thickened and inelastic. The scalp becomes tight and thick, cutting off circulation. In seborrhea and dandruff the follicles are clogged and suffocated by excess oily secretions and accumulated dead cells. The end result, once again, is reduced circulation and hair death.

Many nutritional deficiencies have been found associated with balding. Most of these are part of the vitamin B complex. It is well known that severe malnutrition will cause hair loss. While this extreme of poor nutrition is rare, subclinical vitamin B complex deficiencies are extremely common. Our entire modern society seems to threaten consumption of an adequate B complex supply. The refining of whole grain removes a valuable source of many B vitamins, as does overcooking vegetables in boiling water. Being water-soluble, B vitamins are lost in cooking water. In addition, the ordinary diet usually lacks raw green vegetables, a major source of many B vitamins. Even if intake of B complex is adequate, these vitamins are often utilized excessively to digest concentrated carbohydrates such as sugar, white bread, or other refined grains whose own B vitamins have been stripped away in the refining process. This robs the body of valuable vitamins needed for other purposes.

Hypoglycemia, so common in modern civilization, also requires an excess of B complex to support adrenal function. Any factor, be it hypoglycemia or even simple stress that causes the adrenal glands to work overtime, will deplete the B complex group.

Stress not only depletes B complex as stated above, but also acts directly to reduce blood circulation to the scalp. The hormonal system is particularly susceptible to emotions and may affect hair growth. A sudden shock has often been found to precede sudden hair loss or even complete baldness. Sluggish thyroid function is a common finding in many cases of hair loss.

At certain times a sudden loss of hair is considered normal. During the last few months of pregnancy or for 3 to 4 months postpartum, many women will lose a significant amount of hair. This process usually reverses itself within 6 months after the baby is born. Sudden hair loss is also common following severe illness or high fevers. The hair usually regrows normally.

A major cause of baldness not previously mentioned is improper hair treatment. Strong shampoos, hair dyes, or hot hair dryers may damage the hair and hair follicles. If caught early enough this type of hair loss may be reversed.

The normal lifetime of a single hair is anywhere from 2 to 6 years. It is then replaced by a new hair. In the typical case of balding, we find a larger proportion than normal of shorter, thinner, younger hair. Progressively the follicles produce fine babylike hairs with a short life span and then, in time, cease to function altogether. Hairs found in cuttings of short to moderate-length hair should show blunt ends due to previous hair cuts. If a large proportion show the thin, pointed ends of new hair growth, the balding process may have begun.

Once the hair follicle itself has died, no new hair growth is possible. The fine hair growth found so commonly on a balding head, however, can many times be reversed so that normal hair once again is produced. In some cases, even when no hair growth is present, new hair growth can be stimulated. These cases, however, are less common. I personally have seen several remarkable cases where the follicles did not appear to be producing any hair, and still the patient regained hair development with vigorous therapy.

One case stands out in my mind of an elderly Japanese woman who was 80 percent bald due to diffuse hair thinning. She had dyed her hair black for over 30 years and this was suggested as the possible cause. After 2 months of vigorous application of the treatments below, and no hair dye, all she had to show was a head still 80 percent bald, but now very gray. When I saw her 3 months later, however, to my great surprise she not only had begun to grow new hair, but the new hair was black! With continued treatment for a further 2-month period, she now had regained 80 percent of a normal head of hair and threw away her wig. The new hairs that grew were all black while those that never had fallen were still gray. Needless to say, the patient was very happy with her new head of hair, even though it never got quite as thick as it had been when she was younger.

Treatment

Therapy in all cases must be *vigorous*. Haphazard or occasional therapy will have little or no effect.

Diet

Foods eaten should obviously all be of the best possible nutritional value. Eat only unrefined wholesome food. Certain groups of foods are found especially useful. Sulfur foods, silicon foods, and iodine foods are very beneficial. Eat plenty of onions, horseradish, garlic, egg yolks (not white), watercress, mustard greens, radishes, alfalfa, celery, lettuce, raw greens, carrots, sea foods, kelp, sunflower seeds, pumpkin seeds, seed sprouts, and other whole grains, wheat germ, lecithin, and brewer's yeast. In addition, the diet found under Anemia may be useful.

Physiotherapy

* Crude oil scalp massage

  Twice weekly massage unrefined, undiluted Pennsylvania grade crude oil (Crudoleum—Cayce product) into the scalp vigorously with the fingertips and then massage the entire scalp for 30 minutes with an electric vibrator.

* Pure grain alcohol rinse (20% solution with a few drops of pine oil)—Cayce product

  After massaging the scalp with the crude oil, rinse with this alcohol and pine oil solution.

* Olive oil shampoo

  Shampoo only with a mild olive oil shampoo (Cayce product). Shampoo every 1 or 2 days.

* Biotin shampoo plus biotin cream to scalp

* Alternate hot and cold head sprays

  During the shower, alternate first warm then cold water to the scalp—three to four times, always ending with the cold.

* Scalp massage

  Massage scalp each day vigorously with fingertips or an electric vibrator for 20 to 30 minutes.

  (Note: These vigorous applications will cause an excessive amount of hair to fall in the first 2 to 4 weeks. This should not cause alarm. These hairs were weak and unhealthy and will be replaced with strong, healthy hair.)

* Hair brushing

  Use only a natural bristle brush. Brush hair two times daily, making sure to stimulate the scalp with each stroke.

- Upside-down exercises

  Do head stands, slant board exercises, hang from hips or knees, or any other exercises that stimulate blood flow to the scalp and brain. One nice way to do this is the Back Swing, which is a device to hang from the feet. Another available product is the Gravity Inversion Boots, also used to hang from the feet. This is not to be done by those with high blood pressure or other circulatory disorders.

The essence of therapy for hair loss in most cases revolves around the above local treatments. A good individually prescribed nutritional program is also useful. Emphasis should be placed on nutritional adequacy, good digestion and assimilation, and glandular stimulation.

The following rather broad list may help in your choices. These nutrients have not been decisively linked to baldness, but are general in their use, to increase vitality.

Therapeutic Agents

VITAMINS AND MINERALS

Vitamin E: 400 IU two times per day.*

Vitamin A: 10,000 to 50,000 IU per day. *Use any dose of vitamin A over 50,000 IU per day with medical supervision only.**

Vitamin B_6

Vitamin B complex: 50 mg two to three times daily.*

Vitamin C complex*

Biotin: 5 mg two to three times per day.

Inositol/choline

Niacin/niacinamide: May be used to increase blood flow to scalp. Take at doses needed to give a strong flushing sensation.

Multivitamin/multimineral supplements*

EFA (essential fatty acids)*

OTHERS

Atomodine or 636 (Cayce product): Iodine to be used on doctor's prescription.*

Brewer's yeast

*Asterisked entries indicate the most frequently used therapeutic agents.

Pancreatic enzymes: Take with meals where poor absorption may be causing nutritional malabsorption.*

Kelp*

Lecithin

Raw pituitary: 1, two to three times a day.*

Raw thyroid: Where thyroid disorders are the cause.*

Therapeutic Suggestions

Iodine-containing supplements such as kelp, Atomodine, and 636 are used fairly routinely as thyroid stimulants. Where this is not contraindicated, I usually choose 636 for its tonic qualities. The dose of iodine in it is fairly low (1 drop per teaspoon) and it is taken for 10 days, then stopped for 5 to 10 days, prior to repeating the prescription.

BED SORES (Pressure Sores)

Definition and Symptoms

Ischemic necrosis and ulceration of tissue, especially over bony prominences, due to pressure from prolonged confinement to bed, or from a splint or cast.

Etiologic Considerations

- Prolonged fever
- Emaciation
- Obesity
- Old age
- Paralysis
- Diabetes
- Anemia
- Poor circulation
- Poorly made beds
- Infrequently changed positions

Discussion

Bed sores are a common problem among elderly, weak, or emaciated patients, and for anyone who must remain in one position or be confined to bed due to illness or orthopedic problems. Areas most affected are the overly bony prominences such as the sacrum, hip, heels, elbows, shoulder blades, and back of head.

Treatment

Prevention of bed sores is much easier than treatment. The bed must be kept clean and the sheets without wrinkles. Sheepskin bed covers help disperse weight more evenly, as will air or water mattresses. The patient must be turned regularly and observed for any redness (first stage). Regular massage to increase circulation is useful, as is exposure to sunlight. The following therapies are useful to help remove an established bed sore:

Diet

Plenty of greens and carrot juice three times daily.

Physiotherapy

• Sugar or honey poultice applied continuously.
• Ultraviolet exposure.

Therapeutic Agents

VITAMINS AND MINERALS

Vitamin A: 50,000 to 100,000 IU per day. *Use any dose of vitamin A over 50,000 IU per day with medical supervision only.*

Vitamin B complex: 50 mg one to two times per day.

Vitamin C: To bowel tolerance. Begin at 2 to 6 g per day and increase 2 g per day until loose bowels occur. Reduce dose 2 g and maintain. Vitamin C intravenously will speed healing.

Zinc: 25 to 50 mg two to three times per day.

BED-WETTING (see Enuresis)

BEHAVIORAL DISORDERS, DEPRESSION, STRESS

Definition and Symptoms

Feelings of sadness and hopelessness resulting in reduced desire for socialization or communication. Fear, anger, and guilt may be internalized and directed inward upon the self.

Discussion

When no recognizable situational or psychologically based cause can be found, it is often very useful to look toward nutrition for an answer. The link between nutrition and behavior has been recognized for centuries. From the earliest days of the discovery of the B complex vitamins, it has been observed that deficiency of these nutrients often led to various emotional problems. More recently, many physicians have suggested that diet may play a role in hyperactivity, schizophrenia, and a whole host of other behavioral disorders.

Nutritional deficiency can be caused by consumption of nutrient-deficient foods, or be the result of improper absorption, transport, or metabolism. Not only may nutritional deficiency lead to emotional disorders and stress syndrome, but conversely prolonged stress or severe depression may result in the rapid use of many nutrients beyond the body's normal supply. It is therefore very common for a stressful situation to result in a nutritional deficiency state, even with a normally adequate supply from the diet.

An interesting example of this stress-induced vitamin deficiency state is the now-recognized vitamin B_3 dependency found among former POWs, who lived for long periods under stress and nutritional deficiency. After returning to a normal diet and normal stress, it was discovered that a large percent of these victims could only maintain proper mental and physical health with daily megadoses of vitamin B_3. It appears that stress, or long-term severe deficiency of a single nutrient, vitamin B_3 in this case, has led to a permanent excess need for this nutrient for the remainder of that person's life. Evidence with zinc deprivation in rats has shown some dependency and reduced immune function for up to three generations. It would not be too surprising to find similar conditions of vitamin or mineral dependency induced by severe dependency in past generations, gestation, or early life. This may help explain some psychological similarities between parents and children.

Other causes of emotional disorders are also caused by diet, but along different avenues. Hypoglycemia and diabetes are certainly well-recognized sources of emotional lability and depression. Any sudden drop in the blood sugar level will lead to lethargy and depressive tendencies. Allergy is a less frequently thought of cause of depression or emotional imbalance, but a very real factor. Hyperactivity states due to food additives and sugar is just one of many examples of this type of reaction. Literally any food or food component can be the cause of abnormal emotional states.

Heavy metal toxicity is another frequent cause of emotional disorders. Mercury, cadmium, and lead toxicity are well-documented sources of mental problems.

Endocrine imbalances often affect the emotions. Everyone is familiar with the frequent references to the menstrual cycle and emotional swings. Hypothyroidism also may be a cause of lethargy and depression. Many of these endocrine-related emotional disorders can be corrected through proper nutrition.

Treatment

All cases of depression or emotional problems should first be evaluated for blood sugar abnormalities, food allergy, or endocrine imbalance. If hypoglycemia, hypothyroidism, or diabetes tendencies are discovered, the diet regimens in those sections should be used. Care should be taken to remove as many artificial food additives or chemicals as possible from the diet. Foods suspected of containing heavy metals such as swordfish, tuna, or canned foods, should also be eliminated. Sugar, alcohol, coffee, cigarettes, and any unnecessary drugs should be discontinued. Occupational sources of toxins must be removed. Check the section on Allergy for details on their diagnoses and therapy.

Vitamins and Minerals

Obviously, we are discussing a wide range of disorders and only specific supplementation will be of benefit. The following list, however, represents the most commonly used nutrients for these emotional problems:

Vitamin B_1: 200 to 1000 mg per day. Intramuscular injection may be needed in individual cases.

Vitamin B_3: Megadoses are often needed for B_3-dependent symptoms; 3 to 9 g per day.

Vitamin B_6: Pyridoxine dependency symptoms need megadoses. 250 to 500 mg per day or more are needed, especially where edema exists, or if related to menstrual cycle.

Vitamin B_{12}: 1 mg intramuscularly per week.

Vitamin B complex: 50 mg two times per day.

Folic acid: 400 mcg up to 10 g per day.

Vitamin C: Any stressful condition requires bowel tolerance doses.

Calcium/magnesium: In a 2:1 ratio.

Iron

Manganese

Zinc

Other

Desiccated Thyroid prescription.

Lithium: 2 to 3 mg per day.

L-Tryptophan: 1500 mg two times per day.

DL-Phenylalanine: 250 mg three times per day; or if not effective (with depression), or if it aggravates condition, use tyrosine, 100 mg per kilogram of body weight.

BODY ODOR (Bromhidrosis)

Definition and Symptoms

The secretion of foul-smelling perspiration.

Etiologic Considerations

- Bacteria
- Toxemia
- Liver disorder
- Systemic disease
- Excess saturated fats:
    Meat
    Dairy products
    Hydrogenated fats
    Fried foods
- Fungus
- Chemicals
- Kidney disorder
- Improper diet
- Zinc deficiency
- Essential fatty acids
- Soap and water deficiency

Discussion

Millions of dollars are spent annually in the development and usage of underarm deodorants and antiperspirants. These not only ignore the basic cause of body odor, but in some cases can be detrimental to your health. Offensive body odor may have two basic causes—external or internal.

The external cause of offensive body odor is obviously an acute soap and water deficiency. The oily secretions of sweat accumulate and provide an ideal medium for the growth of bacteria, the accepted cause of this type of body odor. Fungus infections may also contribute to body odor.

Internal causes of offensive body odor are, in general, ignored or simply not understood. The skin acts as a major organ of elimination, releasing toxins through the skin. In certain areas such as under the arms this secretion is most noticeable. However, the entire body sweats. If there is an excessive amount of toxic substance in the body that exceeds the capacity of the digestive system, liver, or kidneys to deal with, it must then exit via the skin. Such toxic substances accumulate due to liver disease or congestion, poor eliminations, kidney disease, uremia, pneumonia, acute rheumatism, scurvy, other systemic diseases, and improper diet.

Improper diet, probably the most ignored cause of foul body odor, is also the number one factor in most cases of internal origin. The main offender is excess saturated animal fats or hydrogenated fats. This not only leads to liver toxicity but causes the sebaceous glands to work excessively, producing a greater media for bacterial infection. When a wet sheet body pack is applied overnight to a toxic, heavy meat eater, the sheet will become both stained and offensive smelling, due to the eliminated poisons in the sweat.

Some cases are due to an unsaturated fat *deficiency* rather than saturated fat excess. These may coincide. A zinc deficiency is also well recognized as a causative factor in many cases.

Treatment

The only real long-term improvement will come from good hygiene, internal cleansing, elimination, and proper diet.

Diet

Various regimens will be effective. The aim of each is to address the major cause for each person. The following have proven useful:

1. 12-to-14-day Elimination Diet:

Days 1 to 3:	Fruit juice fast with an enema nightly.
Days 4 to 6:	Fresh fruit and fruit juices only.
Days 7 to 12:	
Breakfast	Fresh fruit
Midmorning	Fruit or vegetable juice
Lunch	Raw salad
Midafternoon	Same as morning, or potassium broth

Supper   Same as lunch, or three to four steamed vegetables with lemon juice and unsaturated oil.

Evening   Same as afternoon

2. Prolonged fruit or vegetable juice fasting for 7 to 21 days

3. Raw foods diet for 2 to 6 months

4. Vegetarian diets (no dairy products)

5. Liver-cleansing diet (see Gallbladder Disease)

6. Mucus-cleansing diet (see Appendix I)

The best approach is to begin with either the 12-to-14-day elimination regimen, or prolonged fasting, and then adopt the vegetarian diet until symptoms are cleared. Several periods of elimination diets or fasting may be required over a 2-to-4-month period. If, at the end of this procedure, you desire animal products, they may be introduced 5 days a week, with 2 days remaining vegetarian. Red meat (especially pork) is not recommended. Fish is the preferred animal product, then properly raised turkey or wild turkey and chicken. Wild meats contain less fat and are therefore more desirable.

Physiotherapy

• Epsom salts baths

These are useful for body odor due either to internal or external causes. Put 1 to 1½ lb of Epsom salts into a hot tub and soak for 15 to 20 minutes. Finish with a cold spray. Repeat daily the first week, then reduce to two to three times per week until the body odor is normal.

"Salt glow"

Mix 1 lb fine salt in enough water to make a slurry. Begin with a warm shower and then with water off rub salt all over the body firmly. Finish with a cold shower. Your skin will "glow" for hours.*

Alternate hot and cold showers daily to maintain proper skin function.*

Wet sheet trunk packs should be applied nightly during fast and one to two times per week for 4 to 6 weeks.*

Therapeutic Agents

Vitamins and Minerals

Magnesium: 400 to 800 mg per day.

Zinc: 30 to 50 mg two to three times per day.*

*Asterisks indicate the most frequently used therapeutic agents.

OTHERS

Chlorophyll: 2 to 4 tablets three times per day.*

Essential fatty acids: 4 capsules three times per day.*

Lecithin: 2 to 3 tbs granules one to two times per day; or as capsules, 2 to 4 taken two to three times per day.*

BOTANICALS

Burdock (*Arctium lappa*): Alterative, diaphoretic. Helps restore oil and sweat gland function.

Coneflower (*Echinacea angustifolia*): Alterative, blood purifier.

Oregon grape root (*Berberis aquifolium*): Alterative.

Yellow dock (*Rumex crispus*): Alterative.

Therapeutic Suggestion

Zinc, chlorophyll, and EFA are always prescribed in high doses. The botanicals may be of some use as blood purifiers and as general tonics.

BOILS, FURUNCLES, AND CARBUNCLES

Definition

Boils and furuncles: An acute inflammation and infection of a sebaceous gland, hair follicle, or subcutaneous layer of the skin. *Staphylococcus* infection is most common.

Carbuncles: A group of adjacent furuncles with extension of inflammation and infection into the subcutaneous layers of the skin.

Etiologic Considerations

- Toxemia
- Constipation
- Improper diet
  Excess saturated fats
  Excess hydrogenated fats
  Excess sweets, refined carbohydrates
  Chocolate
  Protein deficiency

*Asterisks indicate the most frequently used therapeutic agents.

Acid-forming diet
Unsaturated fatty acid deficiency
- Allergy
- Diabetes
- Liver congestion
- Glandular imbalance
- Poor skin function
- Excess sebaceous gland activity
- Local irritation

Discussion

Even a relatively healthy person may experience a boil or two on rare occasions due to local irritation by a splinter or other foreign object. Systemic or repeated boils, however, are always a sign of internal disorder.

The most common cause of recurrent boils is toxemia. This may be due to reduced function of other organs of elimination and detoxification such as found in constipation or congestion of the liver; or it may be due to an excess burden being placed on these organs that cannot be met. Such congestion occurs on an improper diet with excess saturated fats. The overconsumption of meat, pork, eggs, milk, cheese, butter, or other saturated fats congests the liver, thickens the blood, slows circulation, and increases sebaceous gland activity. Similar mechanisms apply to boils as they do in acne (see Acne).

The overconsumption of sweets and refined carbohydrates is also associated with recurrent boils. Although similar mechanisms as in *Staphylococcus* infections are found (see Staphylococcal Infections), I find the character of systemic or recurrent boils entirely different from those of the typical *Staphylococcus* infection. This may seem paradoxical since both conditions show infections with *Staphylococcus* bacteria. Boils in general differ from a typical *Staphylococcus* infection in that the lesions are more clearly bordered, generally deeper, involving hair follicles or glands, and far less infectious. They are also less likely to be quickly thwarted with external measures alone.

In most cases of systemic or recurrent boils we find glandular disturbances similar, once again, to those found under Acne. Diabetes or food allergy should also be considered as a possible cause in isolated cases.

Treatment

Boils are usually the result of the self-cleansing and self-repairing efforts of the body to regain equilibrium. As such it is important in our treatment to understand the body's aim and assist in making this cleansing more efficient and complete.

Diet

Nearly any diet that encourages internal cleansing will be effective. However, I find the raw vegetable juice fast to be the most effective, followed closely by the citrus juice fast in cases where excess fruit has not been the usual pattern. Either of these diets may be continued anywhere from 7 to 21 days or even longer with care and supervision. Shorter fasts may be used and repeated frequently until the desired result is obtained.

Either of these fasts may then be followed by an all raw diet with an abundance of green vegetables, vegetable juices, seaweed, sprouted beans, seeds and grains, and a little fruit. Until the condition has totally cleared, I suggest adhering to the low saturated fat diet as found under Acne.

Other diets of use in some circumstances are the liver-cleansing diet, apple mono diet, and the mucus-cleansing diet (see Appendix I).

Physiotherapy

- Local

  Ice placed directly on a boil in its early stages will usually abort its development. However, for systemic boils it is better to encourage eliminations.

- Hot Epsom salts compress

  Dissolve Epsom salts in hot water and apply as a compress all night.

- Flaxseed poultice*

  Grind seeds and boil to porridgelike consistency; apply as poultice. Helps mature lesions.

- Clay poultice*

- Chlorophyll poultice

- Cooked hot onion or garlic poultice

- Green papaya poultice

APPLICATIONS

  Aloe

  Dilute calendula tincture wash as an antiseptic.

  Ultraviolet exposure in careful doses.

  Vitamin E: 200 to 400 IU two times per day.

  Tincture of green soap wash, followed by hydrogen peroxide application.*

*Asterisks indicate the most frequently used therapeutic agents.

Tea tree oil: Apply four to six times per day, after green soap and hydrogen peroxide.*

Sugar or honey application for deep, ulcerated sores.*

GENERAL

Hot Epsom salts baths: Repeat daily at first, and then three to four times per week (see Appendix I).

"Salt glow" (see Appendix I).

Alternate hot/cold showers as a general systemic tonic. Regularizes deep and superficial circulation.

Therapeutic Agents

VITAMINS AND MINERALS

Vitamin A: 50,000 to 100,000 IU per day for 2 to 4 weeks; immune support. *Use any dose of vitamin A over 50,000 IU per day with medical supervision only.**

Vitamin B complex: 25 to 50 mg three times per day.

Vitamin B_{12}

Folic acid

Vitamin C: 1000 to 6000 IU per day or more; antibiotic, antioxidant, immune support.*

Vitamin E: 400 to 1000 IU per day.*

Zinc: 30 to 50 mg two to three times per day.*

OTHERS

Atomodine (Cayce product)

Chlorophyll: Local and internal detoxifier.*

Garlic: 2 capsules three times per day.*

Kelp (not with Atomodine): 2 tablets three times per day.*

Propolis (a resinous beeswax): Antibiotic. Dose: 5 to 15 drops tincture, three to four times per day.*

Raw spleen tablets: Immune support.

Raw thymus tablets: 2 tablets four times per day; immune support.*

*Asterisks indicate the most frequently used therapeutic agents.

BOTANICALS

Burdock (*Arctium lappa*): Alterative. Dose: 20 to 40 drops tincture, three to four times per day.*

Coneflower (*Echinacea angustifolia*): Blood purifier, specific for systemic boils. Dose: 15 to 30 drops tincture, three to four times per day.*

Oregon grape root (*Berberis aquifolium*): Alterative. Used in skin conditions due to impure blood.*

Red clover (*Trifolium pratense*)

Yellow dock (*Rumex crispus*)

Therapeutic Suggestions

Immune function supports are useful, including vitamin A, B complex, vitamin C, vitamin E, zinc, and thymus. Garlic is essentially used as a mild antibiotic systemically along with propolis. Some cases benefit with some glandular stimulation using kelp or Atomodine 1 to 2 drops per day for 1 week. Of the botanicals, Echinacea stands out as the most effective. Burdock and Oregon grape also are used frequently, in addition.

BRONCHITIS

Definition

Inflammation of the bronchial tree. May be acute or chronic.

Symptoms

Acute

Symptoms of acute upper respiratory infection

Slight fever
Cough (dry or productive)
Mucopurulent secretions
Flulike symptoms, which may lead to bronchopneumonia
Chest pain and reduced respiratory excursion

Chronic

Cough
Sputum

*Asterisks indicate the most frequently used therapeutic agents.

Difficulty in breathing
Wheezing
Asthmatic episodes
Recurrences of pulmonary infection
Respiratory failure
Exhaustion

Etiologic Considerations

- Diet
    Excess carbohydrates
    Acid-forming diet
    Excess dairy products
    Vitamin A deficiency
- Improper treatments of common colds
- Poor eliminations
- Frequent colds (viral, with secondary bacterial invasions)
- Lowered resistance
- Suppressive treatments of previous health problems
- Exposure, fatigue, malnutrition
- Foci of infection: Tooth or sinus infection acting as reservoir
- Allergy
- Irritants: Occupational inhalants, cigarette smoke
- Asthma and emphysema
- Inadequate circulation
- Spinal: C7 to T4, kyphoscoliosis (spinal curvature)
- Bronchial constriction
- Stomach trouble
- Constipation
- Chronic catarrh
- Lack of outdoor exercise

Discussion

Chronic bronchitis is usually preceded by a series of colds and acute bronchitis. If these two conditions were treated properly, no chronic condition would develop. The most common cause of any chronic lung condition is suppressive treatments for the common cold. These simple eliminations should be allowed to run their course. They act as safety valves to prevent more serious disease from developing from the excessive accumulation of toxic waste within the system. At the first sign of any acute illness, all solid food intake should be halted immediately, and a fruit juice fast, or vegetable juice fast (depending on the condition and patient) should begin. If this were common practice, chronic bronchitis would be rare and restricted to those exposed to lung irritants or cigarette smoke.

Chronic bronchitis is often associated with emphysema. They frequently coexist and are very difficult to differentiate in many cases. In chronic bronchitis, the bronchi becomes thick and inelastic. The mucus becomes thick and dry and the normal cilial action (little hairs that help remove waste and bacteria) is reduced by degeneration, leading to retained mucus. This acts as an ideal medium for infection. As mucus accumulates, the total available oxygen exchange area of the lung is reduced, leading to dyspnea (difficult breathing). Cigarette smoking has a similar action on cilia and reduces their motility.

Coughing in these instances is beneficial. This reflex action aids in removing mucus and waste that the cilia are unable to move further. The cough reflex should therefore not be indiscriminately suppressed. Rather, the causes of excess mucus production and retention should be corrected and the cough will then disappear.

Improper diet and poor eliminations are major causes of excess mucus production. This results in accumulated irritants in the gastrointestinal, lymph, and blood systems. These toxins produce inflammatory changes in the respiratory system.

Spinal abnormalities also predispose the lungs to disease. Kyphoscoliotic changes reduce lung excursion and are a factor in mucus accumulation and downgraded vitality. This also is influenced by decreased lymph, blood, and nervous flow to these tissues. The areas from C7 to T4 are the most commonly involved, causing inflammatory and congestive changes in the lungs and bronchi.

Treatment

There is no quick cure of chronic bronchitis. The causes must first be removed and then the entire respiratory system revitalized. Much attention must also be spent on normalizing eliminations by improving skin and bowel function. Certain herbal preparations have proven useful to help clear the lungs of excess mucus and heal their delicate linings. These herbs should be used in conjunction with other systematic therapies. Too many people rely on herbal therapies in much the same way as most depend on drug therapy. The only true healing comes from within. These external agents should only be used as a temporary aid to help stimulate the body to action.

Diet

The following diets are of use in these cases:

Mucus-Cleansing Diet

On rising	Hot water and lemon juice
Breakfast	Orange or grapefruit
Midmorning	Herb tea, fresh fruit juice, or vegetable juice (carrot)
Lunch	A large plate of boiled or steamed onions. A little natural soy sauce or vegetable seasoning may be used to flavor, but no salt.
Midafternoon	As midmorning, or potassium broth
Supper	Same as lunch
Evening	As midmorning, or potassium broth

Take 2 garlic capsules with all meals. Be sure to drink 6 to 8 glasses of water per day to help thin mucus secretions and aid in expectoration.

Citrus juice fast	Lemon, grapefruit
All-fruit diet	Especially citrus
Alkaline diet	Citrus juice and fruit Green vegetable juice plus raw salads Onions, cooked and raw Hot water, lemon, and honey Onion syrup (see Appendix I) Garlic Herbal teas

Carrot Mono Diet

Breakfast	Carrot juice
Midmorning	Raw carrots and/or carrot juice
Lunch	Raw or cooked carrots
Midafternoon	Carrot juice
Supper	Raw or cooked carrots
Evening	Carrot juice

For more detailed diet advice with mucus conditions refer to the chapter on Asthma.

Physiotherapy

STEAM INHALATIONS

- Pine needles, olbas oil, eucalyptus, and elecampane (for asthmalike symptoms). Add the above inhalants to a pot of boiled water. These may be either the herb or oil form. Make a tent over two chairs with a large towel or blanket. Place steaming pot of herbs under tent and inhale fumes for 5 to 15 minutes. Alternatively, you can simply place the pot on a table or chair and drape a towel over your head and the pot. Inhale deeply. Repeat three to six times daily.

HOT FOMENTATIONS (SEE PART I), COMPRESSES, AND POULTICES TO CHEST

Use any of the following:

- Simple hot fomentations, followed with cold
- Hot ginger* fomentation with or without mustard
- Lobelia hot fomentation for spasmodic cough
- Lobelia, pleurisy root, and mullein hot fomentation
- Camphoderm* (Cayce product)
  Mutton tallow
  Spirits of camphor
  Spirits of gum turpentine
  Rub into chest and apply a hot compress.

POSTURAL DRAINAGE AND PERCUSSION (FOLLOWING HOT CHEST FOMENTATIONS)

Lie with upper torso hanging over a bed and have someone pound with a flat hand over the entire back. Any mucus brought up should be expectorated into a bowl placed near the head. This will help clear the lungs of excess mucus and facilitate healing.

HYDROTHERAPY

Any of the following will help:

- Saunas—two to three times per week, to sweat.
- Chest packs (see Hydrotherapy, Part I).
  Cold wet sheet cross packs over chest, *or*
  Cold wet sheet simple chest pack. Apply nightly in severe bronchitis.
- Alternate hot and cold showers to stimulate respiration and circulation.

*Asterisks indicate the most frequently used therapeutic agents.

BREATHING EXERCISES

- Blow up balloons.
- Increase force of exhalation.
- Diaphragmatic breathing: Begin to breathe by causing the stomach to protrude, followed by the chest. Exhale naturally. It sometimes helps to learn this technique by having someone place the hands over the upper three or four ribs to prevent the chest from rising first. This is important to learn in lung complaints such as bronchitis and asthma. Avoid mouth breathing.

OTHERS

Spinal Manipulation: Respiratory excursion must be increased to clear lungs and restore normal diaphragm movements.

Outdoor Exercises: Swimming is an excellent exercise for those with lung disorders.

Therapeutic Agents

VITAMINS AND SUPPLEMENTS

Vitamin A: Essential for lung health. High doses of micellized A, 25,000 IU two to three times per day, or more in acute cases (up to six times per day for several weeks). *Use any dose of vitamin A over 50,000 IU per day with medical supervision only.* *

Vitamin B complex: 25 to 50 mg three times per day. *

Vitamin B_6: 100 to 250 mg one to two times per day.

Vitamin C: 1000 mg three to six times per day or more; in acute cases up to bowel tolerance (i.e., when diarrhea occurs). *

Garlic: 2 capsules three times per day. Acts as antibiotic and expectorant. *

Zinc: 15 to 25 mg one to three times per day.

Raw adrenal tablets

Raw thymus tablets: 2 tablets three to four times per day. *

Onion syrup (see Appendix I): 1 tsp every 1 to 2 hours in acute cases; four times per day in chronic cases. *

BOTANICALS

Bloodroot (*Sanguinaria canadensis*): Expectorant, bronchial membrane stimulant.

Coltsfoot (*Tussilago farfara*): Demulcent. Soothes irritated bronchial mucous membranes. Use as warm infusion.

*Asterisks indicate the most frequently used therapeutic agents.

Elecampane (*Inula helenium*)

Asthma weed (*Euphorbia pilulifera*): Asthmalike condition with restricted breathing.

Gum plant (*Grindelia squarrosa*): Expectorant, antispasmodic. Used for dry, harsh, and unproductive cough. Dose: Tincture, 10 to 20 drops two to three times per day.*

Horehound (*Marrubium vulgare*)

Hyssop (*Hyssopus officinalis*): For asthmalike condition, with cough.

Ipecac (*Ipecacuanha*): Dose, 5 to 15 drops tincture, two to three times per day for violent, spasmodic cough.*

Lobelia (*Lobelia inflata*): Expectorant, antispasmodic; useful in spasmodic coughs. Dose, tincture 10 to 15 drops two to four times per day.*

Mullein tea (*Verbascum thapsus*)

Onion syrup with wild cherry, horehound, and licorice.

Squill (*Urginea scilla*): Expectorant for dry, bronchial cough. Dose, tincture 5 to 20 drops two to three times per day.*

Wild cherry bark (*Prunus serotina*): For irritable cough.

Therapeutic Suggestions

High doses of vitamin A supplements are usually very effective with lung complaints. Take care to monitor serum vitamin A levels to prevent toxicity. Where high vitamin A is needed, however, higher levels can usually be better tolerated. Vitamin B complex and extra vitamin B_6 are useful, as well as vitamin C, to bowel tolerance. Garlic acts as a wonderful mucus solvent, and should be taken in as many ways as possible (i.e., capsules, food, condiment, and garlic syrup). Onion syrup is also very useful and less offensive. Raw thymus as an immune stimulant is very helpful, as well.

BRUISES (see Wounds)

BURNS

Definition

Tissue damage of skin or mucous membranes in response to heat, chemical, or radiation injury.

---

*Asterisks indicate the most frequently used therapeutic agents.

Symptoms

Burns are classified as *first-degree*, when there is only superficial involvement of the outer layer of the epidermis. Area is pink but blanches white on pressure. Depending on treatment, may or may not blister.

A *second-degree burn* involves the entire epithelium, including glandular structures and hair follicles. Blistering and scar formation occurs.

Third-degree burns involve the full thickness of skin with extensive tissue damage. Areas may be oozing, or in severe cases (*fourth-degree burn*) may be dry and charred.

Etiologic Considerations

- Heat
    Open fires
    Hot liquid
    Ultraviolet rays, sun lamps

- Chemicals, topical or inhalation

- Electricity

- Radiation

Discussion

The rapid and proper treatment of burns is essential to prevent or reduce blistering, scar formation, or contracture of skin. First-degree burns may be treated safely at home. *However, extensive second- or third-degree burns always need to be treated under medical supervision.* These injuries can lead to severe loss of fluids and electrolytes with shock and even death as a possibility. If possible, obtain the services of a doctor familiar with or willing to try the simple measures outlined under the treatment section. Severe burns respond remarkably to these measures. Any extensive second- or third-degree burns should always be treated with medical supervision to prevent scarring and disfigurement.

Treatment

There are a vast number of home remedies or first aid for burns. Of this large variety, however, several stand out as the most effective. They are simple, readily available, and reliable. Most have slowly graduated from the "folk remedy" status to at least the fringe of standard orthodox practice.

Hydrotherapy

The simplest, most effective measure with any burn is to immerse the area in cold water *immediately* after the injury and until all pain has subsided. With a first-degree burn this will often prevent a blister formation. In more severe burns it will minimize tissue damage. If the burn is severe and transport to a hospital necessary, either continue soaking the area if possible, or gently wrap the area with wet sheets and apply water at frequent intervals over this sheeting.

Oil Applications

Just after the injury has been soaked in water, apply a strong concentration of vitamin E. This may be applied to a small area by puncturing a 400-IU capsule and gently covering the burn; or it may be sprayed on with an oil atomizer for larger areas. This needs to be repeated every 1 to 4 hours. Vitamin E has been found extremely beneficial, even in third-degree burns, to promote early healing and prevent scar formation. Vitamin E is used externally with great success with all types of burns. High doses of E should also be taken internally— 800 to 1600 IU per day.

Vitamin C

Between vitamin E applications a 1 to 3% solution of vitamin C should be sprayed every 2 to 4 hours. This reduces pain, accelerates healing, reduces the chance of infection, and decreases local swelling. Vitamin C may also be taken as an injection in severe burns, in megadoses. In all burns vitamin C should be taken orally up to 1000 mg every hour.

These three applications make the best therapy for burns. The following treatments have also been used successfully:

Aloe: Obtain fresh aloe and apply the gelatinous inner contents of the cactus leaves to sunburn and other minor burns. Bottled gel may also be obtained from most health food stores, but is less effective.

Aloe gel and propolis: This combines the soothing and anti-inflammatory effect of aloe with the antibiotic nature of propolis.

Comfrey poultice: Steep comfrey leaves or boil root and apply to burn as a continuous compress.

Comfrey and wheatgrass poultice

Comfrey, wheat germ, or vitamin E oil and honey poultice: This classic poultice combines the beneficial effects of three well-known applications, each individually proven beneficial with burns.

Honey, or honey plus herbs: Apply and cover with gauze (comfrey, marsh-mallow, calendula, etc.).

Honey, propolis, and zinc oxide

Calendula succus compress: ¼ dilution applied to gauze.

Witch hazel (nonalcoholic, dilute)

Bicarbonate of soda plus water: For acid burns flush immediately with water or water plus bicarbonate.

Essential fatty acids (EFA) ointment

Chlorophyll ointment

Therapeutic Agents

VITAMINS AND MINERALS

Vitamin A: 25,000 IU three times per day for 2 to 4 weeks. *Use any dose of vitamin A over 50,000 IU per day with medical supervision only.* *

Vitamin B complex: 50 mg three times per day. *

Vitamin C: Up to 2000 mg per hour; intravenously up to 30 g per day for severe burns. *

Vitamin E: 800 to 1600 IU per day. *

EFA: 2 to 4 capsules three times per day.

Zinc: 30 to 50 mg two to three times per day. *

Calcium

OTHERS

Chlorophyll

Cod-liver oil: 2 to 4 capsules two to three times per day.

Raw adrenal tablets: 1 tablet three times per day with second- or third-degree burns. *

BURSITIS

Definition

Acute or chronic bursitis: inflammation of a bursa (a fluid-filled cavity, especially common where tendons pass near bones).

*Asterisks indicate the most frequently used therapeutic agents.

Symptoms

Pain, tenderness, reduced mobility, swelling, redness, possible fever, muscle weakness.

Etiologic Considerations

- Direct trauma
- Microtrauma (overuse)
- Metabolic disturbance
- Toxemia
- Poor diet
- Infection
- Gout
- Allergy

Discussion

Although most people think of the shoulder (subdeltoid) when bursitis is mentioned, bursitis may affect a number of joints throughout the body. Other fairly common sites are the hip (iliopsoas), ischia (so-called tailor's or weaver's bottom), prepatellar (housemaid's knee), retrocalcaneal (Achilles), olecranon (miner's elbow), semimembranosis (behind knee), trochanteric (bunion), or radiohumeral (tennis elbow). Bursae exist at areas of friction in the body, usually between tendon and bone, acting as cushioning barriers to tissue damage. The two most common causes of bursitis are direct trauma and microtrauma. *Direct trauma*, such as a severe blow to the shoulder, causes the bursa to swell, leading to pain on motion and reduced mobility. This type of bursitis, if well rested after the initial injury, will usually resolve easily within a short period of time. If aggravated and used too soon after the initial injury, this acute bursitis may become chronic, lingering for years.

Microtrauma as a cause of bursitis is the use of the joint and muscles in an "ordinary" activity repeated frequently, such as found in the action of screwdriving or tennis, with rotation (supination) of the forearm against resistance. A similar trauma may occur to the shoulder with repeated hammering. All these actions are within the normal range of expected activity for the body, but many repetitions over a prolonged period of time ultimately cause irritation and inflammation of the bursa and later the joint itself if the bursa communicates directly with the joint as it does with the shoulder. Repeated small blows in the area of the bursa, such as the pushing or stamping on a lever as in some industrial occupations, or repeated kneeling, as in housemaid's knee, will also cause bursitis. Even prolonged or repeated carrying of a heavy purse or shopping bag can initiate bursitis.

Once bursitis has developed there is a tendency for the periarticular structures to become thickened and fibrotic. If the effusion or swelling has been severe, adhesions may form to limit mobility further, causing pain and recurrent swelling.

Much confusion exists regarding bursitis among patients since many physicians use the term fairly loosely. The label of "bursitis" of the shoulder may be used to mean arthritis, a tear in the periosteum at the insertion of the supraspinatus muscle, calcification of the supraspinatus muscle, pain from the third costovertebral joint, other partial muscle tears, or true subacromial/subdeltoid bursitis.

One commonly neglected aspect of bursitis is the possibility that if the nutritional state had been more adequate the same amount of trauma may not have resulted in any symptoms whatsoever. Certainly, high levels of vitamin C are known to help protect against connective tissue injuries. Outside of the athletic injuries resulting in bursitis, the average person I see with bursitis is on a poor, vitamin-deficient diet. Not surprisingly, then, we find the nutritional approach to therapy essential to allow other local therapies to function best.

An interesting consideration with bursitis and other inflammatory conditions is that some people are particularly prone to inflammatory reactions. Two people of similar age and build will respond quite differently to an episode of trauma or repeated microtraumas. One may show only minor symptoms lasting a short period of time, while the other may develop a bursitis that causes discomfort for years, perhaps decades. The difference in these two is that the latter is an inflammatory condition, even before the traumatic incident. I believe the causes of this predisposition are usually dietary or stress-related.* I find cases of bursitis very rare among those who are on a highly nutritious, alkaline (more vegetarian) diet with few obvious irritants, such as coffee, alcohol, refined sugars, salt, and strong spices. This applies to *all* diseases but particularly to such inflammatory conditions as bursitis, arthritis, gastritis, colitis, etc. Stress plays an obvious role in such conditions, working along a variety of negative pathways.

Treatment

Since the average case of bursitis is caused by trauma or repeated use as in tennis, angling, baseball, cricket, hammering, or other activities with repeated

*Levine, S.A., and Kidd, P.M. "Biochemical Pathologies Initiated by Free Radical Oxident Compounds in the Aetiology of Food Hypersensitivity Disease," *International Clinical Nutrition Review*, 5:1 (Jan. 1985).

actions, these are strictly forbidden until full healing is complete. The only cause of chronic bursitis is improper care of acute bursitis, and the best part of this cure is rest.

Acute

- Ice compress: Just as soon as the first symptoms appear, apply cold compresses, leaving them on for 20 to 40 minutes. Repeat this application every 3 waking hours for the first 2 days.
- Restraint: Fix the joint in a resting position and do not use actively. In the case of a shoulder, use a sling if this is necessary to prevent the shoulder's use.
- Passive mobilization (see below) is necessary several times daily.
- Ultrasound: Get ultrasound treatments daily after the first 48 hours for 1 week, then four times per week the second week.
- Alternate hot and cold compresses: After 48 hours of ice-cold applications use ultrasound and alternate hot and cold applications, or use heat followed by joint mobilization ending with cold applications.

Chronic

- Heat compresses
- Alternate hot and cold compresses
- Ultrasound four to five times weekly

Exercises

Passive mobilization, or movement of the injured joint with the help of another person, should be done after the first 48 hours two to six times each day, to the full range of motion *without* the assistance of the patient's muscles. This speeds healing and reduces the possibility of adhesions forming. New machines for this purpose, to mobilize without muscle assistance, have had success in healing joint and soft tissue injuries.

Once all or most of the pain and swelling has subsided, non-muscle-assisted exercises can begin:

1. *Arm swing 1:* Stoop to 90° angle from waist and let arms hang freely, then gently swing arms front and back and then side to side. Do not use shoulder muscles in this action. Then gently swing arms in small circles in both directions, gradually increasing the diameter of the circle as each day progresses.

2. *Toe touch:*   Bend forward at waist and touch toes repeatedly.

3. *Bed exercise:*   Lie in bed and slowly raise arm from the shoulder out from side to point of pain and back.

Begin the following muscle-assisted exercises once the previous two exercises are easily performed without much pain.

1. *Wall creep:*   Stand 1 ft from wall with hands on wall at whatever level is comfortable, say, waist high. Slowly creep your hands up the wall by pulling your fingers forward and back like a spider. Stop when you reach the level where pain increases. Repeat exercises four to five times per day. Mark this level on the wall and over the next few weeks try to exceed this level progressively, going higher until arms can go completely overhead.

2. *Arm swing 2:*   Stand erect and swing arms across body repeatedly in a gentle action. Swing arms in gradually larger swings front to back until full-circle swings can be easily and painlessly made.

3. *Apron tie* repeated by tying and untying an apron.

4. *Collar button-up:*   Attempt to button and unbutton a real or imaginary button behind the collar, repeatedly.

5. *The pickpocket:*   Repeatedly attempt to remove a billfold from the back pocket.

6. *Pulley exercises:*   Arrange a pulley on the wall with a strong rope about 8 to 10 ft long running through. Attach a handle to both ends, or attach through a firm rubber ball with a large knot. If possible, arrange the pulley so that its height from the floor may be freely adjusted. Sit on the floor or on a stool with back to pulley. Begin with pulley close to floor and pull with the injured arm on the rope against the resistance provided from the good arm which is holding onto the opposite end of the rope. Two-pound weights may be used instead. Repeat several times and then raise the pulley 6 in. Repeat these exercises until a height is reached that evokes mild to moderate pain. Do not overdo. The object is to increase both the strength and mobility of the shoulder slowly. Repeat, sitting facing the pulley. Ready-made pulley exercise units are also available at most sports departments. Increase weights slowly.

7. *Stick, rope, ball, and door techniques:*   This simple technique replaces the previous one and is more portable. Attach a wooden handle to one end of a 4-to-6-ft rope and attach the other end through a firm rubber ball with a large knot. The ball end is then slipped behind the door and the door closed so that the rope may be secured at literally any position along the door's perimeter. Stand with back to door, with rope in the near-floor level. Gradually pull the rope against the resistance for 3 to 6 seconds, and relax. Repeat

two to three times, then repeat at higher levels along the door frame. Stop at the level you feel pain and repeat, facing the door.

Poultices

Green cabbage leaf poultice. Apply to tender, swollen bursa nightly.

Comfrey leaf poultice

Apple cider vinegar and salt compress: Prepare a saturated solution of iodized salt dissolved in hot water and add 50% cider vinegar. Saturate a compress and apply hot for 10 to 15 minutes two times per day. Helps with tissue damage, fibrositis, and calcification.

Castor oil packs

Hot Epsom salts packs (with no swelling)

Ice compress (with swelling)

Others

Peanut oil massage to area

Ultrasound therapy daily for first 2 weeks; reduce to three times per week for the next 2 weeks.

Positive galvanism to bursa with magnesium sulfate or oil of wintergreen.

Shoulder mobilization and manipulation to break adhesions in chronic cases.

Therapeutic Agents

VITAMINS AND MINERALS

Vitamin A: 10,000 to 25,000 IU two to three times per day. *Use any dose of vitamin A over 50,000 IU per day with medical supervision only.*

Vitamin B complex: 50 mg three times per day.*

Vitamin B_6: 250 to 500 mg per day.

Vitamin B_{12}: IM 1000 mcg one time per week.*

Pantothenic acid: 250 to 500 mg two times daily.

Vitamin C: 1000 mg six to twelve times per day, or to bowel tolerance.*

Vitamin E: 400 IU two times per day.*

Calcium: 800 to 1000 mg per day.

Magnesium: 400 to 500 mg per day.

*Asterisks indicate the most frequently used therapeutic agents.

OTHERS

Atomodine or other iodine source.

Raw adrenal tablets*

Bromelain (anti-inflammatory): 2 to 4 tablets three to four times per day. Very effective with bursitis. These high doses may cause some gastrointestinal upset in some people. Use with care in history of ulcers.*

DL-Phenylalanine: For pain relief; 500 to 1000 mg two to three times per day.

BOTANICALS

Bryony (*Bryonia alba*): Pain with motion. Dose: Tincture 5 drops two to three times per day, or used as homeopathic dilution.*

Comfrey (*Symphytum officinale*): Use as strong infusion, decoction, or tincture, two to three times daily for 1 to 3 months as therapeutic trial.*

CARBUNCLES (see Boils)

CATARACTS

Definition

Developmental or degenerative opacity of the lens.

Symptoms

Progressive and painless loss of vision.

Etiologic Considerations

• Diet
  Excess milk
  Excess cholesterol
  Galactose intolerance (milk sugar intolerance commonly found in children)
  Fatty acid intolerances
  Protein deficiency
  Deficient nutrition (general, single, or multiple)
  Excess sugar (activates sorbitol pathway)

*Asterisks indicate the most frequently used therapeutic agents.

    Sorbitol (commonly used sweetener for diabetics)
    Vitamin C deficiency
    Vitamin B_2 deficiency

- Improper calcium metabolism
- Hormone imbalance
- Liver disease
- Toxemia
- Mercury toxicity (free radical damage)
- Diabetes (sorbitol accumulation in lens)
- Drugs
- Heavy metal toxicity (mercury)
- Irradiation
- Free radical damage (antioxidants useful to prevent)
- Trauma
- Eyestrain
- Spinal (cervical and upper thoracic)
- Stress and adrenal exhaustion
- Poor eliminations
- Deficient local circulation

Discussion

The common opinion among most cataract patients and physicians is that cataracts are an accepted fact of growing old. Cataracts are so common in the over 60s group that they are considered almost normal. The usual procedure up until recently was to wait until the cataract had "matured" sufficiently to be surgically removed. Newer procedures, however, are able to deal with cataracts at relatively early stages. We can expect future surgical developments to be even more advanced.

Unfortunately, very little research has attempted to link cataract development with dietary habits. I feel that it is along these lines that the cause and prevention of cataracts will most probably be found. Research has already linked some cataracts to the consumption of milk sugar.*† This has been found experimentally in rats and also lactose-sensitive infants. Some researchers strongly feel that

*The Encyclopedia of Common Diseases, Rodale Press, Emmaus, Pa., 1976, pp. 646–656.
†Lancet 1: 355–357, 1984.

excess milk and saturated fat predispose to cataracts. Excess sugar may also affect this picture by potentiating the effects of saturated fats in the body.

Extreme nutritional deficiencies of protein or vitamin C have also been linked to some cataracts, along with improper calcium metabolism, hormone imbalance, liver disease, diabetes, and many drugs.

Toxemia is felt to be a factor in many cases. This is often difficult to prove, but a general toxic devitalized condition is a common finding in many with cataracts. Spinal lesions also are routinely found in the upper cervical region, causing alterations in blood and nervous supply, which can affect the health and integrity of the tissues involved.

Cataracts may also form due to sorbitol accumulation in the lens of the eye. In diabetics (and to a lesser extent hypoglycemics), blood sugar elevations cause the cells of the lens to absorb large amounts of glucose. This is then converted to sorbitol, an insoluble storage form of sugar, which crystallizes out in the eye, forming a cataract.

Treatment

Proper prevention and treatment for cataracts lie in general tonic therapy, where all negative health factors are eliminated, and general vitality is increased to the maximum point for that individual. The actual specifics of therapy differ from person to person.

Diet

Unless the patient is extremely emaciated it is always wise to begin with a 7-day fruit juice and vegetable juice fast. This should be composed of juices from organically grown fruits and vegetables, taken throughout the day whenever the patient is thirsty. No two different juices are to be taken at any one meal. Warm water enemas are to be taken on days 1, 2, 3, 5, and 7. The following vegetable juices or combinations of these are useful:

Carrot	Beet
Celery	Parsley
Watercress	Spinach

This diet should then be followed with 1 to 2 days of a transitional diet of raw fruits and then on to a 7-to-14-day raw foods diet, composed of fresh fruit and fruit juice, vegetable juice and raw salads, sprouts, seaweed, seeds and nuts. This regimen will help cleanse the system of toxins, encourage better eliminations, and supply an abundance of high-quality "live" foods with all their vitamins, minerals, and enzymes. It also gives the body a rest from the toxic effects of animal proteins.

This diet is followed by a good general diet emphasizing more raw foods, seafoods rather than meats, and fewer dairy products. The following is an example:

On Rising	Hot water and lemon juice
Breakfast	Choose from:
	1. Fresh fruit
	2. Fruit smoothie
	3. Fresh or stewed fruit, nuts, honey, and a little low-fat yoghurt
	4. Whole grain cereal
Midmorning	Fresh vegetable juice
Lunch	*Always* a large mixed raw salad, with plenty of greens (keep the vegetables varied). Salads should be tasty and interesting. Include avocado, cooked beans, sprouted beans, artichoke hearts, olives, etc., for variety. If still hungry, choose from the following:
	Whole-meal vegetarian sandwich
	Tofu
	Baked potato
	Any other wholesome vegetarian main dish
Midafternoon	As midmorning
Supper	Salad as lunch or cooked vegetarian protein main meal
	Whole grains
	Conservatively cooked vegetables and seaweed
	Fish (not shellfish)

(*Note:* Absolutely no tea, coffee, sugar, alcohol, or cigarettes should be taken during any of these diets.)

These diets may be alternated repeatedly to encourage further detoxification and increase general vitality. In cases where hypoglycemia or diabetes is a factor, refer to detailed treatment regimens under those headings. Blood sugar regulation is of primary concern with cataracts.

Physiotherapy

The following suggestions may be of use to increase circulation and enhance local nutrition to the eyes.

• Alternate hot and cold showers to stimulate circulation and proper hormonal balance

• Alternate hot and cold sprays to head

- Warm castor oil eye packs
- Cold eye baths: Blink eyes open and closed for 2 to 5 minutes into a container of ice-cold water two times per day.
- Neck exercises
- Bates eye exercises**
- Endonasal technique (see Appendix I)
- Spinal manipulation to cervical and upper thoracic region, one to two times per week for 6 weeks; rest 2 weeks and repeat.
- Sauna baths (weekly)
- Local applications
  Cineraria maritima succus eyedrops: 1 drop two to three times per day in affected eye.*
  Castor oil eyedrops: 1 drop two times per day.
  Honey eyedrops: 1 drop two times per day.

Therapeutic Agents

Vitamins and Minerals

Vitamin A (micellized): 25,000 IU two times per day. *Use any dose of vitamin A over 50,000 IU per day with medical supervision only.**

Vitamin B complex: 50 mg three times per day.*

Vitamin B_2: 15 to 50 mg two times per day (prevention).

Niacin

Pantothenic acid

Vitamin B_6: 50 to 100 mg two times per day.

Vitamin C: 2 to 30 g per day (in high doses increase both magnesium and vitamin B_6 to prevent possibility of increased calcium excretion.*

Bioflavonoids: inhibit enzyme aldose reductase; responsible for conversion of glucose to sorbitol; used to prevent diabetic cataracts.*

Vitamin E: 400 to 800 IU one to two times daily (antioxidant).*

Calcium

Magnesium

Selenium: 200 mcg per day (prevents mercury-induced free radical damage).

*Asterisks indicate the most frequently used therapeutic agents.
**These are found in *The Art of Seeing*, by Aldous Huxley, Chatto and Windus (London) 1974, pp. 6–132.

OTHERS

Atomodine or 636 (Cayce)*

Chlorophyll

Cystine*

Lecithin*

Methionine*

BOTANICALS

Cineraria maritima succus eye drops: 1 drop two to three times per day.*

Therapeutic Suggestions

Therapies for cataracts are general and certainly not well proven. They are mostly tonic therapies. This does not mean, however, that they may not be effective. The true beauty of a systemic rather than a local approach is that the cases due to systemic causes will be dealt with. Good evidence does exist to place some blame on blood sugar abnormalities, as in diabetic cataracts, and any therapy that helps control blood glucose levels has a good chance of at least preventing further cataract formation, and possibly reversing it. I do not suggest that any cataract patient ignore the advice of his or her ophthalmologist, but do encourage a complete nutritional and structural investigation.

The most tried and tested botanical application is *Cineraria* drops, and these should be given a 2-to-6-month trial.

CATARRH (Excess Mucus)

Definition

Chronic excess mucus production affecting tissues, organs, and ducts lined by mucous membranes.

Symptoms

Sinusitis, headaches, runny nose, postnasal drip, sore throat, gastritis, digestive disorders, appendicitis, salpingitis, glue ear syndrome, eustachitis, cystitis, gallbladder disease, prostatitis.

*Asterisks indicate the most frequently used therapeutic agents.

Etiologic Considerations

- Excess carbohydrates (especially refined)
- Excess dairy products
- Allergies
- Excess saturated fats, fried foods
- Sweets, junk foods
- Toxicity
- Green vegetable deficiency
- Overeating
- Local irritation
  Smog
  Fumes
  Chemicals
  Allergens
- Stomach derangement
  Salt
  Spicy foods
  Poor food combinations
  Acidic foods
  Stress
- Hydrochloric acid deficiency, digestive enzyme deficiency
- Poor eliminations
  Skin
  Liver
  Bowels
- Lack of exercise
- Poor circulation

Discussion

The term "catarrh" will be more familiar to our English readers. In the United States it is not used much. What we are speaking about when we use this term is excess mucus production. Most people think of excess mucus in terms of runny noses and sinusitis. Nasal catarrh certainly is a common complaint—however, certainly not the only place in the body where excess mucus may become a problem.

First of all, it is important to appreciate that mucus is a natural and normal secretion of the body. In usual small amounts it lubricates and protects the delicate mucous membranes wherever they are found throughout the body. If, however, this mucus accumulates or is produced excessively, the condition of catarrh is created, which interferes with the normal action of the tissues or organs affected. In addition to the common upper respiratory or nasal catarrh, excess mucus may interfere with the ears, stomach, intestinal tract, fallopian tubes, ducts, or any other mucous membrane-lined part of the body. Often these conditions are treated repeatedly with antibiotics which fail to give relief, since any bacterial infection, if present at all, is merely a result of the internal congestion or inflammation caused by the catarrhal condition, and not its cause. I often see "ear infections" treated with repeated drug prescriptions that can only be relieved when the cause of the body's excess mucus production is corrected. Similar situations frequently occur with salpingitis, which is very important to resolve rapidly for a woman desiring pregnancy.

There are many dietary causes of catarrh. The most frequent problem is an extremely unbalanced diet, with excessive consumption of carbohydrates. Any carbohydrate, even the best unrefined whole wheat bread, if consumed in excess, will tend to create an increase in mucus production. This situation is much more pronounced if the excess is of a refined, devitalized nature such as white bread, white rice, or sugar. If such foods are not more than compensated for by a high vegetable intake, their acidic and mucus-forming nature predominates. One of the most common problems I see in practice is mucus-clogged infants and children who eat mostly starches and very little vegetables, causing chronic or recurrent colds and earaches.

Milk and other dairy products are well-known mucus-producers. Sometimes it is difficult to determine if their mucus-forming characteristics are due to a simple excess, their abnormal and adulterated state (pasteurized, homogenized, and containing many toxic chemicals, pesticides, and hormones), digestive enzyme deficiency (lactose), or a true allergy. As with all things, people respond quite differently to dairy products in their diet. Some seem very well adapted to dairy products, never showing any sensitivity whatsoever. Others find they can only tolerate small amounts before experiencing difficulties. Often we find people who cannot tolerate dairy products from cows, but who can handle goat's products. Others can only eat fermented dairy products, while a much larger percent cannot cope with any dairy substances whatsoever. Orientals are particularly sensitive to dairy products, with up to 85 percent of adults lacking the digestive enzyme lactase necessary to digest lactose, the sugar found in milk.

Any specific allergy or food intolerance may result in a catarrhal condition. The most common food allergies are wheat, yeast, eggs, and dairy products, but literally any food may present a problem.

Another major cause of both general and local catarrhal conditions falls under the classification of "irritants." Local irritants include fumes, smoke, foreign objects, chemicals, drugs, spicy foods, salt, pepper, alcohol, and even poor food combinations. Any factor that irritates a mucous membrane will stimulate excess mucus secretion. An imbalance in the digestive system is a common finding with excess mucus secretion. Gastric catarrh is usually the primary condition in catarrhal conditions elsewhere in the body. Once the digestive organs become inflamed, proper digestion is impossible. If the inflammation reaches the state where toxins seep through the irritated, and in some places thinned mucosa, the stage is set for systemic disease. If the organs of elimination are not working efficiently, or are overburdened by this toxic and irritant excess, a catarrhal condition will develop.

Lack of exercise and poor circulation work together to cause local and systemic congestion, which sets the stage for local accumulation of normal toxic products of metabolism, leading to irritation and ultimately mucus formation.

Treatment

Diet

In the initial stages of any catarrhal condition, wherever its location, it is wise first to eliminate foods most frequently associated with excess mucus production. I routinely eliminate all wheat, yeast, dairy products, and eggs for the first 1 to 2 months, or until progress permits their experimental addition. Obviously excluded from the diet are all refined carbohydrates, sugar, alcohol, coffee, tea, salt, pepper, strong spices, junk foods, and tobacco.

Various elimination regimens are effective with catarrhal conditions throughout the body. Some locations respond better to one or another particular juice, fruit, or vegetable. Citrus fruit (grapefruit and lemon) juices are very useful in some mucus conditions. They are eliminative and help break up congestion. They are not usually employed in cystitis, acute gastritis, or where citrus is known to cause unpleasant symptoms such as sour stomach, rash, etc. An apple juice fast or apple mono diet is well suited for mucus elimination. It is eliminative, but gentle on the stomach and does not usually cause any problems.

Vegetable juice fast (carrot or carrot/beet with or without green vegetables) is usually easily handled by most people. Its effect, however, is much slower, but very gentle and pleasant. Vegetable juices are eliminative, but also act to nourish and rebuild tissues.

The classic onion mucus-cleansing diet as found under Asthma is extremely useful to clear congested mucus conditions. It is excellent for catarrh of the ears, nose, sinuses, throat, and fallopian tubes.

The "master cleanser diet," as popularized by Stanley Burroughs, which advises lemon or lime juice, maple syrup, and cayenne pepper, has some limited value in instances of deep-seated catarrh.

It must be remembered that cayenne pepper is, in itself, a strong irritant, and much of the mucus eliminated was produced as a result of this property. It certainly is not well suited to stomach complaints. Often it is useful in "getting the mucus flowing" in deep-seated chronic conditions.

No general procedural instructions can be given. The individual regimen depends on the patient and the complaint. Usually the regimen will begin with some type of fast for varying periods of 3 to 21 days, followed by a raw foods diet, with only vegetarian proteins, and absolutely no starch or dairy products. Once it is decided to expand the diet, the first grains added are brown rice and millet. Once dairy substances are to be reintroduced, if at all, goat's yoghurt is added first and then goat's cheese if desired. Dairy foods are minimized in the diet for some time. Whole wheat may then be added experimentally, first un-yeasted, and later as home-baked yeast breads. Eggs are also added in poached form. Often several periods of fasting and raw diets are needed to eliminate the condition. If allergy is still suspected, food allergy tests should be performed. Attention must be directed at all times to establishing and maintaining proper bowel function.

Physiotherapy

- Outdoor exercise
- Swimming (particularly ocean bathing)
- "Salt glow" (one to two times per week; see Appendix I)
- Skin brush daily (see Appendix I)
- Colonics
- Alternate hot and cold showers
- Alternate hot and cold compresses locally to site

Therapeutic Agents

VITAMINS AND MINERALS

Vitamin A: 10,000 to 25,000 IU one to three times per day or more in some cases. *Use any dose of vitamin A over 50,000 IU per day with medical supervision only.* *

Vitamin B complex (nonyeast): 25 to 50 mg one to two times per day.*

*Asterisks indicate the most frequently used therapeutic agents.

Vitamin C: 500 to 1000 mg three to six times per day. Use sodium ascorbate form in gastritis.*

Zinc: 25 to 50 mg one to two times per day.*

OTHERS

Garlic: 2 capsules three times per day; not in gastritis.*

Kelp

Onion syrup (see Appendix I): 1 tsp three to six times per day.*

Thymus tablets: 1 to 2 tablets three to six times per day.*

BOTANICALS

Comfrey (*Symphytum officinale*)

Goldenseal (*Hydrastis canadensis*)

Slippery elm (*Ulmus fulva*)

(See also individual topics.)

CELIAC DISEASE (Nontropical Sprue, Gluten Enteropathy)

Definition

A chronic malabsorption syndrome due to gluten intolerance.

Symptoms

Failure to thrive; weight loss; loss of appetite; vomiting in some cases; diarrhea; stools bulky, pale, frothy, foul-smelling, floating; dermatitis; abdominal distension and pain; weakness; anemia; possibly fatal in infants.

Etiologic Considerations

- Gluten intolerance
- Vitamin B_6 deficiency
- Stress
- Other food allergy
- Digestive enzyme deficiency
- Improper weaning

*Asterisks indicate the most frequently used therapeutic agents.

Discussion

Celiac disease may manifest itself very dramatically, causing severe malnutrition and wasting, or else it may act insidiously to downgrade general health and vitality over a number of years. Classic forms of the disorder begin early in life, just as soon as cereal grains containing gluten protein are introduced. In this case the infant fails to thrive, muscular structures begin to waste, especially in the gluteal region, and the abdomen protrudes markedly due to intestinal fermentation. Fat absorption is reduced and fat-soluble vitamin deficiency is common. Other necessary nutrients pass out with the frequent stools.

Adult-onset celiac disease is often diagnosed and may in reality date from childhood, but with only mild or unnoticed symptoms that gradually progressed for multiple reasons.

Gluten is a protein found in wheat, oats, rye, barley, and other grains related to wheat. If these are consumed in these cases the gluten causes severe intestinal irritation and a flattening of the jejunal mucosa, obliterating the small fingerlike villi necessary for proper absorption in the small intestine.

The two main causes of celiac disease are strict gluten intolerance, which may be caused by enzyme deficiency, or other metabolic fault, and improper weaning. Although I know of no solid evidence implicating celiac disease with the early weaning of infants to cereal grains, I suspect this as the single most important factor in most patients. I acknowledge that some infants may have a true gluten intolerance for biochemical reasons, but this is the minority. The introduction of cereal grains before the body's enzymes can digest them can only set the stage for celiac disease by causing gastric irritation, antibody reaction, and intestinal thinning. This seems obvious, since the average infant is approximately 4 months old at the onset of the disorder, a full 2 months before the body has even developed the digestive ability to handle concentrated carbohydrates. Add to this the frequency with which these foods are usually given in the diet and we see how simple irritation can later lead to permanent reaction. The foods mostly commonly found allergic are those given the earliest and most frequently.

Celiac disease may also be complicated by other food allergies such as milk sugar intolerance or yeast. Breastfeeding is a protective factor and may help prevent future food sensitivities.

Associated with celiac disease are several quite serious health problems. Researchers have found a significant percentage of schizophrenics and victims of multiple sclerosis who suffer from a gluten reaction. This may be caused by the malabsorption of vitamins (B_3 and B_6 deficiency are closely associated with schizophrenia) or fat-soluble substances (essential fatty acids found in seeds or nuts are deficient in multiple sclerosis patients).

Treatment

Diet

Therapy is based on instituting a totally gluten-free diet. This can be quite a change for most households and is not easy. Most patients exclude gluten grains permanently, while others are later able to add them in moderation.

It is essential in the early stages of therapy to exclude all grains that contain gluten. This effectively excludes everything except brown rice, millet, and corn. The greatest difficulty of this regimen is in excluding the convenience of sandwiches. These may be substituted for by several soft corn tortillas. Brown rice cakes make a convenient carrier for nut butters and other spreads. Puffed rice, corn, or millet cereals are also available at most health food stores. Another difficulty is in making sure that wheat or wheat flour has not been added to any prepackaged products consumed at home or in a restaurant. Gluten-containing grains are found in a wide variety of restaurant and commercially prepared foods, such as ice cream, candies, salad dressings, luncheon meats, soups, sauces, and even condiments. Great care must be taken to pay attention to all ingredients, especially when eating at restaurants. Read labels religiously. Even an incredibly small amount of gluten in the early stages of the disease can initiate a reaction lasting up to 5 days, so you can see how important it is to be sure gluten is totally excluded.

Some celiacs obtain gluten-free flour for baking. I do not advise this since these products are refined and vitamin-deficient. It is better to exclude these grains once and for all and be done with it. The rest of the diet must be composed only of highly nutritious vegetables, fruits, proteins, and nongluten grains.

Physiotherapy

- Castor oil packs (see Appendix I)
  Since the bowel condition resembles that found in psoriasis (and to which it may often be associated) we advise a similar regimen of abdominal packs (see Psoriasis).

- Spinal manipulation: one to two times per week; midthoracic to lumbar.

- Meditation and relaxation exercises

Therapeutic Agents

VITAMINS AND MINERALS

Vitamin A (micellized): 10,000 to 25,000 IU two to three times per day or more. *Use any dose of vitamin A over 50,000 IU per day with medical supervision only.* *

Vitamin C (buffered): 500 to 1000 mg three to ten times per day, depending on how well it is tolerated.

Vitamin D: Fat-soluble vitamin; malabsorption requires extra D. 400 to 800 IU per day.

Vitamin E: 100 to 400 IU two times per day.*

Vitamin B complex (liquid): 25 to 50 mg two times per day. Intramuscular injection of B_{12}, folic acid, and B complex, one to two times per week.*

Vitamin B_6

Calcium: 800 to 1000 mg per day.

Magnesium: 400 to 500 mg per day.

Zinc: 15 mg two times per day.

OTHERS

Chlorophyll

EFA (essential fatty acids): 2 to 4 capsules three times per day.*

Lecithin

Pancreatic enzymes*

BOTANICALS

Comfrey (*Symphytum officinale*): Use as infusion.*

Slippery elm (*Ulmus fulva*): Soothes inflamed mucosa. Take ¼ to ½ tsp in warm water four times per day.*

Therapeutic Suggestions

The intestine of a patient with celiac disease is extremely thinned and the stomach is irritable. In early stages nutritional supplements may be very poorly tolerated. Try to begin the therapy with a fast of 3 to 5 days, to give the digestive system a chance to rest. Use, as much as possible, intramuscular vitamin injections for the first few weeks and then wean to liquid forms and emulsified forms whenever available.

Due to the prolonged malabsorption, nutritional deficiency is broad-based. Emphasis should be placed on vitamins A, D, E (fat-soluble), essential fatty

*Asterisks indicate the most frequently used therapeutic agents.

acids, B complex, vitamin C, calcium, magnesium, iron, and zinc, but any other supplement may have become deficient in a prolonged case.

CERVICAL DYSPLASIA

Definition and Symptoms

Abnormal cell development of the cervix. As a rule no obvious symptoms exist. Diagnosis is by Pap smear.

Discussion and Treatment

About 30 percent to 50 percent of women with cervical dysplasia later progress to cervical cancer. If there is an abnormality on a Pap smear, a biopsy may be needed to confirm the Pap test and help in clarifying the precise stage. Abnormal Pap smears alert the patient and physician to a problem, and help prevent precancerous lesions from progressing into cancer by allowing the doctor adequate time to perform conization, cautery, or cryosurgery, thus preventing a further and more serious problem from developing.

I find that abnormal Pap smears that do not as yet indicate precancerous or cancerous lesions can usually be reversed with natural therapy. This includes dietary changes to exclude all negative health factors such as coffee, tea, sugar, salt, alcohol, excess animal-based protein, and any unrefined, fried or overcooked foods. The patient is placed on a 6-month's regimen of raw and cooked vegetables, seeds, nuts, beans, whole grains, and low-fat yoghurt (if no dairy allergy exists). Fish is also allowed several times weekly. No other animal-based protein is allowed. Carrot juice, or other fresh vegetable juice combination, should be taken twice daily. Supplement regimens are instituted according to case history and physical indications, but must always include the following:

Folic acid: 5 to 10 mg per day

Vitamin B_{12}: 1 mg intramuscularly one to two times per week

Vitamin A: 25,000 to 100,000 IU per day. *Use any dose of vitamin A over 50,000 IU per day with medical supervision only.*

Vitamin C: To bowel tolerance

Alternate hot and cold sitz baths are very useful if done two to three times daily, to increase local circulation and nutrition. In some cases the vaginal depletion pack is also used (see Appendix I). Periodic follow-up Pap smears are used as a measure of the treatment's success.

CHANGE OF LIFE (see Menopause)

CHICKEN POX (see Childhood Diseases)

CHILDHOOD DISEASES: Chicken Pox (Varicella), Measles (Rubeola), Mumps (Parotitis), Whooping Cough (Pertussis)

Definition and Symptoms

Chicken Pox: A common acute childhood disease caused by a virus. It is characterized by crops of thin-walled vesicles which erupt and crust. Each lesion lasts 2 to 4 days, leaving a pink scar which later disappears. Pock marks may remain. The disease is usually mild.

Measles (Rubeola): An acute viral infection common in children from 6 months to 5 years. It begins with coldlike symptoms and also includes cough, conjunctivitis, and photophobia (avoidance of light). The fever falls after 1 or 2 days, then rises suddenly by day 5 or 6. Associated with this rise is a blotchy rash first appearing on the forehead and behind the ears and rapidly spreading to the trunk. This gradually fades in 3 to 4 days and the skin is then lost. During the first signs of the rash symptoms are at a peak, with a strong fever and bronchitis. Complications include otitis media, loss of hearing, bronchopneumonia, and rarely encephalomyelitis, with later convulsions and rarely death.

Mumps: An acute viral infection characterized by mild fever, malaise and sore throat, with swollen parotid glands, swelling either unilaterally or bilaterally. It may last 2 or 3 days, or weeks. Fever usually lasts only a few days. Complications are rare before puberty, and involve swelling of ovaries or testicles, which may affect reproductive ability.

Whooping Cough: An acute bacterial disease characterized by a severe paroxysmal cough. The organism grows on the trachea and bronchi, producing an endotoxin which sensitizes nerve endings in the respiratory tract, and may have toxic effects on the central nervous system. Symptoms begin with a mild fever, coldlike symptoms, and a cough which gradually becomes more severe, with a prolonged series of expirations, followed by a sudden "whooping" inspiration. This may also induce vomiting. Paroxysms are usually worse at night. The disease lasts 2 to 4+ weeks. Complications include convulsions, hemorrhage from the nose or into conjunctiva or into brain, and bronchopneumonia. Rarely, death occurs.

Etiologic Considerations

- Normal childhood diseases
- Improper diet

- Suppressive treatment of other conditions
- Toxicity
- Complications due to improper treatment

Discussion

These common childhood diseases are contracted by nearly all children, but to varying degrees. Some children show little or no symptoms and the result is that the condition is passed off as a mild cold or cough. Other children, however, suffer and are permanently damaged by complications. It is this individual difference in resistance and vitality that is the single most important factor in our understanding acute disease. Even Louis Pasteur, the father of the germ theory of disease, began to better understand the true nature of disease when he stressed "The *germ* is nothing; it is the *soil* that matters." Germs are not the most important factor in causing disease; the environment must be suitable for them to flourish.

The fact is that germs and viruses are always in our midst. The body normally is capable of maintaining a proper balance of these invaders, both the friendly and the not-so-friendly. The body's self-defense mechanisms attack and remove any dangerous foreign invaders before they may take hold. Its secretions form protective boundaries, its glands act as filters, and the cell walls act as effective barriers. The entire cell, tissue, organ, and body "vitality" is our constant protector. If the "vitality" is maintained all is well, peace prevails, and health reigns. If, however, we let our defenses starve through poor nutrition and deficiency, poor circulation or lack of oxygen, trouble begins. If we further clog our tissues with too many toxins or change the pH (acid/alkaline balance) of the secretions, the "soil" of our body changes, becoming a favorable environment for infection.

There is no single factor that predisposes our children to disease, but rather a multitude of insults on their bodies. Diet certainly takes the most blame. Excess milk and carbohydrates are the two most obvious offenders. Most people are now aware that white bread, refined cereals, and sugar are not an optimum diet, but even excess *unrefined* carbohydrates can alter the body's secretions.

Most children do not suffer from a single vitamin deficiency as much as from a "green vegetable" deficiency. We wean our children *too soon* and *too much* to starches and complex proteins without understanding that the cleansing and balancing effect of vegetables is absolutely essential for good health. Too often I see sick children whose mothers say "He just won't eat vegetables." To this I must ask "And whose fault is that?" Dietary habits are just that—*habits*. You can quite easily get a baby to eat vegetables if that is what he is weaned to. It is easy to give the child a wheat cracker or a bottle of milk to keep him quiet, but certainly not the best choice, healthwise.

A well-fed child will usually be strong enough to deal with infection in a successful way. Well-nourished children either do not catch common childhood diseases, contract only mild cases, or develop strong, healthy reactions that are short in duration, leaving the child feeling none the worse for the experience. It is much more healthy, for example, in measles, to develop a high fever, short in duration, with sweats and good rash formation, than to have a lower fever, little perspiration, and a slowly developed rash. In the first instance, the child is more likely to be over and done with his or her complaint and out playing, while the latter is still being treated for otitis media or bronchopneumonia.

Treatment

The treatment of many of the common childhood diseases is fairly basic. The first priority is a liquid diet in the acute stages (with the later introduction of fruits and vegetables). The fever should not be suppressed, but moderated according to the needs of the patient, with gentle hydrotherapy. The establishment of perspiration with the fever is essential. Bowels must be kept open and herbal laxatives or cnemas may be needed. Various herbal medications are useful at different stages in most of the diseases. Below are a few suggestions useful in each of the complaints:

Chicken Pox

The only real concern with chicken pox is pock scarring. This may be minimized by several simple baths and applications. And, of course, don't scratch.

HYDROTHERAPY
• Tepid baths with
    Starch
    Baking soda
    Apple cider vinegar, *or*
    Oatmeal

• Applications
    Burdock, goldenseal, and yellow dock tea—dab areas frequently.
    Calamine lotion: ⅓ part vinegar, ⅔ part water—dab area then powder.
    Hot bath, to bring out latent rash.

BOTANICALS
    Dwarf nettle (*Urtica urens*): To bring out latent rash.

    Nettle (*Urtica dioica*)

Diet

Fruit juice, vegetable juice

Clear vegetable soups

Vitamin C—take to bowel tolerance.

Propolis

Thymus tablets*: 2 to 4 every 1 to 2 hours.

Even breastfeeding is contraindicated as the child is thirsty, not hungry.

Measles

This disease needs to be treated a little more vigorously. Complications may occur because of nutritional deficiency, suppressive treatments, or overfeeding during the disease.

Hydrotherapy

* Tepid baths and applications for itch, as with chicken pox
* Hot baths to bring out latent rash
* Hot foot baths
* Hot ginger chest poultice
* Steam baths (not packs) to sweat

Botanicals

Burdock (*Arctium lappa*), plus coneflower (*Echinacea angustifolia*) and goldenseal (*Hydrastis canadensis*)

Dwarf nettle (*Urtica urens*): For slow, poorly developed rash.

Garlic (*Allium sativum*)

Garlic (*Allium sativum*) foot compresses (see Whooping Cough)

Lobelia (*Lobelia inflata*)

Onion syrup (*Allium cepa*) (see Appendix I)

Pleurisy root (*Asclepias tuberosa*) and ginger (*Zingiber officinale*) tea.

Wild clover (*Trifolium pratense*) plus sundew (*Drosera rotundifolia*) for cough.*

Yarrow (*Achillea millefolium*) and pleurisy root (*Asclepias tuberosa*) tea, to sweat.*

*Asterisks indicate the most frequently used therapeutic agents.

Chamomile tea (*Anthemis nobilis*): To settle the system, if hyperactive or irritated.

Sundew (*Drosera rotundifolia*): Useful in cough of measles or whooping cough. Dose of tincture 15 to 20 drops three to four times per day.*

Goldenseal (*Hydrastis*) tea and boric acid for painful eyes. Make a strong tea of *Hydrastis* as stock mixture. Take 1 tsp of tea, add to ½ cup of water. To this add 2 to 3 drops of boric acid. Flush eyes every 2 to 4 hours.

DIET

Take fruit juice, lemon juice, citrus juices, vegetable juice, and vitamins A and C to bowel tolerance (vitamin C intravenously in severe cases). *Use any dose of vitamin A over 50,000 IU per day with medical supervision only.**

Mumps

This disease looks much more severe than it really is. The only complications occur during puberty, when swelling of the ovaries or testes can occur, which may cause sterility. The general principles of treatment are those of any other fever, with plenty of fluids and bed rest during the acute phase.

FOMENTATION

Pokeroot (*Phytolacca*) 1 part (highly toxic; see p. 62)

Lobelia (*Lobelia inflata*) 1 part

Mullein (*Verbascum thapsus*) 3 parts

BOTANICALS

Pokeroot (*Phytolacca decandra*) (highly toxic; see p. 62) for hard, painful glandular enlargements.

Pulsatilla (*Anemone pulsatilla*) for ovaritis or orchitis.

Whooping Cough

Of the common childhood diseases, whooping cough deserves the most attention. The cough of even a mild case of whooping cough is extremely disturbing, especially for the parents. Fortunately, with proper naturopathic treatment in an inpatient facility, the disorder may be brought under control and leave the child no worse for wear. Treatments must be vigorous and unrelenting to get best results.

*Asterisks indicate the most frequently used therapeutic agents.

DIET

A light diet is essential. Overfeeding during the whooping cough prolongs the disease and causes complications. In the breastfed overfeeding is also a problem. The child is thirsty, not hungry. Once the disorder has been diagnosed or is suspected, a full fruit juice fast should be started. Citrus juices are especially useful. This may be followed with a diet of fruit juice, vegetable juices (carrot), and clear broth vegetable soup. Later, fruit may be added. Vitamin A and C in large doses should be administered.

APPLICATIONS

Hot fomentations of strong ginger and garlic tea, followed by Camphoderm (Cayce product) applications. Repeat every 2 hours.

Garlic foot poultice (see Appendix I): Mash garlic and apply ¼ in. thick between gauze. Oil soles of feet with olive oil to prevent blistering and apply poultice; then secure with bandage and cover with a sock. Apply all night and one to two times per day if possible for 1 to 2 hours each time. This is a *very* useful application.

SPINAL MANIPULATION AND PHYSIOTHERAPY

• Adjust cervical upper and midthoracic region daily, followed by a deep neuromuscular massage with olive oil, olbas, and myrrh over entire area. (Or rub 20% grain alcohol across shoulders, neck, and diaphragm area.)

INHALATIONS

Use olbas oil steam inhalations with a little extra eucalyptus and pine needle oil.

Therapeutic Agents

VITAMINS AND MINERALS

Vitamin A: 10,000 IU two to six times per day. *Use any dose of vitamin A over 50,000 IU per day with medical supervision only.**

Vitamin C: 250 to 1000 mg up to every hour, or to bowel tolerance. Vitamin C intravenously in severe cases.*

Thymus: 2 tablets four to six times per day.*

BOTANICALS

Black currant leaves (*Ribes nigrum*): Strong tea of leaves; take 1 cup three to four times per day.*

*Asterisks indicate the most frequently used therapeutic agents.

Ephedra: Bronchodilator.

Glycothymoline: 5 to 15 drops daily.

Ipecac: 5 to 10 drops in water three times per day.

Lobelia (*Lobelia inflata*): Antispasmodic, expectorant. Used for whooping cough with difficult expectoration. *

Garlic syrup

Onion syrup (raw)
Place a sliced onion in a bowl with 1 tbs honey. Cover the bowl overnight. In the morning mash and strain. Take 1 tsp every 1 to 2 hours.

Onion syrup (cooked)
Mix 1 lb diced onions with 2 oz honey and 2 pints water. Simmer 1 to 3 hours. Dose is 2 tbs every 1 to 2 hours.

Propolis: Chew frequently; take 2 capsules three times per day.

Senna laxative (Castoria) as needed.

Sundew (*Drosera rotundifolia*): Dose 15 to 20 drops three to four times per day, for spasmodic cough. *

Syrup of squill (*Urginea scilla*): 3 to 5 drops three to four times per day. *

Wild cherry (*Prunus virginiana*)

Also use expectorant, sedative, and antispasmodic herbs as found under Bronchitis. *

COLDS, COUGHS, AND SORE THROATS

Definition and Symptoms

Common knowledge.

Etiologic Considerations

• Diet
Excess acid-forming, mucus-forming foods
Excess carbohydrates
Excess dairy products
Excess sweets
Overeating

*Asterisks indicate the most frequently used therapeutic agents.

Fried foods
Irritants (spices, coffee, tea, alcohol, cigarettes, etc.)
• Toxicity
Improper diet
Stress, lack of sleep
Poor eliminations
• Spinal
Reduced nerve, blood, and lymph supply
• Allergy
See Allergy
• Suppressive treatments for previous acute disorders
• Strep throat (requires antibiotic therapy)

Discussion

The common cold is probably the most poorly understood health complaint. Most of us look upon a recurrent cold as an irritating nuisance, caused by some "virus" going around, and direct all our efforts to eliminate by any means possible and in as short a time as possible, the various uncomfortable symptoms. At the local drugstore we find a bewildering arsenal of weapons to wipe out this enemy, the common cold—antipyretics, antihistamines, decongestants, sedatives, and many more. This is the treatment given us in childhood, recommended daily on TV, and what our doctors recommend. How strange it must sound to hear that this is the worst possible of all courses to follow!

The common cold is *not* an infection that leaps out and attacks an innocent, unsuspecting passerby. It is *not* a disease whose symptoms are best suppressed or shut off like one would a leaky faucet. A cold is not even a disease. It is rather the *cure* of disease.

The most important thing to understand about a cold is that the multitude of symptoms usually present are actions, not reactions, by the body in an attempt to establish internal equilibrium. The body's defense mechanisms are working fast and furiously to reestablish balance. If this can be seen to be true, then to suppress these actions by the body is not a reasonable course of action.

The original causes of the imbalance that the body is attempting to correct may be multiple. *Improper diet* is the single most influential factor. An excess of dairy products and carbohydrates (especially refined carbohydrates) will cause an increase in the amount and quality of mucus formed by the body. Body fluids become more viscous and acidic. Other factors causing acidity are coffee, tea, spices, salt, alcohol, cigarettes, lack of exercise, and stress.

Toxicity is a second major factor. This is a fairly loose term, which implies that something detrimental has accumulated within the body. This may be due to simple excess consumption of normal food elements beyond the body's capacity to deal with effectively. Excess animal fats will certainly cause the liver to work overtime on their metabolism. Other substances are less benign. Blatantly toxic pesticides, food colorings, hormones, heavy metals, and preservatives are found routinely in the average diet. These must be detoxified by the liver or stored in the tissues. The same is true of toxins caused by excess alcohol or drug use. Couple all the above factors with poor eliminations due to constipation and lack of demanding exercise, cigarette smoking, vitamin deficiency, and environmental air and water pollution, and it is easy to see how the body's vitality and ability to maintain inner balance become vitiated.

It is this multitude of factors that the body is trying desperately to counterbalance. Once toxic levels reach an unacceptable level, the body acts to clear the crippling debris. It opens all channels of eliminations and pours forth poisons from all available avenues. The nose begins to run and the excess mucus stimulates both sneezing and coughing to help expel the blockage. Sometimes vomiting and diarrhea are also present to purge the stomach and intestine. Fever increases the general speed of metabolism and circulation, and promotes perspiration to rid the body of toxins and to help burn up and destroy any secondary bacteria or virus that may have taken hold in the more favorable environment created by downgraded health.

If the body is acting out of an innate intelligence (as it must be since neither you nor I direct our body's heartbeat or other life-sustaining activities), then it is reasonable that we encourage, not discourage, its healing actions. Instead of suppressing our cold by the use of drugs, we must stimulate and aid the body's actions.

In a healthy individual a cold needs little or no encouragement. Since general vitality is high to begin with, all one needs to do is, *almost* as the TV advertisement says, "Rest, drink plenty of fluids, and *don't* take aspirin." The body will do the rest. It is simply doing a "spring cleaning" of all the toxic accumulations stockpiled routinely and almost unavoidably in our modern world. Certainly, everyone must breathe and even our very air, in most cases, has become somewhat toxic. In an otherwise healthy individual a cold will be moderately intense, short-lived, and if treated properly, will leave the individual feeling in good health after it is over.

The cold of a healthy individual constrasts sharply with the cold of a sickly person. Rather than the one or two quickly resolving eliminations that are common and acceptable per year, these sickly persons will suffer for weeks with the acute stage and may keep a cough for up to 2 or 3 months. The end result of such an episode is a feeling of weakness and fatigue, which may become chronic. This occurs for two reasons. The first is that the cold usually is treated with drugs, or at least not treated properly (i.e., with fasting, fluids, rest, and gentle herbs, if needed). The second is that due to the severity of the internal congestion and toxicity usually due to chronic self-poisoning and suppression of previous attempts by the body to heal itself, the body is acting out of desperation, rather than desire.

An analogy can be found comparing the normally cleansing effort undertaken each spring with the effort needed after a flood or hurricane. In the latter instance great resources are needed, and in the case of the sickly person these may simply be unavailable. This is the reason these colds are much more sluggish and prolonged, and also the reason these people often need external assistance to aid the body in its attempts at equilibrium. These aids should not be drugs, which are no real aid at all, but simple, gentle measures such as fasting, hydrotherapy, spinal manipulation, and herbs.

The real danger of a cold if handled improperly is not only its prolonged nature, but the possibility of complications such as pneumonia. If colds are actively suppressed the body eventually loses its ability to release internal toxins safely. The end result is the development of chronic disease many years later such as bronchitis, emphysema, and other serious diseases possibly unrelated directly to the respiratory tract.

Often I hear the proud announcement "I *never* get colds" from individuals who show absolute disregard for their health by improper diet, excessive drinking and smoking, and excesses of all kinds. They are, in fact, *too* sick to have a cold! This is precisely the individual who is prone to chronic disease, heart attack, cancer, and the rest of the so-called degenerative diseases. A cold is your friend and ally. Don't try to fight it off.

A final note on sore throats. Group A beta-hemolytic streptococci can have serious complications that can damage the heart. Always have a throat swab done on any serious sore throat, especially if it is accompanied by infected white patches on the throat cavity. Antibiotics should be used for any diagnosed strep throat condition.

Treatment

The proper treatment of colds is to encourage eliminations through all channels so that eliminations through only one channel do not become excessive.

Diet

Liquid fasting is the best diet during a cold. The following fluids have been found most useful:

Citrus (grapefruit)

Hot water, lemon, and honey

Potassium broth

Hot water, apple cider vinegar, and honey

Medicinal herbal teas

In some cases prolonged juice fasting will actually *lengthen* the cold process too long. An overly prolonged elimination is not always in the best interest of the body. In these cases the fruit juice diet may be discontinued after 3 to 7 days and the patient placed on *cooked* vegetables. This will usually moderate the elimination and help establish normal equilibrium.

Another method useful in cases of severe mucus congestion with sinus congestion or excess chest involvement is the 3-day mucus-cleansing diet (see Appendix I). This involves eating oranges or grapefruit for breakfast, a large plate of boiled or steamed onions for lunch and supper, and an orange as dessert. Medicinal herbal teas are taken between meals and either carrot or citrus juices whenever thirsty.

Physiotherapy

- Hot Epsom salts baths plus sweating teas: Take 1 to 2 lb Epsom salts and dissolve in a hot tub. While soaking, consume 2 to 3 cups of hot pleurisy root tea. Immediately after the bath get into bed and cover with plenty of blankets. The object is to sweat profusely.

- Trunk packs: Each evening apply a full cold trunk pack (see Hydrotherapy). The object is to stimulate skin elimination and induce perspiration. Leave this on at least 3 hours or all night.

- Hot mustard foot bath: To increase eliminations and reduce congestion in head and sinuses.

- Salt water nasal douche: To open sinuses.

- Hot ginger chest compress: Followed by application of Camphoderm or olbas.

- Inhalations: Eucalyptus, pine needle, cloves, and thyme. To prepare:

In 1 quart of boiled water place eucalyptus leaves or oil, pine needles or oil, cloves, and thyme. Make an inhalation tent by draping a large towel over the uncovered pot and your head. Place infant on your lap and hold tightly around abdomen (with arms well away from child's teeth!). An infant will naturally protest vigorously and will sputter and cry deeply. This is good as it gets the fumes well into the lungs. Another approach is to make a tent by using two chairs and one or two very large beach towels or a light blanket. This gives more room and is often more acceptable to young children. Repeat application every 2 hours.

- Olbas inhalant
- Gargles (sore throat)
    Hot water and salt
    Hot water, lemon juice, and honey

Hydrastis, myrrh, and water
Sage tea
Sage, cayenne, and honey
Bayberry bark decoction

- Compresses
  Cool compresses to reduce fever as needed (see Fever).
  Apple cider vinegar compresses or rubs (fever control).
  Ice-cold throat compress: Apply and leave on 1 to 3 hours or all night, for sore throat.
  Alternate hot and ice-cold throat compress.
  Hot lobelia and hops throat compress for throat pain.
- Spinal manipulation
- Sweat baths
- Saunas in pine and eucalyptus steam.

Therapeutic Agents

VITAMINS AND MINERALS

Vitamin A: High doses are needed in upper respiratory conditions.* This should be in the form of emulsified vitamin A. Adult doses may be 25,000 IU four to six times per day for 1 to 2 weeks. (This is a toxic dose if taken for several months, but completely safe for short periods.) *Use any dose of vitamin A over 50,000 IU per day with medical supervision only.* Children's dose: Ages 3 months to 1 year—4000 IU two to four times per day for 1 to 2 weeks; ages 1 year to 6 years—10,000 IU two to four times per day. Again, this is a toxic level if prolonged, but entirely safe and sometimes required in acute respiratory complaints for 1-to-2-week periods. Vitamin A is essential for the health of the mucous membranes and increases cilia action to expel mucus.

Vitamin C:
     Adult—1000 to 2000 mg four to eight times per day.
     Child—300 mg four to eight times per day.
     Infant—100 to 250 mg four to eight times per day.*

Pantothenic acid (antihistamine)

OTHERS

Chlorophyll
Garlic: 2 capsules with meals.*

---

*Asterisks indicate the most frequently used therapeutic agents.

Propolis: 2 capsules with meals, or for sore throat chew small amount of raw propolis hourly.*

Raw adrenal tablets

Raw thymus tablets: 2 every hour. Stimulates immunological system.*

BOTANICALS

Boneset (*Eupatorium perfoliatum*): For achy feelings.*

Coltsfoot (*Tussilago farfara*): For cough.

Elder blossom (*Sambucus nigra*): For colds.

Eucalyptus (*Eucalyptus globulus*): For congestion. Use as inhalant.*

Ginger root (*Zingiber officinale*): Useful as tea or hot chest compress (use infusion).*

Goldenseal (*Hydrastis canadensis*): Antimicrobial; useful in staph, strep (with antibiotics), and thrush; use with myrrh (*Commiphora myrrha*) for sore throat. Use tinctures as throat swab; dilute for gargle.*

Cum plant (*Grindelia squarrosa*): For cough.

Licorice (*Glycyrrhiza glabra*): For cough; demulcent, expectorant.

Marigold (*Calendula officinalis*): Use tincture for throat swab.*

Ma-huang (*Ephedra*): For cough (bronchodilator).

Mullein (*Verbascum thapsus*): For cough.

Mustard (*Brassica* spp.)

Peppermint (*Mentha piperita*): Hot tea for sweating.

Pleurisy root (*Asclepias tuberosa*): For sweating.*

Squill (*Urginea scilla*): For cough.

Sundew (*Drosera rotundifolia*): For cough.

Wild cherry bark (*Prunus serotina*): For cough; a sedative expectorant.*

Wild clover (*Trifolium pratense*): For cough.

White pine (*Pinus strobus*): Expectorant.

Yarrow (*Achillea millefolium*)

USEFUL PRESCRIPTIONS

Onion syrup (see Appendix I): Dose: 1 tsp per hour.

Garlic syrup

*Asterisks indicate the most frequently used therapeutic agents.

Mother Earth cough syrup (Cayce product):
  Wild cherry bark
  Horehound
  Rhubarb
  Wild ginger
  Honey

Mustard chest plaster
  1 part mustard, 4 parts flour, white of egg or 1 tsp olive oil. Add water
  to form thin paste. Place between cloth and apply to oil-covered chest.

COLD SORES (Herpes Simplex of the Face and Mouth)

Definition and Symptoms

An infectious viral disease caused by herpes simplex *(Herpesvirus hominis)*
and characterized by thin-walled vesicles which have a tendency to recur in the
same area, usually at the junction of skin and mucous membranes such as the
border of the mouth. They may also affect the gums, mouth, or conjunctiva.

Etiologic Considerations

• Stress
• Immune deficiency
• Diet
• Local irritation

Discussion

Some people have regular outbreaks of cold sores, while others seem relatively
immune, even when exposed. Those susceptible often find stress is a major factor
in instigating an outbreak. Some women notice a relationship between their
menstrual cycle and outbreaks. Local irritants, such as excess ultraviolet exposure
or acidic foods, can instigate an outbreak. Dietary factors often are related. It is
a common finding that a cold sore outbreak will follow episodes of drinking or
improper diet. The common denominator seems to be a condition of immune
deficiency related to stress or dietary indiscretions, with local irritation as an
instigating factor.

Treatment

Physiotherapy

• Thymus ointment: Apply six times daily.

• Ice application: Apply ice at first sign of tingling for 15 to 20 minutes; repeat frequently throughout the day. Apply vitamin E between applications.

• Zinc: .025% (topical).

• Myrrh tincture (topical).

• *Hydrastis* (goldenseal) tincture (topical). Alternate with aloe vera.

Vitamins and Minerals

Vitamin A: 50,000 to 100,000 IU per day in acute stages. *Use any dose of vitamin A over 50,000 IU per day with medical supervision only.*

Vitamin B Complex: 50-mg dose one to three times per day.

Niacinamide: 500 to 1000 mg per day.

Pantothenic acid: 250 to 500 mg per day.

Vitamin B_{12}: 1 mg intramuscularly per day in acute stages.

Bioflavonoids: 1000 mg per day.

Zinc: 25 to 50 mg one to three times per day.

Other

Lysine: 2 to 4 g per day.

Superdophilus or megadophilus: 1 tsp four to six times per day.

COLIC, ADULT OR INFANT (see Flatulence)

COLITIS: Spastic Colitis, Ulcerative Colitis, Irritable Colon, Mucous Colitis

Definition

Ulcerative Colitis: A chronic, inflammatory disease of the colon characterized by ulcer formation, with passage of blood and mucus.

Spastic Colitis, Irritable Colon, Mucous Colitis: A chronic motor disorder of the colon, characterized by pain, constipation, diarrhea, or alternating episodes of each.

Symptoms

Ulcerative Colitis: Attacks of bloody diarrhea, cramps, blood in stool, and mucus. May be symptom-free between episodes.

Spastic Colitis: Abdominal pain, abdominal distension, cramps, gas, constipation, diarrhea, mucus, but no blood in stool.

Etiologic Considerations

* Primary intestinal flu episode common
* Chronic constipation (irritating residue adhering to walls of intestine)
* Food allergy from additives, lactose, or gluten intolerance
* Refined diet (fiber deficiency)
* Fried foods
* Sugar, coffee, spices, irritants, salt
* Aluminum cookware
* Hurried meals
* Emotional—stress, overwork, anxiety, irregular habits, lack of sleep, hurried lifestyle, frustration
* Abuse of laxatives
* Previous antibiotics
* Intestinal parasites

Discussion

The occurrence of colitis almost exclusively in civilized nations places it in the class of so-called "civilized diseases." This stems from its main causes, which are dietary and lifestyle. A refined diet, with its fiber-deficient foods, causes habitual constipation which eventually leaves toxic residues adhering to the intestinal lining. These toxic substances lead to irritation, inflammation, and eventually ulceration of the delicate membranes. This in turn causes a lymphatic disturbance due to local irritation and the absorption of these toxic forces into the lymphatic channels. The chronic use of laxatives to correct poor eliminations further irritates these membranes and by the action of the law of dual effect, causes reciprocal bowel statis after their initial stimulating action is completed.

The emotions also have a direct effect on the digestive system. Both motor and secretory functions of the gastrointestinal tract are influenced by the autonomic nervous system. It is stimulated by the parasympathetic and inhibited by the sympathetic nervous system. Any strong emotion, stress, or anxiety will be interpreted by the body more or less as an emergency situation, with the result that the sympathetic nervous system takes control. Among its actions is diverting energy away from digestive functions and instituting defense actions. The digestive result of these actions is a slowing or stopping of all digestive activities, including peristaltic action. This causes constipation.

Occasionally, if the stress or sympathetic action is particularly strong, the result may be quite the opposite, with a powerful and expulsive peristaltic action causing sudden diarrhea. Thus we see the commonly occurring symptoms of alternate constipation and diarrhea, so frequently seen in colitis.

Many cases of colitis follow an acute bout of intestinal flu. This is more common in ulcerative colitis. This initial irritation may then be very difficult to heal if the body is already downgraded in health and vitality by poor diet and any of the other possible causative factors. Food allergy, especially to milk or wheat, is commonly the main cause of the intestinal irritation and when the offending substance is removed from the diet healing commences immediately.

Treatment

Diet

Roughage is the key consideration in the dietary regimen. Roughage does not cause colitis, as many seem to believe who place patients on permanent low-fiber diets in an attempt to cure the condition. A high-fiber diet is the best prevention and cure. However, it is true that in the initial stages a bland, low-fiber diet is often necessary due to bowel irritation and devitalization. Later, a high-fiber diet is instituted to complete the healing process and prevent recurrence.

In most cases an initial period of liquid fasting is the treatment of choice. The length of the regimen depends on the ability of the patient to abstain from solid food and the general health picture, vitality, weight, etc.

The following liquids are especially useful for the fasting period of from 3 to 14 days:

Carrot juice
Apple juice
Slippery elm tea (warm, not hot)
Comfrey tea (warm, not hot)

An enema is to be taken nightly on days 1, 2, 3, and every other night thereafter during the liquid fast (or less, at the discretion of the physician). This fast should be broken slowly, adding ripe mashed banana with slippery elm powder, unsweetened apple sauce or baked apple (no skin).

An alternate initial plan beneficial in some cases is to begin with a mono diet of raw grated apples plus apple pectin and slippery elm powder three to four times a day, with apple juice between meals. Some patients respond best on a strict well-cooked brown rice diet for up to 10 days.

After either of these initial phases, a bland diet follows, composed of carrot juice, stewed or baked apple, apple sauce, raw grated apple (eaten alone), ripe bananas, avocado, yams, sweet or white potatoes, and a few steamed vegetables such as carrots, parsnips, or squash. Meals must be kept as simple as possible. As improvement becomes apparent, further steamed vegetables are added, and well-masticated cooked brown rice, and if no soy allergy exists, tofu, and steamed fish. At this point the gradual introduction of raw and high-fiber foods is the goal. The first aim is the introduction of a salad for lunch. Raw grated carrots are best to begin with, and slowly all other raw vegetables are added until a large salad is well tolerated.

At this point cure is at the doorstep. The only further hurdle is to experiment with the common allergic foods—dairy products and wheat. It is best to begin with goat's yoghurt. If this is well tolerated for a week, other dairy foods may be tried, such as low-fat cottage cheese. Wheat should be tried last. Should any of these foods cause any adverse reaction whatever, they should immediately be stopped and tests performed for food allergy and lactose or gluten intolerance. Dairy allergy is very common in cases of colitis.

The final diet should be meat-free for several months. Fried foods are absolutely forbidden.

Hydrotherapy

- Cold compress: Apply over abdomen to reduce inflammation.
- Colon irrigation with a few drops of glycothymoline, to be done to remove adherent fecal waste. This may be done in special cases one to six times in a series of one to two times per week, and then stopped and normal bowel movements established through diet.

Spinal Manipulation

Thoracic and lumbar.

Psychological Factors

Since colitis is so frequently influenced by the emotions, all patients should pursue a program of relaxation therapy and meditation. The lifestyle must be altered so that the patient may learn how to relax. All activities must be analyzed and any that evoke stress, destructive emotions, or require a hurried pace must be avoided or dealt with differently. Activities may not need changing, only the attitude. Even the best of foods will become indigestible when the mind and emotions are in turmoil.

Therapeutic Agents

VITAMINS AND MINERALS

Multivitamins: give intramuscularly daily in early part of therapy.

Vitamin A: 25,000 IU one to four times per day in micellized form. *Use any dose of Vitamin A over 50,000 IU per day with medical supervision only.* *

Vitamin B complex: Liquid B complex is best, taken one to three times per day. Yeast-free sources are needed if yeast allergy exists. Intramuscular injection of B complex with high doses of B_{12} (1 ml per day for 10 to 14 days) are essential in the first few weeks of therapy. *

Calcium pantothenate: 200 to 1000 mg per day. *

Vitamin C (buffered): Take vitamin C in powdered form diluted in water. Dose: 1 to 2 g three to four times per day, or more if well tolerated. Intravenous injections of vitamin C may be very useful in early stages. *

Vitamin E: 400 IU one to two times per day (prevents scarring and encourages healing). Some cases require much higher doses.

Calcium: 800 to 1000 mg per day. *

Magnesium: 400 to 500 mg per day.

Zinc: 25 to 50 mg one to two times per day.

OTHERS

Atomodine*

Apple pectin*

Chlorophyll

Cod-liver oil

Garlic (with care): Used in cases where infection or bacterial overgrowth is suspected.

Lactobacillus: Do *not* use if dairy allergy is suspected, which is very common with colitis.

*Asterisks indicate the most frequently used therapeutic agents.

Mucozyme (Nutridyne): 1 to 2, three times per day.*

Raw adrenal or lymph tablets: 2, two to three times per day.*

Raw bran: 1 tbs with water before meals in later stages of diet; not to be used in cases where wheat allergy exists, or if aggravation occurs.*

BOTANICALS

Comfrey tea *(Symphytum officinale)**

Goldenseal *(Hydrastis canadensis)**

Marshmallow root *(Althaea officinalis)*: An excellent demulcent. Use powder, 10 to 30 grains, three to four times per day.*

Peppermint oil: 2 to 6 drops with meals.*

Slippery elm *(Ulmus fulva)*: Excellent for healing mucous membranes. Steep ¼ to ½ tsp of powder in cup of hot water; cool and drink 1 cup four to six times per day.*

Spotted cranebill *(Geranium maculatum)*: Especially astringent with bloody stools.

Wild ginger *(Asarum canadensis)*

Aloe *(Aloe vera)*: 2 oz juice three times per day.

Therapeutic Suggestions

Due to the extreme irritability of the bowels and prolonged malabsorption syndrome most vitamins, minerals, and essential fatty acids are usually deficient. In early stages use vitamin injections to bypass the bowels and ensure introduction into the system. Liquid or liquefied supplements are better absorbed than intact pills, which may be used later in therapy. Micellized fat-soluble vitamins are better handled in these cases than oil forms.

CONSTIPATION

Definition

Difficult and/or infrequent bowel movements.

Symptoms

Infrequent and/or difficult bowel movements, headaches, coated tongue, tiredness, bad breath, mental depression, and mental dullness.

*Asterisks indicate the most frequently used therapeutic agents.

Etiologic Considerations

- Diet
  Fiber deficiency
  Refined foods
    White flour
    White rice
    Sugar
    Boiled vegetables
  Excess
    Meat
    Milk
    Fried foods
    Coffee, tea, alcohol
    Acid-forming foods
  Overeating

- Inactivity
  Lack of exercise
  Sedentary existence
  Bedridden

- Long-term laxative use

- Liver dysfunction
  Gallbladder disease
  Fried foods

- Stress
  Overwork
  Anxiety

- Spinal
  Lesions
  Poor mechanics
  Visceroptosis, prolapsed colon

- Avoiding call of nature

- Appendectomy

- Spastic colitis

- Food allergy

- Pregnancy

- Hypothyroidism (associated with hypochlorhydria and constipation)

- Anemia

- Partial intestinal obstruction
  Adhesions
  Scars
  Cancer

- Hirschsprung's disease—absence of normal nerve plexus and ganglia on the wall of the colon.

- Dehydration

- Hydrochloric acid deficiency

Discussion

Constipation is more than a troublesome condition. It is an insidious drain on the health of millions of people. As bowel transit time is increased, the stool becomes hardened and difficult to pass due to dehydration. The body slowly reabsorbs the fluid content in the feces and along with it many soluble toxins. This autointoxification is the reason people suffering from constipation have coated tongues, foul breath, lack of energy, and difficulty in thinking. These poisons affect every area of the body.

Fiber deficiency and constipation are associated with diverticulitis, appendicitis, and colon cancer. The small, hardened feces are very difficult for the normal intestinal peristaltic actions to deal with effectively. With the lack of bulk added by fiber in the diet, the intestine resembles a tube of toothpaste that is almost empty. The same difficulty you have in getting out that last bit of toothpaste is exactly the problem your intestine has. The peristaltic contractions are more forceful but less effective and tend to create small outpockets or diverticuli in the intestinal walls (see Diverticulitis).

Associated with both diverticulosis and constipation is a change in the normal bacterial flora. As a result, bile acids normally found in the feces and excreted are altered by prolonged exposure to these abnormal bacteria, and become carcinogenic. Thus we see the cause-and-effect relationship behind low-fiber diets and colon cancer.

Most people habitually use laxatives to regulate bowel movements when constipation is a chronic problem. In many cases this causes a strong intestinal action due to the irritant qualities of the laxative. The unfortunate aftereffect, however, is that the bowel reacts to this unusual stimulation by becoming less active just after its use. The result is that in 2 to 3 days when no further bowel movement has occurred, a second dose of laxative is used—and on and on for years, even decades!

Enemas will also have a similar effect. Laxatives which contain mineral oil not only cause the bowels to become overstimulated and weakened, but actually rob the body of all fat-soluble vitamins.

Constipation can have its beginnings very early. The normal breastfed child will have a bowel movement approximately 20 minutes after the start of a feed. This is quickly learned by mothers who breastfeed their infants without first making sure they have diapers on! This bowel action is a true physiological reflex.

Over time, as solid foods are introduced, this reflex becomes less sensitive and can be affected by the type of foods consumed. Mothers soon become aware of these effects and use foods such as bananas to harden the stool and slow transit time, or prunes and papayas to soften them and encourage a bowel movement. Later, as the child is weaned and cow's milk is introduced, bowel movements become less regular and more difficult to regulate. Once the child is toilet-trained, less attention is placed on regularity in some cases, and constipation may take hold with a strong hand. Unless the child is weaned to proper foods such as whole grains, fruit, and raw vegetables, the early years can set up a lifelong constipation problem.

In the early years, and also with adults on hectic schedules, the call of nature may be habitually ignored or postponed. This causes the body to discontinue sending these messages to the brain until it has no further choice, due to bowel overload, but to obey.

Regularity has become a meaningless expression in describing or diagnosing constipation. In the past I routinely asked my patients if they were regular until I realized that to some people once a week was "normal." It is far more useful to know the consistency of the bowel movement and how often a bowel movement occurs. If the bowels move once or twice a day and the stool is hard or difficult to pass, the patient is constipated, no matter how regular he or she is. This can occur with what we call "loaded bowel syndrome," where nearly the entire transverse and descending colon are filled with hard feces.

Another useful index is bowel transit time, or the time it takes for food to pass through the body. In diets composed of unrefined cereals, fruits, and plenty of raw vegetables the transit time is usually 12 hours or so. On a refined diet this may extend to 24, 48, or 72 hours or longer, as in our example of the once-a-weeker.

Certainly, factors other than diet play a role in many cases of constipation. Lack of exercise removes the mechanical action of the muscles on the intestinal contents, thus slowing bowel action. This also reduces normal circulation throughout the digestive tract. The presence of spinal lesions in any of the segments from the midthoracic region through the lumbar plexus is another major factor.

Eating while under any stressful emotion basically paralyzes all digestive functions, including peristaltic action. Still, all these factors mentioned and those listed under Etiologic Considerations account for a very small proportion of cases of constipation. Diet and diet alone stands most prominent as both cause and cure of this disorder.

Treatment

Obviously, if the main cause of constipation is a fiber-deficient diet, then both prevention and cure must lie in an unrefined high-fiber diet. If constipation is habitual and of long duration, the weakened bowels must first be strengthened and reeducated, even before a high-fiber diet will stimulate regularity. Often, specific short cleansing fasts or mono diets with herbal aids, hydropathic applications, and spinal manipulations are required to retonify intestinal actions. In the case of long-standing constipation, it is usually beneficial to begin the regimen with a 3-day fruit juice fast with nightly enemas. This is done even where the habitual use of laxatives or enemas is a main contributing factor in causing intestinal weakness. This may or may not be accompanied by colonic irrigation, depending on the case. Following this fast is a 3-day apple mono diet. This consists of four to five meals of raw apples with apple juice between meals. On the evening of the third day, the patient takes 2 tbs of raw, unrefined olive oil. No enemas or laxatives are taken during this mono diet or after in the full anticonstipation diet which follows below.

During the apple mono diet the patient should begin taking 25 drops of cascara sagrada tincture diluted in water four times per day. When taken regularly in low doses cascara acts as a bowel tonic, not a laxative. In the right doses it helps strengthen bowel action, not weaken it. This is continued for 2 to 3 weeks, then reduced to three times daily for another 2 weeks. If the bowel movements are now regular, the dose is reduced to two times daily for 2 weeks, one time daily for 2 weeks, and then stopped entirely.

Follow this fast with the diet below:

On Rising	Fig, prune, and raisin tea (see Recipes)
Breakfast	Choose from the following:

1. Soaked or simmered dried fruit (do not use water in which soaking takes place) with 2 to 3 tsp of wheat germ and a little soymilk, nutcream, or fruit juice.

2. "Mummy food" (see (Recipes)

3. Granola with yoghurt and wheat germ (not on first day following fast). Soak overnight to soften if desired. Chew well.

4. Prunes or figs (stewed or simmered) with yoghurt and wheat germ. Milled nuts may be added.

	5. Fresh fruit and any whole meal cereal.
Midmorning	Fig, prune, and raisin tea or fruit-bran tea (see Recipes).
Lunch	A large raw salad with milled nuts (no peanuts) or cottage cheese and a slice of 100 percent whole wheat bread (brown bread is *not* sufficient) or two crispbreads with tofu, miso, cottage cheese, or nut spread. Stewed apple or soaked or simmered raisins for dessert with wheat germ or bran topping.
Midafternoon	Herb tea, fig, prune, and raisin tea, apple or prune juice.
Supper	Choose from the following:

1. Any vegetarian savory meal with baked potato (eat the skin also) and two other vegetables. Any fresh fruit or fruit dessert such as prune whip, stewed fruit with nut-cream and wheat germ, etc.

2. Lean meat, fish, or fowl with two to three vegetables other than potatoes and brown rice. Fruit-bran pudding (see Recipes).

3. Salad, same as lunch.

On Retiring	Fig, prune, and raisin tea or herb tea (see Recipes).

Items in diet of special usefulness:

Raw fruit and vegetables, especially apples and celery
Unrefined grains
Bran: 1 to 2 tbs with water at mealtimes
Prunes, raisins, and figs
Molasses
Olive oil
Fluids: 4 to 8 glasses per day

Recipes

• *Fig, prune, and raisin tea*
Cut up about 10 to 12 figs and place in a saucepan together with 10–12 cut-up prunes and about 2 tbs raisins. Cover with 2 pints of water and simmer for about 30 mintues. A little more or less water may be used according to taste, but do not make the juice too weak. If desired, lemon juice may be added to vary the flavor.

- *Fruit-bran tea*
Put 2 heaping tbs of cleaned bran and ¼ lb of chopped figs or prunes or raisins in a jug. Pour on 1 pint of boiling water, cover the jug and allow to stand all night. In the morning, strain the essence and take either hot or cold. A stronger drink may be made by simmering the ingredients for 1 hour and then straining and drinking the essence.

- *Mummy food*
This is excellent to increase and regulate bowel function and increase eliminations. Take 1 cup black or Assyrian figs chopped fine, 1 cup dates chopped fine, ½ cup coarse yellow corn meal and cook to mush in 2–3 cups water. Eat slowly and in moderation. 1–2 tbs may be taken with any meal or separately as a meal in itself.

Physiotherapy and Hydrotherapy

- General tonic
    Sitz baths—alternate hot and cold
    Castor oil abdominal packs (see Appendix I)

- Spastic colon
    Hot enemas of chamomile tea
    Hot compress to abdomen
    Hot sitz baths

- Exercises
    General exercise of any nature
    Abdominal exercises
    Slant board exercises

- Spinal manipulation
    General thoracic and lumbar one time per week for 4 to 8 weeks.

- Habits
    Don't eat under stress
    Don't drink with meals
    Drink 4 to 8 glasses fluids daily
    Visit toilet 20 minutes after each meal to establish habit reflex

- NO, until bowels are normal
    Refined foods
    Spicy foods
    Coffee
    Sugar
    Tea
    Alcohol

Therapeutic Agents

VITAMINS AND MINERALS
   Vitamin B complex
   Vitamin E

OTHERS
   Bran: 1 tbs with 1 to 2 glasses water before or with meals.*

   Brewer's yeast

   Cod liver oil: 3 capsules twice daily.*

   Flaxseed

   Garlic

   Hydrochloric acid

   Lactobacillus (mega dophilus or superdophilus): 1 tsp three times daily.

   Psyllium seeds or husks: A bulk laxative and lubricant.
   Dose: 5 to 7.5 g in water.

BOTANICALS
   Agar agar

   Aloe (*Aloe vera*): 2 oz juice three times per day.

   Cascara (*Cascara sagrada*) in tonic doses, not laxative doses*

   Chamomile (*Anthemis nobilis*)

   Dandelion (*Taraxacum officinale*)

   Goldenseal (*Hydrastis canadensis*)

   Guar gum: Bulk laxative: 2 to 4 tbs per day.

CORONARY DISEASE (see Heart Disease)

COUGHS (see Colds)

*Asterisks indicate the most frequently used therapeutic agents.

CRADLE CAP

Definition and Symptoms

Seborrheic dermatitis of the newborn, characterized by thick, yellow, crusted lesions appearing on the scalp, and sometimes the face and behind the ears.

Discussion

Cradle cap is an extremely common childhood problem due to overproduction of sebum, a waxy, oily substance that may plug the sebaceous glands, leading to inflammation and acne formation. The entire scalp may become covered by a thick accumulation of sebum and dead skin cells.

Treatment

Physiotherapy

• Oil applications: Most oils will work. Apply oil and follow with a scalp massage for 5 to 10 minutes; leave oil on for 30 to 60 minutes. Brush scalp vigorously (take care not to cause inflammation or bleeding) and then shampoo. Repeat one to two times per week until cleared.

• Vinegar scalp massage

Vitamins and Minerals

Vitamin B_6: 5 to 10 mg per day; topical vitamin B_6 salve may be useful. See Dandruff.

CROUP (see Colds)

CYSTITIS AND URETHRITIS (Urinary Tract Infection)

Definition

Inflammation of bladder and/or urethra; infection of either structures.

Symptoms

Frequency and burning on urination; pain and tenderness over bladder area; intense desire to pass urine even after bladder has been emptied; strong-odored urine, which may be cloudy.

Etiologic Considerations

- Thirty times more common in females: The short female urethra and close proximity of urethra to anus are predisposing factors.

- *Escherichia coli* infections most commonly found in bacteria: This is a normal inhabitant of the intestine. Poor toilet technique in young females is a major cause of transfer to the vagina.

- Reiter's disease: Urethritis, arthritis, and conjunctivitis as a triad is diagnostic.

- Sexual activity: "Honeymoon" cystitis is common due to local irritation.

- Lack of lubrication in elderly may be a cause.

- Obstruction: An enlarged prostate will block urethra, causing reduced urine flow and congestion. Stricture (narrowing of urethra) may act similarly.

- Venereal disease

- Irritants
    Emotions (anger, fear, stress, worry)
    Alcohol
    Drugs; antibiotic use
    Chemicals; spermicides
    Preservatives
    Diet

- Spinal: T6 to coccyx lesions may cause reflex irritation, congestion, poor circulation, and tissue degradation, leading to infection.

- Poor eliminations: Poor bowel functions cause toxins to be retained and recirculate into the blood, to be handled by the kidneys.

- Liver congestion: Poor liver function causes excess kidney function as accumulated toxins pass to the kidneys.

- Urine stasis: Inadequate fluids, or improper fluids.

- Following childbirth: The bladder position may favor urine retention if postnatal exercises are not performed.

- A prolapsed transverse colon due to poor abdominal tone, multiple births, or poor spinal mechanics may put pressure on the pelvic organs, causing poor local circulation, congestion, and tissue degradation.

- Allergy

- Birth control pills

Discussion

Confusion exists as to the real cause of cystitis. The most common assumption is that bacterial pathogens enter the urethra and ascend into the bladder where they grow and multiply, causing a clinical infection. While I don't wish to deny that bacteria may be isolated from the bladder or urethra in a case of urinary tract infection or that proper hygiene is important, I feel the primary cause of these complaints usually lies elsewhere. The mere presence of bacteria will not cause an infection. If this were so, then *everyone* would have thousands of infections, both inside the body and out. Bacteria are an ever-present part of life.

The bacteria found in urinary tract infections are the *result* of disease, not its cause. Under normal circumstances, with a healthy body or tissue, bacteria can have no harmful effect. The body's resistance or vitality is so strong that bacteria are immediately dealt with and destroyed, or at least kept under control so that rapid reproduction is impossible. Only when the environment is more favorable for the bacteria will disease result.

Diet

Much of what has been written about diet and cystitis is either misleading or incorrect. We are told by many authorities that cystitis is caused by a too-alkaline diet, which, to correct, we should avoid fruits and vegetables and eat plenty of grains, nuts, fish, cheese, and anything else that will make our urine (and system) strongly acid. The common explanation is that bacteria cannot live in an acid environment. This is true, by the way, and a very useful fact in the treatment of acute genitourinary infections. However, it is *not* the cause of cystitis. The dietary causes of cystitis go much deeper and are more complex than the acidity/alkalinity question alone implies.

Our greatest concern should be the health and integrity of the tissues of the genitourinary system. To maintain these tissues, a balanced diet composed of an *abundance* of fresh and conservatively cooked vegetables, whole grains, protein (preferably more vegetarian than animal), essential fatty acids (unsaturated oils), and a small amount of fresh fruit should be eaten. The fluids consumed should be abundant and as natural as possible. Choose from water, fruit juice, vegetable juice, and mild mint teas. (Pure fresh water is the only really natural drink.) This diet should, if at all possible, be based on organically grown foods. On such a diet, and possibly with the addition of a general vitamin and mineral supplement regimen, all the essential nutrients should be available for absorption by the body to nourish these vital organs.

Rather than an acid-reacting diet being healthy for the genitourinary system, this average acid diet so prevalent today along with lack of raw vegetables is what causes many nutritional problems, *including* the predisposition to cystitis. Once tissues are downgraded by improper nutrition, short-term dietary regimens may be necessary for healing.

Digestion and Eliminations

Too little emphasis is placed on the role of assimilation and eliminations in causing cystitis. If the digestion is weak, even the best of foods cannot provide real nourishment. What good are the best vitamins and minerals if they are never absorbed? Eliminations, too, are very important. Constipation and liver congestion both cause toxins to be recirculated and cause the kidneys excess work. Once the kidneys are overworked, the rest of the genitourinary system becomes irritated. Stress also profoundly affects digestion and elimination, and should always be considered a factor in disease causation.

Spinal Imbalances

One of the most ignored factors in internal complaints, especially those thought to be caused by infection, are spinal lesions. Any injury that causes a lesion in the area from the midback (T6) all the way down to the tailbone (coccyx) can set up what is called a somaticovisceral reflex. This is mediated by nervous and hormonal pathways and may cause reflex irritation, poor circulation, congestion, and tissue degradation in the kidneys, bladder, urethra, uterus, ovaries, prostate, or any other internal structures. This may then cause these structures to become more susceptible to infection by lowering their tissue vitality. Antibiotics and the birth control pill are also important factors in upsetting the body's ecology, producing a predisposition to cystitis.

These factors, and to a lesser extent the rest of the etiologic considerations, should all be weighed carefully in each case of genitourinary disease, to diagnose the real cause of the complaint and not just relieve the immediate symptoms with antibiotics or other artificial measures.

Treatment

Diet

Purify kidneys, bladder, and urethra.
Stage 1: Liquid fast (5 to 7 days) on the following fluids:

Potassium broth (heals and nourishes; see Appendix I)
Parsley tea (diuretic action)
Watermelon seed tea (purifies)
Cranberry juice (slightly acidifies urine, increases urine flow, and reduces the adherence of bacteria to the mucous membrane walls; drink 4 glasses per day)*

*Asterisks indicate the most frequently used therapeutic agents.

Apple cider vinegar, water, and honey (1 cup three times per day)

Stage 2 (7 to 10 days), until condition clears:

Noncitrus fruits and juice
Watermelon and watermelon juice
Cranberry juice
Salads and vegetable juices
Asparagus
Apple cider vinegar plus honey
Vegetarian meals (no eggs or dairy products)
Whole grains
Baked potatoes
Kidney beans
Garlic
Parsnips
Carrots and carrot juice
Fluids: 8 or more glasses per day

Hydrotherapy and Physiotherapy

- Hot sitz bath (pain relief)
- Hot compress
- Trunk packs
- Hot glycothymoline packs over pubic area with 50% water, 50% glycothymoline
- Short wave over bladder for 15 to 20 minutes

Eliminate toxic elements by encouraging good bowel function (see Constipation):

Enemas with liquid fast
Laxative foods with Stage 2

Therapeutic Agents

VITAMINS AND MINERALS

Vitamin A: Essential for mucous membrane health. 25,000 IU two to six times per day, for short periods. *Use any dose of vitamin A over 50,000 IU per day with medical supervision only.*

Vitamin C: 500 to 1000 mg three to six times daily, or to bowel tolerance.*

Folic acid: 40 to 80 mg per day.

Pantothenic acid: 100 mg two times per day (with a B complex).

Niacin: 100 mg two times per day (with a B complex).*

Vitamin E: 400 IU one to two times per day; healing factor.*

OTHER

Acidophilus: 2 capsules three times per day if no dairy allergy exists.

Chlorophyll

Garlic: 2 capsules three to four times per day.

BOTANICALS

Bearberry (Arctostaphylos uva-ursi): Diuretic and gastrointestinal antiseptic. Dose: Tincture, 20 to 30 drops four to six times per day.*

Buchu (Barosma betulina): Diuretic, urinary tonic, antiseptic. Dose: tincture, 10 to 15 drops three to four times per day.*

Comfrey (Symphytum officinale)

Couch grass (Agrophyrum repens): Demulcent, diuretic. Dose: Tincture, 5 to 20 drops three to four times per day.*

Goldenseal (Hydrastis canadensis): Tea three times per day.*

Juniper berries (Juniperus communis): Diuretic.*

Marshmallow root (Althaea officinalis): Excellent demulcent, diuretic. Use powder in warm water, 10 to 30 grains, three to four times per day.

Parsley root and seed (Petroselinum sativum): Use as tea or tincture, 5 to 15 drops three to four times per day.*

DANDRUFF

Definition

A chronic scaling inflammation of the skin occurring on the scalp and eyebrows.

---

*Asterisks indicate the most frequently used therapeutic agents.

Symptoms

Diffuse scaling of the scalp; variable itching.

Etiologic Considerations

- Seborrheic dermatitis:
  Dysfunction of the sebaceous glands with increased oil production.
- Acidity/Diet
  Excess carbohydrates and deficiency of green vegetables
  Excess alcohol
  Excess citrus
  Salt
  Sugar
- Allergy
  Wheat
  Dairy products
  Citrus
  Other
- Excess saturated fats; fried foods
- Stress
  Hormonal
  Acidity
- Poor eliminations
- Essential fatty acid deficiency
- Other vitamin and mineral deficiency
  Vitamin A
  Vitamin E
  Vitamin B complex
  Vitamin B_6
  Zinc
- Fungus
- Strong irritant shampoos or hair treatments
- Digestive enzyme deficiency

Discussion

Most people consider dandruff of cosmetic importance only. The usual mode of treatment is to attack the offending white scales with various shampoos and other topical agents. This rarely is successful in permanently removing the problem and is a clear example that symptomatic treatments are useless.

Dandruff is a symptom that may be caused by many different factors. Although this condition is commonly considered the result of what is called seborrhea, or an excess secretion of oil by the sebaceous glands, this tells us very little. Many patients with dandruff have excess sebaceous gland activity. This oil in fact is what binds the dead skin cells together to form visible plaques. The excess oil itself must have some unusual irritant quality not normally present if this is the major cause. In some cases this can be found from dietary errors such as excess acidity, allergy, improper fat consumption, or other irritants such as salt, sugar, or alcohol. This will cause irritant elements to be excreted in the body's oily secretions and may cause the body to react with an irritation and rash.

Another possibility is that nutritional deficiency may cause improper function of the sebaceous glands and scalp. Evidence of various forms of dermatitis is readily available in most severe B complex deficiencies as well as in essential fatty acid and zinc deficiency.

Scalp irritation and rash may also develop from the use of strong acid or alkaline shampoos, very hot hair dryers, or unnatural and strong hair treatments or dyes. Hormonal factors also may play a part.

Treatment

Diet

A common finding in cases of dandruff is improper diet. This many times is an excess consumption of citrus. As a first step in treatment I forbid the consumption of any but the blandest of fruits and allow only papaya, avocado, and a very few bananas. Later I add other fruits but exclude the entire citrus family until complete cure has been attained. Since most cases show a diet high in carbohydrates and animal fats and low in green vegetables, I restrict or entirely eliminate carbohydrates and saturated fats for a time, and advise a diet primarily of raw and cooked vegetables and vegetarian proteins. These include sunflower seeds, pumpkin seeds, a few nuts, beans, and tofu.

It is best to begin this regimen with 1 to 3 days of vegetable juice fasting and enemas. This is followed for 1 to 2 weeks by a diet made up of a small amount of bland fruits and a great quantity of both raw and conservatively cooked vegetables, plus raw vegetable juices. For a further 2 weeks it is useful to continue to restrict the diet to a purely vegetarian cuisine. This may then be followed by a diet similar to that found under Acne, a condition to which dandruff is closely associated. This diet severely restricts saturated fats.

Physiotherapy

- Scalp massage
  To 4 oz pure distilled water add 20 drops of 85% grain alcohol and 2 to 6 drops of oil of pine. Massage into scalp and then follow this by massaging a small amount of white vaseline into the scalp.

- Shampoo
  Use pine tar shampoo or alternate with olive oil shampoo.

- Crude oil scalp massage
  2 times per week (see Baldness)

- Vinegar scalp rub

- Vitamin B$_6$ cream application

Therapeutic Agents

VITAMINS AND MINERALS

Vitamin A: 25,000 IU one to two times per day. *Use any dose of vitamin A over 50,000 IU per day with medical supervision only.* *

Vitamin B complex: 50 mg two to three times per day. (If yeast allergy exists, use nonyeast source). *

Folic acid: 2 mg per day.

Vitamin B$_6$: 100 mg two times per day.

Vitamin B$_{12}$: 1 mg intramuscularly per week. *

Oil of evening primrose: 1 to 2 capsules two to three times per day. *

PABA (Para-amino benzoic acid): 100 to 200 mg per day.

Zinc: 25 to 30 mg three times per day. *

OTHERS

Atomodine (or other iodine source)*

Cod-liver oil: 2 to 4 capsules two times per day. *

EPA (Eicosapentaenoic acid): 2 to 4 capsules three times per day.

Kelp

Biotin

Hydrochloric acid

*Asterisks indicate the most frequently used therapeutic agents.

Lecithin: As much as possible. 4 capsules three times per day and/or as granules in food.*

Raw thymus: Immunological support.

Therapeutic Suggestions

Although saturated fats in the diet are avoided, essential fatty acids are encouraged. EFA, EPA, GLA, and oil of evening primrose may show very good responses along with the rest of the suggested supplements. The scalp treatments outlined in detail under the section on Baldness must be an essential part of therapy.

DEPRESSION (see Behavioral Disorders)

DIABETES (Diabetes Mellitus, Sugar Diabetes, Adult-Onset Diabetes)

Definition

A disease characterized by carbohydrate intolerance of varying degrees, due to inadequate production of insulin by the beta cells of the islets of Langerhans, or insulin insensitivity of the body cells, but also involving other glandular organs and body tissues.

Symptoms

Sugar in urine, raised blood sugar, excessive thirst, polyuria (excess urination) and frequency of urination, excess hunger, muscle wasting, weight loss, weakness, electrolyte loss, dry skin, itching, rashes, paresthesia, numbness, tingling of hands and feet, neuropathy with severe pains, vascular degeneration, atherosclerosis, retinopathy, loss of sight, kidney disease, gangrene in dependent limbs due to poor circulation leading to amputation, ketosis, acidosis, coma, and premature death.

Etiologic Considerations

- Diet
    Excess refined carbohydrates and sugar consumption
    Excess saturated fat consumption
    Nutritional deficiency

*Asterisks indicate the most frequently used therapeutic agents.

- Adrenal exhaustion
- Pancreatic insufficiency
  Refined foods, coffee, alcohol, cigarettes, stress, nervous exhaustion
- Sudden severe shock causing constriction of blood flow to vital organs causing damage
- Obesity
- Lack of exercise
- Sedentary existence
- Hyperthyroid
- Hyperadrenocorticism
- Liver damage, toxicity, or congestion
- Pancreatitis or other pancreas damage due to trauma, tumor, or infection
- Toxemia
- Spinal: T6 to T10 lesions causing imbalance of function of liver, pancreas, spleen, adrenals, and other organs with congestion and sluggishness
- Poor eliminations
- Heredity
- Pregnancy and severe infection: Latent diabetes appears, due to increased insulin requirements at this time
- Allergy

Discussion

Diabetes affects up to 5 percent of the people in the United States, with many more undiagnosed. The most obvious physiological abnormality recognized in the past is a deficiency of secretion of insulin by the beta cells of the pancreas. Elevated insulin levels also may occur where the body has developed a decreased sensitivity to insulin. In general, high-insulin diabetics tend to be overweight, while insulin-deficient patients become thin and emaciated. The high-insulin diabetic may simply be at an earlier stage of the disease, later to become insulin-deficient with sudden weight loss.

Insulin's role in the body is to facilitate uptake of glucose from the bloodstream by the body's cells for energy utilization. In diabetes the pancreas either does not produce enough insulin, or the body has become less sensitive to it, causing a wide range of metabolic results.

The normal level of glucose in the blood is kept within the narrow range of 80 to 120 mg %. If, due to insulin deficiency or insensitivity, this rises to 170 to 180 mg %, sugar spills over into the urine, carrying with it vast amounts of water, water-soluble vitamins, and minerals. This causes a severe electrolyte imbalance and dehydration, stimulating excessive thirst. Since the body's glucose fuel cannot make its way into the cells where it is needed, the body begins to convert fats and protein into sugar as an emergency measure. This results in wasting of the body with weight loss and dehydration. As excess fats are broken down ketone bodies accumulate, resulting in ketosis, dizziness, nausea, vomiting, hyperventilation, and eventually coma. Excess protein breakdown also leads to a general acid condition of the body's fluids.

Characteristic changes occur within the cardiovascular system, leading to atherosclerotic changes which reduce blood flow to the feet, causing slow healing, tendency to infection, ulceration, and finally gangrene, leading to amputation of the toes or feet. Small vessels in the eye are weakened, leading to rupture and blindness.

Not all cells of the body require insulin for glucose uptake. Certain cells called "insulin insensitive," found in the eye, kidney, myelinated nerves, and red blood cells, take up glucose passively along concentration gradients. Therefore, as glucose increases in the blood, these cells take up large amounts of glucose. Since this amount absorbed is far in excess of the energy needs of these cells, the body must convert it to fructose and then sorbitol to get it out of the way. These two sugars are relatively insoluble and soon exceed their solubility, tending to crystallize out within the cell. In the eye this results in the typical cataract formation found in diabetes. In the kidney it reduces glomerular filtration, causing kidney damage. It damages the nerves, leading to diabetic neuropathy, and reduces the oxygen-carrying capacity of the red blood cells.

The pancreas not only produces insulin, but also secretes digestive enzymes and bicarbonate essential for the breakdown of the basic food groups. When the pancreas is functioning at a low ebb due to overstimulation, it not only may have a reduced insulin output, but also will secrete less digestive enzymes. This sets up a vicious cycle when it comes to protein metabolism. Due to insufficient proteolytic enzymes, protein is not efficiently broken down into its amino acid components.

Since digestive enzymes and hormones (i.e., insulin, cortisol, adrenalin, etc.) are composed of amino acids, this maldigestion may eventually lead to further digestive enzyme deficiency and reduced hormone output, resulting in an aggravation of the diabetic syndrome.

In addition to this undigested protein, molecules may pass into the bloodstream, initiating allergy or allergy-like hypersensitivity reactions. (See Allergy for more discussion on results of this protein maldigestion.)

The deficiency of fat-digesting capability is also a problem that may be directly related to the complications of arteriosclerosis and other cardiovascular problems associated with diabetes, by altering the relative lipid ratios.

In short, diabetes is a terrible disease, responsible for one in every eight deaths in the United States, and one in every three cases of blindness. The saddest part of this disease is that it is almost entirely preventable.

Diabetes is clearly a disease of civilization. Studies of various populations show that as the consumption of sugar and refined carbohydrates such as white bread and white rice increases, so does the incidence of diabetes. In groups where no refined sugars are consumed and the diet includes unrefined whole grains, little or no diabetes can be found.

Diabetes is closely associated with obesity. At least 80 percent of all diabetics are or were obese. The consumption of refined carbohydrates seems to be the major contributing factor in this obesity. It is possible to consume a large amount of refined carbohydrates in the form of sugar or refined grains such as white bread, macaroni, or white rice in a short time, since the bulky fiber has been removed. If, however, carbohydrates were taken in their natural, unrefined state, it would be impossible to consume even one-fifth of this amount. For example, if a person drinks only one soda drink in 5 minutes (which may contain up to 7 tsp of sugar), it would have taken him or her hours to eat the equivalent carbohydrate value found in apples, carrots, or whole grain bread. Refined carbohydrates, especially in their disaccharide form (i.e., sucrose, which is composed of one molecule of fructose and one molecule of glucose), are especially a problem since they stimulate triglyceride formation associated with the cardiovascular complications of diabetes.

Adult-onset diabetes normally has an incubation period of about 20 years before it becomes manifest. As our children are exposed earlier and earlier to a vast amount of refined cereals, sweets, and soda, we are now finding what would be considered "adult"-onset diabetes in younger age groups.

Although many nutrients have been found that when deficient can, in experimental situations, induce diabetes in animals, no single nutrient deficiency is the real cause, nor will there be a real cure. Diabetes is not simply a disorder of the pancreas, but affects the entire body, especially the liver, nervous system, circulatory system, thyroid, spleen, kidney, hypothalamus, pituitary, and adrenal glands. It is not just a disorder of carbohydrate metabolism, but also affects utilization of both fats and proteins. The entire metabolism is upset, as well as all the hormones that normally control it.

Although consumption of refined carbohydrates is one of the major causes of diabetes by causing the pancreas to secrete excess insulin, or the body to become insensitive to insulin, and overworking the pancreas and eventually weakening it, other factors play their part. Stress and adrenal exhaustion are factors in many cases of diabetes. Although the pancreas, with its production of glucagon which causes an increase in blood glucose levels, is the major antagonist to insulin in the control of blood sugar levels, the adrenal glands are also involved. Normally food is consumed and converted into glucose, raising the blood sugar level. The pancreas secretes insulin to remove the glucose from the blood. If the sugar level falls too low (as in hypoglycemia) the adrenal glands secrete hormones that trigger the conversion of stored sugar in the liver and muscles in the form of glycogen back to sugar for use. These glands, the pancreas, liver, and adrenals, are all under stress with either *hypo- or hyper*glycemia. Stress is interpreted in the body as an emergency situation and the adrenal glands respond by secreting adrenalin to derive energy to deal with the supposed threat. If this is too often repeated, or too prolonged, as in chronic nervous tension, the pancreas, adrenal glands, and liver become severely depleted and fail to respond properly and hypoglycemia or diabetes may result. Vitamin deficiencies such as B complex and vitamin C may be the result of this situation since the adrenal glands need large amounts of these nutrients to function.

Refined carbohydrates, stress, coffee, nicotine, and alcohol or recreational drugs all cause the adrenal glands to work in excess, and as we have already seen, overstimulation eventually will lead to inhibition of function. Thus we see that the civilized way of life is the largest factor in the causation of pancreatic and adrenal malfunction leading to diabetes.

Another recent and very interesting clinical observation is that blood sugar levels react differently for different people in response to the same food. Although consumption of refined carbohydrates is considered a primary factor, many seemingly safe foods can cause similar reactions depending upon individual sensitivity. The same endocrine reactions of high or low blood sugar levels, along with pancreative and adrenal gland depletion, can occur following ingestion of literally any food or food group, including protein, fats, and even unrefined carbohydrates, as well as chemicals or tobacco. These reactions can be considered as an allergy, or probably more appropriately, may be labeled hypersensitivities. In such cases, where standard high complex carbohydrate regimens fail to control the blood sugar level adequately, the individual must have his or her blood sugar reactions tested for all commonly ingested foods, or undertake a rotation diet where individual foods are not eaten more frequently than every 4 days.

Other glands and organs are related to diabetes as well. The liver, where sugar is stored in the form of glycogen as an energy reserve, is found to suffer fatty degeneration in diabetes. Liver disease may be either the result or one of the causes of diabetes. Liver damage, toxicity, or congestion all seem to be associated with the onset of diabetes.

Spinal lesions in the midthoracic region are a common finding in diabetics. These may cause imbalances of function between the liver, pancreas, spleen, adrenal glands, and other organs, causing congestion and sluggish function or hyperactivity.

Insulin, discovered in the early 1920s, has been used in various forms to treat diabetes and has been clearly lifesaving in the short term and does help control the blood sugar level in diabetes.

The insidious cardiovascular changes characteristic of this disease may be more difficult to deal with. These changes in the arteries can cause loss of sight and limb, and may result in early death.

The problem with insulin use is that it is very difficult to prescribe it so that it mimics exactly the body's own production of insulin. In the past, insulin was given in rather large doses, one or two times a day. This causes elevated levels of insulin in the bloodstream for longer than usual. Normally the body secretes insulin in response to food, causing an elevation of blood sugar, and feedback controls moderate its level. With injected insulin, the problem is even more complex. Normally, insulin secreted from the pancreas goes first to the liver, where over half of it is used up, the rest then going into the general circulation. With insulin injections, however, all the insulin courses through the bloodstream before reaching the liver. The result is a temporary hyperinsulinism.

The problem with too much insulin in the blood is that excessive insulin levels stimulate the synthesis of cholesterol in the blood vessel wall, and may be a factor in arteriosclerosis.*†

Newer methods of insulin administration are currently being introduced which may correct this serious problem, and many physicians are now attempting to prescribe insulin along more physiological lines. There certainly is no question, however, that if diet can control glucose levels, it is a far safer and more desirable form of therapy than is insulin.

Treatment

Diabetes is a chronic degenerative disease. As such, by definition, vital organs and tissues have begun to be destroyed. The possibility of cure by natural means depends on the severity of the case and the length of insulin dependency. While some forms of diabetes, such as congenital or juvenile-onset diabetes, can never be corrected through diet alone and will always require insulin, even in these cases diet does help moderate the problem.

Certainly, mild cases of adult-onset diabetes are usually easy to correct. Even once insulin has been taken, if not for too prolonged a period, cure is fairly simple. Prolonged cases, however, require much more effort and total cure may not be possible if the pancreas has been so deranged over years of improper diet and drug suppression that it has literally ceased to function. Exogenous insulin certainly does not cause diabetes; however, the body can become dependent upon it and reduce its own insulin production. Sometimes the best that can be done in these cases is to reduce the insulin need through proper diet and the consumption of insulin-like substances found naturally in some foods.

*Lowenstein, B. E., *Diabetes*, Harper & Row, New York, 1976, pp. 39–40.
†Philpott, William H., *Victory Over Diabetes*, Keats Publishing Co., New Canaan, Conn., 1983, pp. 56–57.

Diet

Until very recently diabetics were routinely counseled to reduce carbohydrates. No distinction was made between refined or unrefined, except that sugar and products with sugar were reduced. The typical diabetic then reduced carbohydrate consumption but continued to eat all manner of devitalized foods. To derive needed energy which normally would have come from carbohydrates, most ate far more animal fats and proteins. These saturated fats only aggravated the dangerous cardiovascular disease from which most diabetics suffer (see Heart Disease). The type of diet prescribed by most naturopathic physicians for adult-onset diabetes for years has recently found favor. Rather than a low-carbohydrate diet being the best approach, a high *unrefined* carbohydrate diet is the most beneficial. In a recent study* 70 percent of the diet was composed of high-fiber unrefined carbohydrates. The average insulin requirement fell drastically during this regimen. Even more surprising was the fact that nearly all the overweight patients *lost* weight while those at a normal weight remained stationary. Many of the patients were able to discontinue insulin therapy altogether.

A good diabetic dietary regimen excludes any and all refined foods such as sugar, sweets, pastry, white flour products, and white rice, and replaces them with natural, high-fiber carbohydrates that take longer to be digested. The key is to supply the body with slow-burning fuel that will not cause a sudden increase in sugar in the blood and therefore require excess insulin. Most of the fats eaten should be vegetarian or unsaturated in nature. No red meats are allowed, and even chicken and fish are restricted to several times per week. The best proteins are vegetarian, with special emphasis on soy proteins due to their high concentration of lecithin, which is a fat emulsifier and contains large amounts of choline, found useful in preventing and treating neurological complications of diabetes. Acid and subacid fruits are allowed in moderation in some cases if eaten with some protein to slow digestion. Many diabetics, however, must strictly avoid all fruit and fruit juice, at least initially. All sweet fruits and dried fruits are forbidden. Meals should always be kept small and taken six times per day. As much as 75 percent of the diet should be composed of raw foods.

Some foods have an insulin-like action in the body, or other specific usefulness, and should be included in the diet regularly. These include:

Jerusalem artichokes	Fiber (i.e., wheat bran, oat bran, and guar gum)
Brussels sprouts	
Cucumbers	Oatmeal or oat flour products
Green beans	Soybeans and tofu
Garlic	Avocado

*Anderson, J. W., "High-carbohydrate, High Fiber Diets for Insulin-treated Men with Diabetes Mellitus," *American Journal of Clinical Nutrition*, 32:2312, 1979.

> *Spirulina*   Wheat germ
> Brewer's yeast   Buckwheat
> Raw green vegetables

The following is a sample diet that has been very useful in diabetes:

On Rising	1 tsp *Spirulina* in warm water
Breakfast	Choice of one of the following:

        1. Whole grain cereal (i.e., oatmeal, whole wheat cereal, etc.), *or*

        2. Fruit, yoghurt, and nuts (not peanuts) and wheat germ,* *or*

        3. Yoghurt, nuts and wheat germ, *or*

        4. Once or twice per week, poached eggs on whole wheat toast, *or*

        5. ½ grapefruit or other citrus with some protein*

Midmorning   Whole grain snack (i.e. bread, crackers, biscuits, etc.)
1 tsp *Spirulina* in warm water

Lunch   *Always* include a raw salad composed primarily of green vegetables such as lettuce, cucumber, celery, watercress, parsley, spinach, broccoli, brussels sprouts, garlic, avocado, cabbage, sprouted alfalfa, beet tops, onions, cauliflower, etc. Carrots may be included in small amounts only in the early stages of the diet, with larger portions later in the diet regimen. Also, any of the following:

        1. Cottage cheese

        2. Crispbreads, 100 percent whole grain bread or other unrefined starch

        3. Nuts (i.e., almonds, walnuts, brazils, hazels, etc.)

        4. Beans or tofu, fish, fowl, or lean meat

Midafternoon   Same as midmorning

Supper   1. Same selection as lunch, *or*

*On doctor's approval.

2. A selection from the following conservatively cooked vegetables: green beans, onions, spinach, brussels sprouts, green peppers, zucchini, kale, artichokes, cabbage, broccoli, okra, beet tops, or other vegetables, especially those that grow above the ground.

3. Soybeans in any form (beans, tofu, etc.)

4. Whole grain (especially buckwheat or oats)

5. Fish

6. Fowl or lean meat

7. A small Jerusalem artichoke (hen's egg size) five times per week, cooked in its own juices in patapar paper

8. Low-fat dairy protein

Evening   Same as midmorning and midafternoon
Take 1 tsp brewer's yeast and 1 tsp raw bran three times daily.
A large portion of each meal should include a slow-burning carbohydrate.

POTASSIUM BROTH RECIPE:
(may be taken at any time)

Take washed, unpeeled carrots and chop fine, the ¼-in. outer peelings of potatoes with the skin, parsley, large amounts of onions and garlic, cabbage and other greens, celery, and any other vegetables on hand.

Prepare broth by washing and chopping the vegetables and then simmer in a large covered pot of water for not more than 30 to 40 minutes. Strain and drink the essence only, flavored if desired, with pure vegetable concentrate. Excess may be stored in glass containers in refrigerator for up to 2 days. Very useful to help restore lost electrolytes and minerals.

Physiotherapy

- Spinal manipulation to midthoracic area and any other specific lesions one time per week for 6 to 8 weeks; rest 2 to 3 weeks and repeat one to two times.

- Alternate hot and cold compresses over pancreas.

- Castor oil packs (see Appendix I) over entire abdomen from lower ribs to pubis.

- Increased exercise is essential, along with normalization of ideal weight to lean body mass.

- Daily "salt glow": Mix 1 to 2 lb of salt with water until soupy. Stand in shower and rub the mixture vigorously all over the body. Rinse with cold water and dry briskly with a rough towel.

• Alternate hot and cold showers to increase circulation.

• Alternate hot and cold leg baths to increase local circulation.

Therapeutic Agents

VITAMINS AND MINERALS

Vitamin A: 25,000 to 50,000 IU per day. *Use any dose of vitamin A over 50,000 IU per day with medical supervision only.* *

Vitamin B complex: Balanced 50 mg two to three times per day; essential for proper carbohydrate metabolism and adrenal function. Needed with any stress. Lowers need for insulin. *

Vitamin C + bioflavonoids: 3,000 to 12,000 mg per day; strengthens capillary walls, essential for adrenal function, needed in excess in stress. Potentiates action of insulin, therefore reduces insulin need. Bioflavonoids (1000 mg per day) help prevent and help stop progression of diabetic cataracts. *

Vitamin E: 400 IU two to three times per day. Beneficial in heart disease, essential for healing, lowers insulin need, improves ability of muscles to take up glucose and store as glycogen. *

Essential fatty acids: 2 capsules three times per day; use EPA, GLA, or oil of evening primrose. *

Vitamin B_6: 250 mg two times per day, especially useful in pregnancy-onset diabetes and to prevent complications of arteriosclerosis. Vitamin B_6 is specifically useful to help diabetic neuropathy. A daily intramuscular dose of 50 to 100 mg vitamin B_6 along with 1 mg of vitamin B_{12} and 500 mcg folic acid is used until pain reduces in intensity; then the dose and frequency is gradually reduced. *

Inositol: 500 to 1000 mg three times per day; helps prevent and treat diabetic neuropathy. *

Chromium [best source is glucose tolerance factor (GTF) yeast tablets]: 2 mg one to two times per day. Needed in small amounts as catalyst for insulin, to act in the uptake of glucose. *

Zinc: 15 to 30 mg two times per day; essential for insulin secretion. *

Manganese

Potassium

*Asterisks indicate the most frequently used therapeutic agents.

OTHERS

Garlic: 2 capsules three times per day.*

Kelp: 3 to 4 tablets two to three times per day.

Lecithin: 2 tbs granules (or more).*

Concentrated phosphatidylcholine: 2 to 4 capsules three times a day, or 1 tbs liquid three times per day.

Brewer's yeast [glucose tolerance factor (GTF)]: Necessary for proper production and utilization of insulin. Animals on GTF-deficient diet soon get diabetes. 1 tsp three times daily.*

EPA (Eicosapentaenoic acid): 1 capsule two or three times per day.

Spirulina: Lowers insulin need. 1 tsp three times per day.*

Bran: 1 tsp three times per day.*

With doctor's prescription:
    Raw pituitary tablets
    Raw adrenal tablets*
    Raw thyroid tablets

Pancreatic enzymes: Take 1 to 3 tablets with, or just following, meals. The exocrine function of the pancreas (the secretion of digestive enzymes and bicarbonate) is often even more inhibited in pancreatic exhaustion and insufficiency than is its endocrine function of insulin secretion.*

Atomodine (do not take with other iodine-containing foods such as kelp): 1 drop two times per day, increasing 1 drop per day until 3 to 5 drops two times per day are taken; then decrease 1 drop per day until back to original dose. Rest 1 to 2 weeks and repeat, only with doctor's prescription.*

BOTANICALS

Jambul (*Syzygium jambdlanum*)*

(*Note: Diabetes is a serious disorder and should always be monitored by a physician.* Sudden change of diet, especially the introduction of brewer's yeast and other factors that tend to reduce insulin need, can cause an unexpectedly *low* blood sugar unless insulin needs are frequently monitored. No diabetic should ever reduce or stop his or her insulin without being under the care of a physician well aware of the consequences of uncontrolled diabetes.)

*Asterisks indicate the most frequently used therapeutic agents.

DIAPER RASH (Napkin rash, Irritant contact dermatitis, Ammoniacal dermatitis)

Definition

A common dermatitis of infants affecting the diaper region with or without secondary infection with bacteria or fungus.

Symptoms

Redness, tenderness, edema, inflammation, thickening of skin, raw, oozing skin; secondary yeast infection appears bright red with well-defined borders, and often has distinct red papules.

Etiologic Considerations

- Irritant chemicals
    Ammonia and urea from urine
    Fecal enzymes from stool
    Detergents
- Moist heat
- Plastic diaper covers or plastic diapers
- Allergy
    Citrus
    Cow's milk
    Fruit
    Wheat
    Other
- Abrasion
- Antibiotics
    Allergic reaction
    Secondary yeast infection
- Vitamin B complex deficiency
- Essential fatty acid deficiency
- Saturated fat excess
    Cow's milk
    Formulas

Discussion

Diaper rash affects most babies to some degree periodically throughout infancy. The most common cause is prolonged contact with irritants such as urine, stools, or detergents in the moist, warm environment created by not changing the diaper frequently enough. A local irritation or contact dermatitis develops, confined to the diaper region and thighs, which may be complicated by fungal or bacterial infection.

Although prolonged contact with irritants does play a part in the average case of diaper rash, these rashes frequently are the most obvious symptom or manifestation of a primarily dietary problem. Certainly, direct irritation of the baby's delicate skin by diapers washed with strong detergents and not rinsed well will cause a rash. This type of diaper rash, however, is fairly uncommon. If a mother leaves her baby for prolonged periods in a wet or dirty diaper, a rash will also develop, due to the continual maceration of the skin and the normal urine and fecal irritations. This type of rash is perhaps more common than a detergent-caused rash, but still it is uncommon to find a mother so busy or unconcerned about her baby's comfort as to leave the child too long in such an unpleasant condition.

I feel that the real problems causing diaper rash are not usually local hygiene, but dietary. Breastfed infants may respond with a diaper rash to something the breastfeeding mother eats or drinks, or to any new food or drink added in her diet. Unless the mother becomes aware of this relationship, a slight rash can develop into a chronic one which is impossible to remove by normal external measures. The offending food in the mother's diet may be literally anything, but citrus or acid foods are the most common. Nearly every infant will develop a diaper rash if the mother eats an excess of vitamin C, pineapples, or oranges. Later, as weaning begins, a diaper rash usually indicates a food sensitivity. This may be due to adding a food too rapidly to the diet, or in too concentrated a form. It may, however, be a true allergic reaction. In either case, this reaction must be carefully watched for and the offending food totally eliminated for 4 to 6 weeks or longer, and then slowly reintroduced. Often no reaction will occur the second time, but if it does, discontinue the food and introduce it much later in the weaning process.

Cow's milk is another common offender and may represent a true allergy or a reaction to excess saturated fat. In general I suggest discontinuing cow's milk permanently. Goat's milk seems to be much better tolerated and may be used as a dairy source by most infants and children.

Wheat or gluten grains are always suspect with diaper rashes. I usually advise that these grains, especially any yeasted preparations, be added as one of the last foods in the weaning process, sometime after the first birthday.

Formula-fed infants who develop a rash may have a specific allergic reaction to the type of formula, or may be suffering from exposure to excess saturated fat, Vitamin B complex deficiency, or essential fatty acid deficiency.

Many diaper rashes that follow the use of antibiotics for any reason have the possibility of being an antibiotic reaction, or a secondary fungal infection. These occur fairly commonly since antibiotics destroy many friendly bacteria that act to prevent normal and ever-present bacteria and fungi from gaining too strong a foothold.

Treatment

Obviously, cure will come only when the cause is removed. No amount of exterior medication will be of lasting benefit if the conditions favorable for the rash development are not removed. I often see unfortunate infants who have received a barrage of corticosteroid creams, nystatin (for *Candida albicans* infection), and even oral antibiotics. Often the distressed parents have taken the child to nearly every pediatrician in town, receiving conflicting diagnoses of anything from simple diaper rash to ringworm complicated with yeast infection and staph. These cases are very upsetting, especially since the rash is usually of internal dietary origin and could have been treated easily and rapidly in its early stages. Once the local skin has been severely inflamed and thickened, a chronic condition settles in, which can take months of proper therapy to remove. From my experience, the use of corticosteroid creams should be forbidden for the treatment of diaper rash. All that it does is calm the inflammation down for a short period, and once its use is discontinued, the rash flares up again with a vengeance.

Diet

Once a rash has been allowed to develop for any extended period of time, great difficulties arise in finding which particular aspect of the mother's (if breastfeeding) or baby's diet is at fault. Sometimes the infant must be totally reweaned, a very painful process for baby and mother alike. Before this is resorted to, it is often sufficient to analyze both mother's and infant's diet to first attempt to exclude the probable offender. This is usually easier than it sounds. The mother is placed on a highly nutritious, mostly vegetarian diet, excluding citrus fruit, citrus juices, tomatoes, strong spices, alcohol, coffee, and any junk foods. Fruit and fruit juice, even noncitrus juice, is either excluded or drastically reduced. Raw salads are encouraged at least two times per day. One to two glasses of carrot juice should be taken daily. All supplements are discontinued except for vitamin A, vitamin B complex, Vitamin E, essential fatty acids, and zinc. The infant's diet must be analyzed individually, depending on age and progression in the weaning process. The most commonly offending foods are fruits and fruit juices, especially citrus; also tomatoes, and wheat or other gluten grain, although literally any food may be a factor. The above foods are totally excluded from the diet. Little or no fruits are allowed. The bulk of the diet should be vegetables and brown rice, if grains have already been introduced. Carrot juice is also encouraged, one to two times per day. Formula-fed infants are converted to goat's milk. The infant supplements are the same as for the breastfeeding mother, except in much smaller doses.

Physiotherapy

Although the most common cause of the problem is internal and dietetic, attention must still be given to local therapy.

- Diapers   The best diaper for an infant with a rash is no diaper at all. Keep the child bare and exposed to air and sunlight as much as the climate will permit. When diapers must be worn, make sure that the diaper is antiseptically cleaned and well rinsed or use disposable. Change the diaper frequently. Wash the area with cool water and gently dab dry using a soft cotton diaper. Apply prescribed powder, oil, or cream as discussed below, depending on the type of rash. Make sure the area is completely dry before applying cream or oil medication, to prevent water from being trapped below this layer.

- Ultraviolet light or sunlight   Expose the infant to small daily doses of sunlight or ultraviolet light. Be careful not to burn the baby's very thin and sensitive skin. No ocean swimming is allowed until the rash is gone. Fresh pool water, especially rainwater, is fine. If the climate is agreeable, let the child play for hours in the pool, under supervision, of course. It is best if the water is very cold. This should only be done on a warm and sunny day to prevent the onset of hypothermia. Vinegar added to the pool water is useful.

Therapeutic Agents

VITAMINS AND MINERALS

> Vitamin A: 25,000 IU three times per day for the mother; 2000 to 5000 IU three times per day for the infant. *Use any dose of vitamin A over 10,000 IU per day for infants with medical supervision only.**

> Vitamin B complex: 50 mg three times per day for the mother; 10 to 25 mg two to three times per day for the infant.

> Vitamin E: 400 IU two times per day for the mother; 25 to 40 IU two times per day for the infant.

> Essential fatty acids: 4 capsules three to four times per day for the mother; contents of 1 to 2 capsules two to three times per day for the infant. GLA (gamma-linoleic acid) is a good source.*

> Zinc: 30 mg two to three times per day for the mother; one-fourth to one-half of a 15-mg tablet two times per day for the infant.*

> Oil of evening primrose: 1 capsule two times daily for the infant.*

*Asterisks indicate the most frequently used therapeutic agents.

OTHERS

Local applications

Different combinations of local therapies are effective in individual cases. Sometimes trial and error is the only way to determine which will be most effective. As a naturopathic physician, I tailor each medication to the individual, using a little more or less of a particular ingredient, depending on the case history and how the rash presents itself.

The following applications or combinations of these are effective:

Powders
    Calendula powder
    Clay
    Slippery elm powder
    Comfrey powder
    Peruvian balsam powder
    Zinc stearate powder
    Goldenseal powder
    Lycopodium powder

Ointments and oils
    Calendula cream
    Tea tree oil (antibiotic, antifungal)
    Vitamins A and D ointment
    Liquid lecithin
    Lanolin
    Gentian violet (for yeast infection). Apply two times per day.
    Combine:
      3 parts castor oil
      1 part tea tree oil
      ½ part Peruvian balsam tincture
    Apply every 2 hours after a mild green soap wash.

Another approach is to powder by day and oil at night. A useful combination of powders includes:

Clay	4 parts
Zinc stearate	½ part
Peruvian balsam powder	½ part
Slippery elm powder	½ part

| Comfrey powder | ½ part |
| Calendula powder | ½ part |

Powder after each diaper change, at least every 2 hours. At night apply the above oil or calendula cream, liquid lecithin, or other water-repellent medicinal ointment.

A further useful approach is to apply liquid lecithin day and night every 2 to 4 hours.

A useful preventative (and part of many treatment regimens) is to wash the diaper region with dilute vinegar (1 to 2 tbs per quart of water). Repeat with each diaper change. Often this is the only treatment needed.*

OTHERS
Aloe
Cod-liver oil*
Vitamin E
Pokeroot *(Phytolacca)* ointment (for ringworm) (highly toxic, see p. 62)
Oil of evening primrose*
Tincture of green soap

BOTANICALS
External
Aloe *(Aloe vera)*
Calendula *(Calendula officinalis)*
Comfrey *(Symphytum officinale)*
Peruvian bark *(Cinchona* spp.): Combined with castor oil for ringworm
Pokeroot *(Phytolacca decandra)* (highly toxic; see p. 62)
Slippery elm *(Ulmus fulva)*
Tea tree oil

Therapeutic Suggestions

If the rash has a definite bacterial infection, begin therapy with a mild tincture of green soap wash, hydrogen peroxide rinse, and tea tree oil applications repeated every 2 to 3 hours for about 1 week to 14 days. I find this an effective procedure for use in bacterial and fungal rashes.

Mild, uncomplicated diaper rash usually responds to changes in mother's diet, or possibly a change of diaper type. (Some diaper service diapers are good to prevent rashes, while others cause diaper rashes; and some infants do better

---

*Asterisks indicate the most frequently used therapeutic agents.

with cloth diapers, others with disposable diapers.) I rarely use therapeutic supplements for infants with mild rashes; more prolonged or severe rashes may need them. Vitamin A, B complex, zinc, and essential fatty acids are often useful. The most useful powder and cream is calendula for mild rashes. A cod-liver oil and zinc oxide ointment such as Desitin is also useful. *Be sure to change diapers frequently.*

DIARRHEA

Definition and Symptoms

Frequent loose and watery stools with or without gas or abdominal discomfort.

Etiologic Considerations

Infant

- Overfeeding
- Allergy
- Mother's diet
- Bottle feeding (rare in breastfed infants)
- Teething
- Infection (viral or bacterial)
- Or other causes, as adult

Adult

- Food allergy
    Milk (lactose intolerance)
    Wheat (celiac disease, others)
- Gastritis, colitis
- Food poisoning
- Infection (viral or bacterial)
- Water supply
- Overeating
- Intestinal parasites
- Digestive enzyme deficiency
- Heavy metal poisoning

- Toxicity
- Stress, fear, emotional upset
- Pancreas, adrenal malfunction
- Anemia
- Excess vitamin C
- Antibiotic use

Discussion

Nearly every person will suffer an occasional bout of diarrhea. This may be due to gastric flu, mild food poisoning, or simply injudicious eating. These acute episodes are usually of short duration and are the result of the body's attempts at internal cleansing and purging. As such they should not be suppressed, but encouraged. If, however, a loose bowel condition becomes chronic, a serious problem exists. With each passing day of chronic diarrhea nutrients are lost in the stool, lowering general vitality and creating a vicious cycle of downgraded health.

It is extremely important to resolve acute diarrhea of infants as soon as possible, to prevent severe dehydration with catastrophic results. Episodes of infantile diarrhea occur much more frequently among bottle-fed babies, with gastroenteritis being a serious threat to the bottle-fed child under 6 months of age. Most children at some time will suffer periods of diarrhea with colds, gastric flu, or even teething. Many food sensitivities, intolerances, or allergies will first manifest themselves with bouts of diarrhea which may later become chronic, or paradoxically, disappear altogether if the condition is not attended to. In this case the more superficial reaction of loose bowels has been replaced by progressively deeper symptoms.

Breastfed infants may respond with diarrhea to foods in the mother's diet. Severe dehydration from violent or prolonged diarrhea (six or more watery stools a day in the absence of oral fluid intake) may occur rapidly in infancy or childhood. *These cases require hospitalization for intravenous replacement of fluids. Never attempt to treat severe diarrhea at home without medical supervision.*

Diarrhea occurring later in life may have many possible causes. Food allergy is one of the commonest factors, with gluten (see Celiac Disease) or lactose (milk sugar) intolerances being fairly common. Other foods may cause similar reactions. Gastritis and colitis are also a cause of loose bowels. Improper diet and stress are the usual factors involved in these cases. A digestive enzyme deficiency will cause food to pass undigested into the lower bowel, causing fermentation and diarrhea. This may be congenital or acquired, due to overeating, stress, glandular imbalance, or old age. Severe B complex deficiencies and anemia will also result in diarrhea. On the other hand, excess supplementation with vitamin C and sometimes zinc will cause intestinal irritation and diarrhea. Many cases of chronic bowel irritability can be traced to parasitic infection and is corrected once these are removed. Acute and chronic diarrhea is also frequently found to be caused by the water supply, especially in areas on water catchment systems. A history of previous antibiotic therapy just prior to the onset of diarrhea pinpoints this as a cause of altered internal ecology, a frequent cause of loose bowels.

Treatment

Obviously, the treatment chosen will depend on the type of diarrhea, acute or chronic, and its cause.

Acute diarrhea is an action by the body to reestablish internal equilibrium. This purging action is a self-defense mechanism to rid the body of unwanted and possibly dangerous material as rapidly as possible. This acute internal cleansing should never be suppressed. One of the oldest and most effective therapies for acute diarrhea is to fast and encourage further elimination with a purge and an enema. By fasting, the irritated digestive system is given a chance to rest and heal. Occasionally an enema may help flush the system rapidly. This should not be done if colitis is suspected. Diarrhea of infancy can be extremely dangerous. Any diarrhea in infants that does not clear in 24 hours should be seen by a physician.

Be sure enough fluids are taken to prevent dehydration. This is extremely important. Several foods and drinks have been found useful to control acute diarrhea after the initial fasting period of 1 to 3 days. These include the following:

Green apples (no skin)

Bananas (remove central vein of banana)

Carob powder (rich in pectin) and amaranth powder

Barley water

Carrot and cabbage juice

Carrot soup

Yoghurt

White toasted bread (this is an old treatment I found while reading the original works of Hippocrates). I have found it quite useful. Eat only well-toasted 100 percent *refined* white bread for 1 to 2 days. This is just about the *only* use I have ever found for white bread.

Slippery elm tea

Blackbery leaf tea or juice

Sauerkraut and tomato juice: 1 tbs of each every hour.

Acute diarrhea should not last longer than 2 to 3 days. If it is not getting better with only clear fluids at this time, it may be considered *chronic diarrhea*, which may be much more difficult to treat. The source of the loose bowel condition must be traced and eliminated. Refer to Colitis, Digestive Disturbances, Celiac Disease, or other related topics in this book. The following dietary suggestions may be useful in individual cases:

Green apple mono diet (no skin)
Bananas plus carob powder
Yoghurt
Yoghurt plus carob powder (equal portions)
Brown rice mono diet
Blackberry juice and gelatin

Therapeutic Agents

VITAMINS AND MINERALS

Vitamin A (micellized): 10,000 to 25,000 IU one to four times per day. *Use any dose of vitamin A over 50,000 IU per day with medical supervision only.*

Liquid B complex: 25 to 50 mg two times per day, plus B complex and B_{12} intramuscular injection one to three times per week. *

B_3 if long-term or pellagra-type syndrome exists.

OTHERS

Pancreatic enzymes: When chronic, due to digestive enzyme deficiency.

Bran: May aggravate acute cases or chronic cases due to irritable bowel or wheat intolerance; however, can be very beneficial in some chronic cases.

Roberts Formula (Naturopathic Formulations)

Lactobacillus: 1 tsp powder three to four times per day. Useful in correcting proper bowel ecology. Will aggravate cases due to dairy intolerance.

Mucovata (Seroyal): A useful bulking agent.

Pectin: A bulking agent, useful in most cases. The apple mono diet is high in pectin, and is the basis for its use.

Chlorophyll: To heal mucosa.

Garlic capsules for infective causes.

*Asterisks indicate the most frequently used therapeutic agents.

DRINKS

Distilled water: Water is always the best for short duration cases where fluid loss has not been too severe, resulting in extreme electrolyte loss.*

Carrot juice and cabbage juice

Peppermint tea

Chamomile tea

Slippery elm tea

Blackberry juice or tea

Raspberry leaf tea and cinnamon (or oak if severe); ½ tsp four to six times per day for patient under 1 year.

Barley water

BOTANICALS

Amaranth (*Amaranthus hypochondriacus*): Astringent.

Blackberry tea (*Rubus* spp.): 3 to 4 cups per day; astringent.*

Cinnamon (*Cinnamomum zeylanicum*): Astringent, hemostatic. Use strong tea, four to six times per day, or 10 to 30 drops tincture in warm water.

Oak bark tea (*Quercus*): Astringent.

Peppermint essence (*Mentha piperita*): 3 to 15 drops every 2 to 3 hours.*

Raspberry juice (*Rubus villosus*)*

Spotted cranebill (*Geranium maculatum*): Used especially with blood loss (*note: blood loss could be an indication of a serious problem and anyone with this symptom should always be seen by a doctor*).

Tormentil (*Potentilla tormentilla*)

Witch hazel (*Hamamelis virginiana*): Astringent; used as dilute retention enema.

Therapeutic Suggestions

Be careful not to give too many medications and thus further irritate the condition. Keep therapy simple whenever possible. Use all supplements with caution in this and other irritable bowel complaints. The best therapy is a water fast for 1 to 3 days for both acute and chronic cases. Chronic cases require intramuscular vitamin injections and the use of botanicals. Diarrhea due to parasites may be best treated with orthodox measures.

*Asterisks indicate the most frequently used therapeutic agents.

DIGESTIVE DISORDERS (Gastritis, Heartburn, Indigestion)

Definition and Symptoms

Acute or chronic abdominal discomfort, pain, irritation, bloating or gas, often accompanied by general malaise, headache, nausea, and sometimes vomiting.

Etiologic Considerations

* Improper diet
    Refined carbohydrates and sugar
    Poor food combinations
    Overeating
    Insufficient chewing of foods
    Hurried meals
    Too-frequent meals (snacking)
    Strong spices; salt
    Coffee, tea, alcohol, carbonated beverages
    Drinking with meals
    Acid-forming foods
    Excessively hot or cold foods
    Food additives, preservatives, colorings
    Food allergy or digestive incompatibility (milk, wheat, etc.)
* Digestive enzyme deficiency
    Hydrochloric acid deficiency common in older age groups
* Constipation
* Cigarettes
* *Candida albicans* overgrowth
* Bacterial overgrowth
* Drugs
    Aspirin and others
* Spinal lesions
* Stress

- Psychological
- Heavy metals
  Aluminum cookware
  Water catchment systems
- Obesity
- Pregnancy
- Hiatal hernia
- Gallbladder disease
- Hypothyroidism (hydrochloric acid deficiency associated)
- Liver disease
- Ulcer
- Lack of exercise

Discussion

Indigestion, heartburn, and gastritis are not really diseases in themselves, but are symptoms of abnormal digestion. The usual treatment for these common problems is the prescription of antacid medications aimed at removing the unpleasant symptoms without attempting in any way to treat the cause. Sodium bicarbonate preparations are the most frequently used antacids. This rapidly neutralizes gastric acid and will relieve heartburn caused by excess acid. Used on a regular basis, however, it disturbs the body's acid/alkaline balance, creating a condition of alkalosis. Sustained alkalosis with a substantial intake of calcium in the form of milk or calcium-containing antacids creates milk-alkali syndrome, causing irreversible kidney damage. Clearly this "cure" is not as benign as the commercials would have us believe.

The real causes of these digestive disorders are usually very simple to diagnose and treat. The largest number of factors, obviously, center around diet. I am constantly amazed at the incredible combinations some people cram into their mouths. I begin the treatment of all digestive complaints by asking the patient to compile a list of everything he or she eats—solid or liquid—for a 3-day period. The results are usually quite revealing.

Following is a summary of the most common dietary mistakes:

Consumption of refined carbohydrates (especially sugar): Refined carbohydrates cause a rapid secretion of gastric acid. This acid is normally buffered by the protein content of a food substance. In this case the bran and fiber have been removed through the refining process, with the end result being excess gastric acidity. Sugar is the worst offender in this class since it is devoid of any real substances whatsoever for the acid stimulated to work upon. (For more detail see Peptic Ulcer.)

Poor food combinations: The average person pays absolutely no attention to proper food combinations. Often a meal will consist of raw fruit, cooked fruit, raw vegetables, cooked vegetables, soups, several types of protein, starch, coffee, alcohol, and sweets. Indigestion, here we come! Always keep meals simple and never combine:

> Fruit with vegetables
> Fruit (especially citrus) with starches
> Liquids with solids

(*Note:* Some nutritional advisers warn against eating starches with proteins due to their different requirements for digestion. This, however, does not seem logically possible since many foods are composed of a large percent of starch *and* protein. With specific reference to concentrated starches and concentrated protein, Airola suggests in *How To Get Well* and *Everywoman's Book* to eat proteins first. This allows for their normal exposure to the stomach's hydrochloric acid, which is essential in protein digestion, but not that of carbohydrate. The average healthy stomach, however, can ignore this rule.)

Excessively large meals: When the stomach is overloaded the amount needed to be digested can exceed the body's supply of digestive enzymes. Food then passes into the lower small intestine, is only partly broken down, and causes fermentation, indigestion, and gas. Never eat until completely full.

Too-frequent meals: If food is eaten too soon after a previous meal its normal digestive process is disturbed. It is usually best to allow at least 1½ hours after a fruit meal, 2 to 2½ hours after a vegetable meal, and 3¼ to 4 hours after a combined meal with proteins, carbohydrates, and fat. Be especially careful to allow complete digestion of a starchy meal before having any fruit, especially citrus.

Insufficient chewing of foods: The digestive enzyme salivary amylase (ptyalin) initiates carbohydrate digestion of starch in the mouth and continues to act for 20 to 30 minutes in the stomach before it is inactivated by gastric acid production. Chewing stimulates salivary amylase secretions, breaks food down into smaller particles for more complete exposure for enzymatic digestion, and also stimulates secretion of digestive enzymes in the stomach, pancreas, and small intestine for further digestion. Chewing is especially essential to break down the indigestible walls of cellulose found in all vegetables, to expose their inner food substances to digestive juices. The habit of bolting down food in hurried meals is a major cause of indigestion.

Drinking with meals: Any liquids taken with solid meals dilute the action of digestive juices, making complete digestion more difficult. This applies to any drinks, even soup. These should be taken at least 15 minutes before other foods are eaten and not sooner than ½ hour afterwards.

The use of strong spices or other gastric irritants: Salt is the most common irritant to the stomach. It causes extreme acidity and irritates the delicate mucous membranes. Other irritants include sugar, pepper, curries, coffee, soda, and alcohol.

Excess acid-forming foods: The overconsumption of refined carbohydrates, sugar, and other acid-forming foods is a common finding. Green vegetables are the best alkaline elements for proper pH balancing.

Excessively hot or cold foods: These irritate the delicate stomach linings which cannot cry out with pain since they have little sensation of temperature. This is why food that burns your mouth or esophagus no longer hurts once it reaches the stomach. If done repeatedly the stomach becomes deranged and poor digestion results.

Eating while under stress: When food is eaten under stressful conditions, or when anxiety, anger, or other similar emotions are present, digestion is severely disturbed. The emotions cause the parasympathetic branch of the nervous system, responsible for normal digestive enzyme secretion and gastric motility, to cease functioning so that the sympathetic branch of the nervous system may prepare for what it interprets as an emergency situation. Always spend 10 to 15 minutes in some quiet, soothing activity before meals. Prayer or a few minutes of meditation before meals is also advisable.

Eating when sick: All animals fast during an illness. This is nature's law and should be followed.

Fried foods: Deep frying makes any food difficult to digest and may be a factor in the high incidence of stomach cancer in civilized nations.

Although disregard of the above rules of eating are the major causes of indigestion, other factors may exist.

Food allergy is a fairly common cause of digestive upset. Milk and wheat are the two most frequent offenders, but any food may be at fault. This disturbance may be caused by a true allergy or simply a food intolerance due to a specific digestive enzyme deficiency such as the lactase deficiency of milk intolerance.

Other digestive enzyme deficiencies can cause gastric disturbances in the digestion of carbohydrates, proteins, or fat. These may be associated with a disorder of the pancreas, liver, or gallbladder. *Hydrochloric acid deficiency* is a common problem (especially in the over-50 age group) causing gas, bloating, poor protein digestion, and chronic malabsorption of most minerals and some vitamins. Although we frequently associate hyperacidity with heartburn symptoms, hypoacidity is a much more common cause of this condition. Hydrochloric acid deficiency is also associated with many other digestive complaints, as well as with hypothyroidism, asthma, allergies, rheumatoid arthritis, osteoporosis, lupus, pernicious anemia, diabetes, systemic candidiasis, chronic hepatitis, intestinal parasites, eczema, vitiligo, and others. Milk consumption is a common cause or aggravating factor in many cases, since it takes so much hydrochloric acid to acidify milk, leaving little or no reserve for other protein in the meal. The result is incomplete breakdown of protein, causing gas, bloating, and such other more systemic problems as allergy.

Emotional causes of indigestion are also fairly common. As discussed above, stress and other destructive emotions upset the normal digestive cycle, making even the best of food indigestible. Prolonged stress, anger, or worry also create an acidic condition of the entire body.

Spinal lesions in the thoracic region can alter the nerve and blood supply to the stomach or other organs of digestion, making normal function impossible. This area should always be treated in cases of chronic indigestion.

Heavy metal poisoning may be a factor in some cases. Certainly the use of aluminum cookware is to be avoided, especially if indigestion is a problem. Many other heavy metals may produce the same effects (see Heavy Metals).

Some indigestion during pregnancy is normal. This may be minimized by proper diet with plenty of alkaline foods such as vegetables and proper exercise. Avoid large meals if this is a problem, in preference to four to six smaller ones.

Treatment

Diet

For acute or chronic indigestion the first course of action is always to fast. Any of the following fasts are used with this complaint:

Water with a twist of lemon
Dilute apple juice
Carrot juice
Carrot and cabbage juice
Slippery elm tea

These may be followed by a mono diet regimen such as:

Apple mono diet
Carrot mono diet
Brown rice diet

In severe cases strict regimens similar to those found under Colitis or Peptic Ulcer are needed.

In cases where *Candida albicans* overgrowth is suspected from the case history and symptomatology (gas, bloating, rectal itching, ear itching, vaginitis, constipation, diarrhea, nail bed fungus, infantile colic, depression, fatigue, skin rashes, allergies, psoriasis, autoimmune diseases, antibiotic use, and birth control pill use) the dietary regimen and supplement plan are a bit different. The emphasis still is to avoid refined carbohydrates and excess fruit or fruit juice, since yeast grow best in a highly refined carbohydrate diet. A yeast-free diet is also recommended, even though the yeast in foods is a different type of yeast than *Candida*. A significant proportion of patients report aggravation of a yeast infection upon consumption of yeasted foods. Yeast-free vitamin supplements are to be used as well. The main portion of the diet should be vegetables and proteins. Nonglutinous grains (such as rice, millet, or corn) seem to be better tolerated during the regimen. Garlic is useful, in the diet and in supplement form. Acidophilus in the form of yoghurt or in supplement form (superdophilus or megadophilus) is beneficial when taken several times each day. Used to inhibit yeast growth are biotin, garlic, caprillic acid, aloe vera juice, olive oil, and the anti-yeast herb taheebo. Many cases require nystatin for 2 to 6 months. However, with a change of bowel ecology from proper diet, and possibly hydrochloric acid supplementation (yeast grows poorly with adequate hydrochloric acid secretions), this may sometimes be avoided, but the treatment program is prolonged, and the diet must be adhered to rigidly.

Therapeutic Agents

VITAMINS AND MINERALS

Vitamin A: 10,000 to 25,000 IU one to two times per day. *Use any dose of vitamin A over 50,000 IU per day with medical supervision only.* *

Vitamin B complex (liquid): 25 to 50 mg one to two times per day.*

Vitamin B$_{12}$ (may require intramuscular injection if hypoacidity is a problem).*

Folic acid*

Vitamin C: Sodium ascorbate if hyperacid; ascorbic acid if hypoacid.

Vitamin E: 400 IU two times per day.*

OTHER

Bromelain enzyme*

Charcoal tablets: 1 every 1 to 2 hours in acute cases.

Pancreatic digestive enzymes*

*Asterisks indicate the most frequently used therapeutic agents.

Aloe vera juice: 2 oz three times per day.*

Mucovata (Seroyal) bulking agent

Fiber

Hydrochloric acid: If hypoacid. Capsules work best when 20 to 40 grains are taken before meals as the adult dose, 10 to 20 grains for children. If this causes discomfort, begin with a 5-to-10-grain dose and increase after 3 to 5 days. Some cases need very slow acid increase and may require the gradual introduction of lemon juice and water (1 to 8 oz), gradually increasing to a 50/50 mixture, to accustom the stomach to acid before hydrochloric acid capsule supplementation.

Kelp*

Lactobacillus or acidophilus: To normalize bowel ecology.*

Lemon juice

Papaya enzyme

Pepsin

Sodium alginate*

Soured milk or yoghurt

BOTANICALS

Angelica *(Angelica archangelica)*

Anise *(Pimpinella anixum)*

Chamomile *(Anthemis nobilis)*

Comfrey *(Symphytum officinale)*

Dandelion *(Taraxacum officinale)*

Fennel *(Foeniculum vulgare)*

Ginger root *(Zingiber officinale)*

Goldenseal *(Hydrastis canadensis)*

Peppermint *(Mentha piperita)*

Slippery elm *(Ulmus fulva)**

Therapeutic Suggestions

Begin therapy with fast and diet changes. Only use supplements and botanicals later if still required. Often, they are not.

*Asterisks indicate the most frequently used therapeutic agents.

DIVERTICULITIS AND DIVERTICULOSIS

Definition

Diverticula:　Spherical pouches protruding from the lumen of the intestine through the bowel wall. Most commonly found in the sigmoid colon.
Diverticulosis:　Uncomplicated diverticula.
Diverticulitis:　Diverticula with inflammation present.

Symptoms

Diverticulosis often causes no symptoms or may cause irritable colon symptoms (may be coincident).
Diverticulitis:　Symptoms of "left-sided appendicitis."

Pain in lower left quadrant.
Nausea, vomiting, abdominal distension, colic.
Constipation and/or diarrhea (may alternate).
Tenderness, fever if infection is present.

Etiologic Considerations

* Fiber deficiency: Refined diet, white bread, white rice.
* Nutritional deficiency: Muscular weakness in intestinal wall.
* Constipation
* Obesity
* Visceroptosis: Poor abdominal tone, prolapse, poor spinal mechanics.
* Spinal: Poor abdominal circulation of blood and lymph.
* Stress: Reduced peristalsis
* Poor bowel habits
* Thyroid deficiency
* Adhesions due to previous appendectomy
* Spastic colon
* Allergy (especially to dairy products)

Discussion

Diverticulitis is another of the "civilized diseases." While 30 percent of Americans over 45 suffer the discomfort of diverticular disease, it is extremely rare in undeveloped nations living on a diet of unrefined foods. It has become increasingly obvious that our low-fiber diet of highly refined foods is the major cause of diverticulitis and colon cancer.

Diverticulitis occurs when the neck of the diverticulum becomes blocked by swelling or feces. This causes a condition of stasis which favors bacterial invasion. An abscess may form and spasm may result in intestinal destruction. This in itself may require surgery. Perforation of the abscess may also occur, leading to peritonitis, a severe surgical emergency. Healing of any of these complications may result in fibrosis and narrowing of the colon. This in turn may later require surgery. As you can see, prevention in this case is much better than cure.

Diverticula become filled with bacteria in many cases and these consume a large amount of B vitamins. Occult blood loss also may occur, explaining the commonly associated condition of anemia found so often in diverticular patients.

Clearly, since a lack of fiber is the major cause, the commonly employed low-fiber diet is not the best cure. Lack of fiber in the diet causes chronic poor eliminations and constipation. This constipation in turn causes an increase in the gas pressure against the colon walls. To make the situation even more conducive to diverticula formation, the low-residue, low-fiber diet takes two to three times as long to pass through the colon. This encourages excessive water absorption and leaves a very concentrated small stool, which is very difficult to expel and demands more forceful peristaltic contraction to move it along its course. The excess work puts increased pressure on the colon walls, helping to produce outpouchings of diverticula.

A high-fiber diet composed of unrefined grains, raw fruits, and vegetables helps prevent diverticular disease and favors proper intestinal action in several ways. On such a diet the stools are two to three times as bulky as those formed on a low-fiber diet. The fiber absorbs water, making a softer stool that is passed easily with less forceful peristaltic contractions. Transit time is also reduced, with an average of 12 to 24 hours as compared to 36 hours (or significantly longer) on a low-residue diet.

Contrary to the situation with a low-fiber diet where the excess abnormal bacteria produce harmful carcinogenic substances from normal bile acids, cellulose actually encourages friendly bacterial development, which in turn produces several of the B complex vitamins for use by the body. In addition, while a low-fiber diet with its sticky feces tends to cake the intestinal membrane, fiber will help clean these walls and stimulate local circulation.

Treatment

While a low-fiber diet is the major cause of diverticular disease, often the initial stages of treatment do require adherence to a low-fiber diet. This, however, is of short duration, lasting only as long as it is necessary to be able to reduce local irritation. Once the inflammatory stage of diverticulitis is under control, the gradual introduction of high-fiber foods is essential to reach maximum results.

Diet—Acute

Choose from any of the following, consuming only one type of liquid at any single meal:

Water (best fast, but most difficult)

Carrot juice

Carrot and lettuce juice

Celery and lettuce juice

Beet root juice

Watercress juice

Grape juice

Apple juice

Slippery elm tea *(Ulmus fulva)*

Comfrey tea *(Symphytum officinale)*

Marshmallow tea *(Althaea officinale)*

Chlorophyll liquid

Spirulina liquid drinks

This liquid diet (fast) should be continued until all painful symptoms have subsided. At this point semisolids may be added slowly and carefully, watching for any adverse reaction. Add papaya, mashed banana, steamed carrots, baked yams, or sweet potatoes.

Once it becomes apparent that these foods are well tolerated, other cooked and puréed foods of higher fiber content may be added. Some people at this stage can handle grated raw foods. Begin with raw grated apple and raw grated carrot. It still will be necessary to avoid fruit skins and fruit, and fruit and vegetables with small hard seeds such as tomatoes, cucumbers, figs, strawberries, raspberries, guavas, etc.

The next stage includes addition of grains and proteins. Brown rice well cooked and well masticated is a good initial choice of grains. Tofu and steamed fish are good proteins. Once these are well tolerated the diet can rapidly be expanded to include all natural unrefined food. Thorough mastication is absolutely essential in the initial stages of this diet.

Most patients can be weaned to a high-fiber diet fully in 6 to 8 weeks. This diet will then help heal the intestinal walls and prevent further severe attacks of diverticulitis. In long-standing cases the diverticula may remain, as shown by x-ray, for years. Others simply never go away. Most cases, however, remain symptom-free irrespective of the presence of old diverticula as long as the high-fiber diet is adhered to and bowel eliminations remain regular.

Physiotherapy—Acute

- Castor oil packs (see Appendix I).
- Alternate hot and cold sitz baths are very beneficial for long-term cure.
- Cold trunk packs for tonic effects.
- Hot moist compress for pain relief.
- Hot sitz bath for pain relief.

Spinal Manipulation

Two times per week for 3 to 4 weeks; 2 weeks off, then repeat three times or as required.

Therapeutic Agents

VITAMINS AND MINERALS

Vitamin A: 10,000 to 25,000 IU two to six times per day in acute cases; for maintenance one to two times per day. *Use any dose of vitamin A over 50,000 IU per day with medical supervision only.**

Vitamin B complex: 25 to 50 mg one to three times. A good *liquid* B complex may be best in these conditions.*

Vitamin E: 400 to 800 IU per day.*

Vitamin C: 250 to 1000 mg two to six times per day.*

OTHER

Atomodine, at doctor's prescription:*
    1 drop for 7 days; 5 days off
    2 drops for 7 days; 5 days off
    3 drops for 7 days; 5 days off (repeat two to three times)

Bran flakes three times per day (8 to 10 tsp each day). (Do not use with wheat sensitivity.) Helps normalize bowel function and therefore establish more normal bowel ecology.*

*Asterisks indicate the most frequently used therapeutic agents.

Pancreatic enzymes: With meals where digestive enzyme deficiency exists.

Garlic

Hydrochloric acid: If hypoacid.

Lactobacillus capsules: 2 capsules three times per day. Helps correct bowel ecology.

Liquid chlorophyll

Molasses: Helps correct bowel function.

Molasses, mashed banana, and low-fat yoghurt.

Mucozyme (Nutridyne): 2, three times per day.*

Raw, unprocessed, finely milled bran and soaked prunes.

BOTANICALS

Comfrey *(Symphytum officinale)* with slippery elm as a warm tea, three to four times per day.*

Marshmallow *(Althaea officinalis)*

Slippery elm *(Ulmus fulva)*: ½ tsp in warm water three to four times per day. Demulcent; soothes mucous membranes.*

Wild yam root *(Dioscorea villosa)*: For colic.

Therapeutic Suggestions

In general, the diet change is 90 percent of the solution. Bran helps add fiber and speeds up normal bowel function. Stick to the high-fiber approach even with 7 to 10 days of gas or discomfort. Your body is readjusting. Add supplements later in the regimen. Mild botanicals such as slippery elm may be taken early on without aggravation. The daily consumption of six to eight large glasses of water is a very useful aid to proper bowel function, especially in conjunction with the bran.

DROPSY (see Edema)

DUODENAL ULCER (see Peptic Ulcer)

*Asterisks indicate the most frequently used therapeutic agents.

EARACHE: Otitis Externa and Otitis Media

Definition

Otitis externa: Inflammation and infection of external ear.
Otitis media: Inflammation, infection, or serous congestion of middle ear.

Symptoms

Infective:
  Pain
  Fever
  Throbbing
  Discharge

Serous:
  Feeling of fullness
  Loss of hearing acuity
  Little or no pain
  Ringing in ears

Etiologic Considerations

- Lowered immunity
    Diet
    Stress

- Allergy
    Cow's milk
    Wheat
    Other

- Excess mucus-forming foods

- Green vegetable deficiency

- Refined diet

- Excess sugar

- Preceding infection
    Colds
    Measles
    Mumps
    Pneumonia
    Tonsilitis, etc.

Enlarged adenoids (common before puberty)
Localized boil, external

- Improper treatment of acute disease

- Bacterial infected swimming water

- Excess earwax
EFA deficiency

- Impacted wax
"Q-tip syndrome"

- Forceful cleaning of nose

- Breastfeeding while lying down

Discussion

Ear infections affect most people at some time in their lives, usually following an upper respiratory infection. They are often the result of blocked eustachian tubes, which allow mucus to accumulate within the ear, acting as a medium for bacterial proliferation. Infants are particularly susceptible to this problem and may develop an ear infection with nearly any viral or bacterial upper respiratory infection. Other less commonly related agents are allergies, nursing while lying down, and second-hand smoke. I have found that many chronic or recurrent middle ear infections have a nutritional basis.

The average case presents with a diet high in refined mucus-forming foods and a deficiency of raw green vegetables. This is certainly true with children. Allergy often is related—not the type most doctors blame (dust, molds, grasses, etc.) but *food* allergies. Dairy and wheat allergies or excess are often a factor with ear problems.

Chronically enlarged adenoids may cause blockage of the eustachian tubes, leading to congestion and fluid exudation into the middle ear, creating serous otitis media, which may remain uninfected, or act as an ideal medium for bacterial proliferation. Although the adenoids are the immediate and obvious cause of eustachian tube blockage and therefore ear congestion, the enlarged adenoids, which you cannot see without special equipment, are in reality only *symptoms* of a deeper disorder. Tonsils or adenoids do not enlarge without a cause, and it is in correcting the conditions that led to their enlargement that a true cure may be found (see Tonsillitis).

Another aspect of improper diet directly related to recurrent infections is decreased immunity. If the diet does not supply essential nutrients for the immunological system, or if stress depletes the body's vital reserves, resistance to infection is reduced. The body is then very susceptible to colds, flu, tonsillitis, and other acute diseases, which may eventually affect the ears. Once a weakness is established in the ears due to damage from an infection, it makes recurrent infections more likely.

External ear infections are generally less obviously related to diet and nutrition, and more readily influenced by changes in the local environment of the external ear. "Swimmer's ear" is a common disorder caused by repeatedly wetting and softening the earwax, which then becomes an ideal medium for bacterial development. This is very common where the swimming water is stagnant or polluted. There is a local thermal swimming pool near where I live commonly called "hot pond," but which I refer to as the "staph pond" since such a large number of people get ear or skin infections after they swim in its stagnant waters. Most communities have similar areas.

The people most often affected by external ear infections are heavy wax producers. This seems to be at least partly related to diet and it is the proportion of saturated vs. unsaturated fats that are implicated. To reverse the tendency to produce excess wax I advise restricting saturated fats and taking daily doses of essential fatty acids in capsule or liquid form.

It is crucial to begin treatment for all ear infections at the very first sign of a problem. If you are attentive to the early signs or sensations that indicate infection (fullness in the ear, loss of hearing, pressure or mild pain, or the inability to clear your ears), it is possible to treat many of these problems with natural means. Once the infection has progressed to acute pain, it is very likely that you will require antibiotics. Whenever you have an upper respiratory infection, it is essential to begin a mucus-cleansing diet immediately, and to make certain that your ears can be cleared frequently, especially after blowing your nose.

Treatment

Diet

Minor ear congestion or infection may benefit by the mucus-cleansing diet detailed under Asthma.

Recurrent cases of infective or serous otitis media require a diet very high in raw vegetables, with little or no starch or dairy products. This should be combined with intermittent periods of 3 days on the mucus-cleansing diet. Similar regimens to those found under Asthma and Tonsillitis will be useful.

Physiotherapy

Local applications

• Mullein essence:* This is the most effective application for all ear infections.

*Asterisks indicate the most frequently used therapeutic agents.

Apply 6 to 10 drops in affected ear three to four times per day and insert cotton. It will relieve pain almost instantly and is anti-infective. Mullein oil preparations are better where fungus is a factor.

- Garlic oil and propolis ear drops

- Garlic foot compress (see Appendix I): Very useful for children who refuse or cannot adhere to a mucus-cleansing diet.

- Probe palatal end of eustacian tube with index finger. Apply *Hydrastis* tincture or olbas oil to this area with tip of finger.

- Onion poultice (raw or cooked), plus heat. Apply to ear.

- Chamomile, hops, and lobelia fomentation, plus heat (for pain).

- Botanical ear oil: 1 part lobelia, 1 part myrrh, 1 part mullein, ½ part sassafras, ½ part hemlock, 4 parts olive oil. 4 drops in ear three times per day.

- Hydrogen peroxide plus oils; then ear lavage; for excess wax.

- 70% isopropyl alcohol: 1 drop in ear following swim, to prevent infection.

- Hot compresses for acute pain

- Alternate hot and cold compresses for chronic pain

Therapeutic Agents

VITAMINS AND MINERALS

Vitamin A: 10,000 to 25,000 IU three to four times per day for acute cases; two times per day for chronic cases. *Use any dose of vitamin A over 50,000 IU per day with medical supervision only.* *

Vitamin B complex: 25 to 50 mg two times per day.

Vitamin C: 500 to 1000 mg up to every hour.*

Zinc: 15 to 30 mg two times per day.*

EFA and EPA: For chronically hardened earwax.

OTHERS

Garlic: 2 capsules three times per day.*

Thymus: 1 to 2 per hour in acute; 2 three times per day in chronic.*

Sour apples: Serous otitis.

*Asterisks indicate the most frequently used therapeutic agents.

BOTANICALS

Mullein *(Verbascum thapsus)*: Antibacterial. 4 to 6 drops in ear four times per day.*

Therapeutic Suggestion

In my experience most acute earaches are immediately helped by mullein essence, 4 to 6 drops four times per day in the affected ear. This will give nearly *instant* pain relief, and is effective against both external and middle ear infections. This should always be accompanied by the mucus-cleansing diet (onions) and plenty of carrot juice, raw green apples, garlic, vitamins A and C, zinc, and thymus.

Chronic ear infections may be very obstinate. A trial of nutritional therapy is suggested prior to allowing tubes to be placed in the ears. This is a last resort.

EDEMA

Definition

Excess fluid retention locally or systemically.

Symptoms

Swelling of hands, ankles, feet, face, abdomen, or other areas of the body. Premenstrual syndrome, headaches, leg ulcers.

Etiologic Considerations

- Congestive heart failure
- Kidney disease
- Poor circulation
- Severe protein deficiency
- Anemia
- Adrenal malfunction
- Liver disease
- Hypothyroidism
- Premenstrual

*Asterisks indicate the most frequently used therapeutic agents.

- Pregnancy
    Physiological
    Toxemia
- Diet
    Excess salt, meats, dried fish
- Potassium deficiency
- Varicose veins
- Vitamin B complex deficiency
- Vitamin B_1 or B_3 deficiency
- Vitamin B_6 (premenstrual fluid retention)
- Oral contraceptives
- Drugs
    Steroids
- Sprain
- Obesity
- Constipation
- Allergy
- Lack of exercise

Discussion

Edema may be a symptom of an extremely severe internal disorder. At the first onset of unusual fluid retention, a complete physical examination is suggested. Once serious problems such as congestive heart disease, kidney disease, or liver disease are ruled out, more subtle causes may be safely dealt with.

Severe anemia and protein deficiency are rarely a cause of edema, except under extreme conditions. The only such case I personally have seen was a young lady of 22 who followed a strict fruit and raw vegetable diet for 14 months. She consulted us not for her lack of energy, cardiac irregularity, emaciation (69 lb), or hair loss, but because she was now having difficulty in getting her shoes on over her extremely swollen feet. I was shocked to find how ill-informed she was regarding general nutrition. She was actually surprised that her various symptoms were due directly to her no-protein diet. I explained that she was 2 to 3 months from death due to liver, kidney, and heart failure and placed her on a new diet *with* protein. Within 4 weeks her edema was almost completely gone. I emphasize this case since it clearly demonstrates the lack of knowledge that some people show in relation to their health. She had read somewhere that protein was harmful to the body, causing all kinds of poisons to accumulate and lead to disease. She had further read of people living for long periods on all-fruit or all-fruit-and-vegetable diets to cleanse themselves and increase their vitality. I hope her case makes clear that these diets are for *short-term use only*, and are not intended for people to live on indefinitely.

Other more common causes of edema are related to the menstrual cycle. Premenstrual edema is extremely common and is dealt with in detail under Premenstrual Tension Syndrome. The use of birth control pills has also been found to cause fluid retention. The pill severely depletes many of the B complex group, especially vitamin B_6, which is given with great success as therapy for many cases of edema. Fluid retention during pregnancy also occurs in many women. This can be due to an increase by 50 percent of the blood volume during pregnancy, pressure exerted by the fetus which restricts venous return from the legs, or constipation, which also may restrict blood flow. Obesity during pregnancy exaggerates these effects. Toxemia of pregnancy is also characterized by edema.

Diet may also play a role in fluid retention. The habitual consumption of excess salt as a condiment or salt-containing foods such as dried meats, fish, and pickles, and canned and restaurant foods (especially Chinese) upsets the body's fluid equilibrium, favoring fluid retention. Potassium deficiency will act in the same manner. This can really be a problem with older people who consume vast amounts of salt (salt taste dulls over a period of years, requiring more and more to be used). These people also tend to eat less potassium-containing vegetables due to denture problems, get much less exercise, and sit for prolonged periods of time. Each of these factors plays a part, along with the general tendency toward reduced heart and kidney function, to produce the common edema of old age.

It is important to remember that edema may be the body's response to internal toxins which it attempts to dilute.

Treatment

The common treatment for edema is the use of powerful diuretic drugs that help get rid of accumulated fluids. This only treats the symptom without attempting to find or correct the cause. Not only is fluid excreted, but many vitamins and minerals are lost, causing generalized weakness, mental dullness, and reduced vitality. The only cure for edema is finding and removing the cause. For edema of heart, kidney, or liver origin, consult those chapters for detailed treatment. The therapy given below is fairly generalized to help as many with edema as possible. Many cases of edema are serious and are best treated in conjunction with a sympathetic physician.

Diet

Nearly any fluid retention problem can be benefited by a vegetable and fruit juice fast emphasizing vegetables, as carrot or carrot and beet juice. This may be continued anywhere from 3 to 21 days with supervision. Another useful regimen is the all-watermelon diet for 2 to 3 days.

Follow this regimen with an all raw foods diet with plenty of raw green vegetables. A good salt-free lacto-vegetarian diet should then be followed until complete cure is established. Absolutely no animal proteins other than fermented dairy products (yoghurt, kefir) are allowed. (*Note:* This diet does not apply to edema due to anemia. See Anemia if this is the main cause.)

Physiotherapy

- Slowly increase general exercise
- Hourly leg and calf exercise
- Alternate hot and cold sitz baths*
- Alternate hot and cold leg sprays
- Alternate hot and cold hip sprays
- Alternate hot and cold showers
- Sauna (if no contraindication) to induce perspiration

Therapeutic Agents

VITAMINS AND MINERALS

Vitamin A: 25,000 IU one to two times per day. *Use any dose of vitamin A over 50,000 IU per day with medical supervision only.*

Vitamin B_3: 50 to 400 mg one to two times per day.

Vitamin B_6: 50 to 250 mg one to two times per day; diuretic.*

Vitamin B complex: 25 to 50 mg one to three times per day.*

Vitamin C: 500 to 1000 mg three to six times per day.

Bioflavonoids: Reduce capillary permeability.*

Vitamin E: 400 IU one to two times per day.*

Potassium*

Apis (*Apis mellifera*) homeopathic dose: For edema due to stings or swelling similar to this clinical picture (i.e., trauma).

BOTANICALS

Aphanes (*Aphanes arvensis*): Edema of kidney or liver origin.

*Asterisks indicate the most frequently used therapeutic agents.

Broom tops (*Cytisus scoparius*) and lily-of-the-valley (*Convallaria majalis*): With weakened heart.

Buchu (*Barosma betulina*): Diuretic.

Cactus (*Cactus grandiflorus*): Edema of heart origin.

Cleavers (*Galium aparine*): Diuretic.

Cola syrup (Cayce): Kidney origin.

Dogbane (*Apocynum androsaemifolium*): Edema of heart origin.

Hawthorn berries (*Crataegus oxyacantha*): Edema of heart origin. Dose: 10 to 20 drops tincture three to four times per day.

Juniper berries (*Juniperus communis*): Diuretic.

Lily-of-the-valley (*Convallaria majalis*): Edema of heart origin.

Pareira root (*Chondrodendron tomentosum*): Edema of kidney origin.

Parsley (*Petroselinum sativum*): Diuretic.

Pipsissewa (*Chimaphila umbellata*) and poplar bark (*Populus tremuloides*)

Wahoo (*Euonymus atropurpureus*): Edema from convalescence.

Watermelon seed (*Citrullus vulgaris*): Diuretic. Use infusion of dried seeds.

EMPHYSEMA

Definition

A degenerative disease of the lungs characterized by enlargement, distension, and destruction of the alveolar spaces.

Symptoms

Wheezing, chronic nonproductive cough, expectoration, shortness of breath, foul breath, cyanosis, and difficulty in exhalation.

Etiologic Considerations

- Cigarettes
- Diet
  Excess refined carbohydrates
  Excess dairy products
  Deficiency
  Allergy

- Pollution
    Smog
    Radioactivity (nuclear)
- Cadmium exposure
    Industrial
    Auto exhaust
    Cigarettes
    Galvanized pipes
- Occupational
    Glassblower's lung
    Metal worker's lung
    Miner's lung
    Others
- Poor body mechanics
- Spinal
- Lack of exercise
- Poor circulation
- Obesity
- Toxicity
- Poor eliminations

Discussion

Emphysema literally means "inflation," which accurately describes the condition of the small air exchange sacs (alveoli) in the lungs which become over-distended, filled with mucus, and inelastic. This destruction of the alveoli reduces the effective oxygen exchange surface of the lung, so that the victim is in a state of slow suffocation. This general lack of oxygen and consequent increase in carbon dioxide within the system causes the patient to breathe more rapidly. Due to loss of tissue elasticity in the lungs, air is difficult to expel, leaving the patient with expanded chest and great difficulty in exhaling. As the air sacs break down, mucus accumulates, which further reduces the active oxygen exchange surface. The cough reflex is stimulated but is not efficient enough to remove mucus from the lower parts of the lung. The small cilia, whose job it usually is to waft mucus toward the throat to be expelled, have also been destroyed, in most cases by smoking, and so do not function. The result is extremely difficult breathing, chronic cough, and inability to perform even mild tasks. Over time this progressive degeneration may lead to lung infection, high blood pressure, enlargement of the heart, and heart failure.

Emphysema is commonly associated with bronchial asthma and chronic bronchitis, and often follows a history of either. In general, the same factors are responsible for all these conditions, with special importance being placed on one or another aspect, depending on the condition.

Cigarette smoking is more related to chronic bronchitis and emphysema than it is to asthma, which often has more of an allergic or psychological basis. Certainly, cigarette smoking is central to most cases of emphysema, unless other inhalants are a factor. Cigarettes dry and irritate the delicate mucous membranes, destroy available sources of vitamin C, increase the need for vitamin B complex and vitamin A, and destroy the delicate cilia essential for cleansing the lungs of unwanted foreign matter. Apart from these well-known effects, cigarettes have also been found to contain a large amount of the toxic element cadmium, which has been found to cause emphysema in laboratory animals. It is also found in high concentrations in the lungs of humans with emphysema. Other sources of cadmium are air pollution, auto exhaust, and galvanized water pipes.

Air pollution and radioactive fallout have both been implicated in the rapid rise in emphysema. Any irritant inhalant from industrial pollution can be a factor, as well as any occupation that exposes the lungs to irritants. Well-known occupational emphysemas are miner's lung, glassblower's lung, and metal worker's lung.

With emphysema, diet plays a role similar to that in chronic bronchitis and asthma. A common fault is an excess of refined carbohydrates and a general lack of raw green vegetables. This mucus-forming diet predisposes to minor lung ailments which, if too often repeated or improperly treated, may become asthma or bronchitis and later emphysema.

Poor body mechanics can affect the respiratory excursion, reducing oxygen exchange by the lungs as well as local circulation and nutrition. Kyphosis, a forward bending in the midback, or scoliosis, a side-bending deformity in the midback, both may reduce the space allowed for the lungs to expand. Lack of demanding exercise and habitual shallow breathing allow the ribs to become less mobile, reducing the vital capacity or lung excursion, predisposing to lung disease.

Spinal lesions in the upper and midback can also severely upset local nerve, blood, and lymph supply to the lungs, resulting in downgraded tissue vitality.

Treatment

Emphysema is a degenerative disease. It comes at the end of years of abuse and results in tissue breakdown and scar formation. Even early cases of emphysema already have permanent lung damage that can never be totally corrected.

Prevention is obviously the best way of avoiding lung damage, but even advanced cases may be improved significantly with proper care. In a case of emphysema so severe that the patient can barely walk without complete breathlessness and prostration, sometimes improvement to the point of being quite active can be achieved.

Diet

Similar dietary regimens to those found under Asthma and Bronchitis are very useful with emphysema. In advanced cases vitality is usually very low and therapy must be moderated accordingly. Mucus solvents such as onions and garlic should always be included in the diet, as well as citrus fruits with their pulp, these being high in vitamin C and bioflavonoids. Foods high in vitamin A are essential for lung health and should be included regularly. The bulk of the diet should be raw vegetables. Dairy products, wheat, and excess starches are to be avoided. Alternate the diet with periods of citrus or vegetable juice fast (especially carrot juice and watercress). Also, 3 to 4 days on the mucus-cleansing diet (see Appendix I) strictly or modified to include carrots as well as raw salads is beneficial. Results will be slow but steady, and perseverance is essential.

Physiotherapy

- *Postural drainage with percussion:* Hang from the waist over the edge of a bed with a bowl placed at the head for easy expectoration. Apply a hot, moist compress to the back repeatedly for 5 to 10 minutes and then have a friend pound vigorously on the back with open palms. As mucus is loosened it should be expectorated. Repeat one to three times per day.

- *Alternate hot and cold chest packs:* To stimulate circulation, respiration, and mucus elimination.

- *Alternate hot and cold showers* as above, and also to improve general skin function.

- *Exercise:* Progressively increase the amount and speed of whatever exercise you are capable of. Exercise is best done in a warm, moist environment, not outdoors on a cold day, which would cause drying of the mucous membranes. Stationary bicycling has been used in various studies to great benefit, although any exercise that requires progressively more exertion will do.

- *Inhalation therapy:* Inhalations of various herbal steam mixtures are beneficial to help heal the lungs and aid expectoration. These include:

Mixture 1:   Eucalyptus oil
                 Fir balsam
                 Tolu

Benzoin

Mixture 2:   Sage
              Thyme
              Rosemary
              Cloves

Other: Olbas inhalation and chest compress

- *Diaphragmatic breathing* (See Asthma)
- *Breathing exercises* (See Asthma)
- *Spinal manipulation:* Weekly manipulations to entire thoracic region, including ribs and intercostal deep muscle massage.

Therapeutic Agents

VITAMINS AND MINERALS

Vitamin A: 25,000 to 100,000 IU per day, with supervision. Essential for health of mucous membranes. *Use any dose of vitamin A over 50,000 IU per day with medical supervision only.* *

Vitamin B complex: 50 mg two to three times daily. *

N,N-Dimethylglycine (DMG): 50 mg two times per day.

Vitamin C and bioflavonoids: 3000 to 12,000 mg of vitamin C per day. *

Vitamin E: 400 to 1200 IU per day; reduces oxygen needs; antioxidant; healing agent. *

OTHERS

Adrenal tablets*

Amino acids

Carrot juics: 1 glass one to two times per day. *

Cayce expectorant #49

Chlorophyll

Garlic: 2 capsules three times per day. *

Lecithin

Onion syrup (see Appendix I): 1 tsp three to six times per day. *

Protein supplements

Raw thymus tablets: Immunological support.

*Asterisks indicate the most frequently used therapeutic agents.

BOTANICALS

Boneset *(Eupatorium perfoliatum)*

Comfrey *(Symphytum officinale)*

Quebracho blanco *(Aspidosperma quebracho-blanco)*: Respiratory stimulant. Dose: 5 to 25 drops tincture three times per day.*

Refer also to Bronchitis.

Therapeutic Suggestion

Emphysema responds slowly due to its degenerative nature. Mucus solvents (garlic, onion syrup) are very useful. Very high doses of vitamin A are needed, along with B complex, C, and especially E. The patient must stop smoking and avoid exposure to occupational inhalants.

ENURESIS (Bed-wetting)

Definition

The involuntary loss of urine that may occur beyond the age when urinary bladder control is usually acquired (around age 3 to 4).

Symptoms

Involuntary loss of urine while sleeping.

Etiologic Considerations

• Urinary tract disorders
  Urinary infection
  Obstruction to urinary tract
  Urethral stricture or stenosis
  Ectopic urethral insertion into bladder
  Immature bladder, lack of neuromuscular development and control, small bladder with reduced capacity.

• Diet
  Food allergy
  Excess sugar

*Asterisks indicate the most frequently used therapeutic agents.

Excess liquids
Excess spices
Excess salt
Excess irritants, chemicals, pesticides, strong spices, etc.

- Hypoglycemia
- Diabetes
- Spinal lesions
- Psychological

Discussion

Development of bladder control is gradual. Usually a child will be able to stay dry by day during the second year of life and stay dry at night late in the third year of life, with only occasional accidents. By age $3^1/_2$ 75 percent of all children have acquired bladder control both day and night. By age 5 over 90 percent have bladder control. The incidence of bed-wetting continues to fall so that by age 15 less than 1 percent still suffer from enuresis. The frequency of bed-wetting is still fairly high up until the fifth year due to immaturity of the bladder and neuromuscular system.

Organic causes of bed-wetting usually involve the genitourinary system. These include conditions such as chronic infection, urethral stricture or stenosis, obstruction, and ectopic urethral insertion into the bladder. Only 3 percent or less of all children with enuresis have an organic cause to their condition. The incidence of organic causes becomes much more frequent in the older groups, where up to 75 percent of all adolescents who suffer enuresis *do* have an organic cause. Organic lesions are more common among long-term primary enuretics (those who have never gained bladder control). They also usually suffer loss of urine during the day.

The most commonly accepted finding with young children with enuresis is that they have very small bladders. Not only do they wet the bed, but they also have frequency of urine all day long. Their bladders simply do not have the capacity to hold all the urine formed at night and enuresis results.

Some authorities feel that part of the problem in enuresis is due to a deeper than usual state of sleep. This has been associated with hypoglycemia, which can give a deep comalike sleep. This deep state does not allow the part of our brain responsible for social awareness to receive the signal of a full bladder.

Other cases are linked to dietary factors. Hypoglycemia has already been mentioned, but food allergy has also been found as a causative factor in some children. Dairy allergy is always the first suspect. Literally any food may cause an allergic reaction and literally any part of the body may be affected. Some respond with a stuffy nose, others have itchy eyes or skin rashes, while still others become enuretics. Once these food allergies are traced down using the cytotoxic test, RAST test, or pulse test and eliminated, the enuresis disappears. Other foods are also suspected, perhaps not as pure allergies but rather as irritants. These include strong spices, salt, sugar, pesticides, and chemicals.

Probably the most important cause of enuresis, which is so often neglected, is spinal lesions. These may be caused by birth trauma or any one of the serious falls that all children seem to take so frequently. These lesions may disrupt the normal flow of both nerve impulses and circulation to the bladder. This is such a common finding that all children suffering enuresis should receive a spinal examination as part of a complete history and comprehensive physical examination.

The psychological causes of bed-wetting are fairly well understood. They are also more common in secondary enuretics (those who gained bladder control and then lost it) over age 5. One common finding is that an older child will develop enuresis on the arrival of a second child. This is a method to gain attention, or a desire to return to an earlier stage of development with more parental care. Other emotions causing enuresis are fear, anxiety, resentment, and the desire to "get even" with the parent for some reason.

Psychological causes are found frequently in children of split marriages or those in institutions. Too-rapid or strict toilet training may actually cause enuresis (also, too little attention to toilet training may lead to bed-wetting. After the age of 4 toilet training becomes very difficult). Anxiety due to parental disapproval or teasing children may slow the learning process. Punishment will usually make the situation worse rather than better.

Treatment

It is important to remember that all children do not develop bladder control early. A child should not be suspected of enuresis unless, in spite of steady, consistent but gentle attempts at toilet training, persistent bed-wetting occurs after age 4. During treatment, the aim should be to make the child feel secure and understood and that with a little help cure is expected. He or she should know, however, that bed-wetting is not normal or desirable, but not made to feel guilty. He must be encouraged to make his needs known by day. The child's urine volume should be measured several times to determine the bladder's capacity. If 250 to 300 ml can be passed, the problem is not a small bladder. Liquid intake should be stopped after 3 to 4 P.M., including all drinks, fruits, or soups. The bladder should then be fully emptied before going to bed. The child should be on his back while a story is read to him for $1/2$ hour. Then the bladder is emptied once again. A towel may be tied around the waist so that a large knot protrudes from the back. This will prevent the child from comfortably sleeping on the back. This position has been found to be the worst for enuretics.

The parent must then wake the child just before going to bed or at 10 P.M. and possibly again in 3 hours.

Hypnotism has been found to be very useful in these cases. Mild forms of positive suggestions may be all that is needed. As the child is just falling asleep, tell him in a soft, reassuring, and positive tone that when he needs to urinate he will awake all by himself and go to the bathroom and urinate all by himself, and return to his nice dry bed. Tell him that each time he does this it will make it that much easier to do it again the next time until before he knows it his bed will be dry every night. Tell him also that when he awakes in a dry bed he will feel very happy. This procedure must be repeated every night. Never include any mention of *not* wetting the bed or any other suggestion that is negative. Suggest only the positive behavior that you wish him to develop. If you wish you may also consult a trained hypnotist for more complete self-hypnotic instructions.

Ask the child to keep a record of the dry nights and reward him for a high weekly score. Do not punish or in any way consider wet nights. Reward only the positive.

Exercises

BLADDER STRETCHING

If the urine output and bladder volume is reduced but the frequency is high, the child may be suffering from a small bladder. Bladder capacity may be stretched by giving an excess amount of liquids during the day and asking the child to refrain from urinating as long as possible. Tell him that if he has an accident he should not be embarrassed. Explain what you are doing. You must also expect an increase in the frequency of bed-wetting during this bladder-stretching procedure. When the bladder can void 250 to 350 ml, bed-wetting will usually cease.

KEGAL EXERCISE

This exercise is performed by using the voluntary muscles to slow down and stop urine flow. During each urination stop the flow several times and hold 1 to 2 seconds. This is a very effective method. Once the child has learned which muscles to contract he should be instructed to do the Kegal exercise at other times throughout the day as well.

Physiotherapy

COLD SITZ BATHS

These are essential to tone the bladder and associated organs. They stimulate both circulation of blood and lymph as well as nervous flow to these areas. A further benefit is the strengthening of both voluntary and involuntary muscles in the pelvic region.

Begin the bath with *just* cool and add colder water progressively until the temperature is as cold as the child will bear without undue complaint. The object is to stay immersed from hips to midthigh in very cold water for up to 5 minutes.

The duration of the sitz bath should begin with short immersions, gradually increasing the treatment time to the maximum of 5 minutes. If the child is willing, it is more therapeutic to immerse directly into very cold water rather than decrease the temperature gradually. Repeat this cold sitz bath one to two times daily for several months or longer, as needed. Follow the bath by vigorously drying with a rough towel until the child feels warm. (*Note:* If the cold sitz bath is too severe for your child, try the alternate hot and cold sitz, remaining in the hot water 1 minute and the cold water for 2 to 3 minutes. Repeat three times, ending with cold water.)

Spinal

Weekly lumbar, lumbar/sacral, and sacroiliac manipulation is helpful in some cases.

Therapeutic Agents

VITAMINS AND MINERALS

Vitamin A: 5000 to 10,000 IU one to two times per day. *Use any dose of vitamin A over 50,000 IU per day with medical supervision only.**

Vitamin B complex: 25 to 50 mg per day.*

Vitamin E: 100 to 200 IU one to two times per day.*

Magnesium: 100 mg two times per day.*

Calcium: Tranquilizes. 200 to 300 mg, one to two times per day.

OTHERS

Celery

Cranberry juice: One glass three times per day.

Raw bran (before bed)

BOTANICALS

Cinnamon *(Cinnamomum zeylanicum)**

Goldenseal *(Hydrastis canadensis)*

*Asterisks indicate the most frequently used therapeutic agents.

High bush cranberry or cramp bark *(Virburnum opulus)*

Queen of the meadow *(Eupatorium purpureum)*: Kidney involvement.*

St. John's wort *(Hypericum perforatum)**

Therapeutic Suggestion

The single most effective tonic for the bladder is the alternate hot and cold sitz baths. These should be accompanied by specific nutritional therapy according to the needs of the patient. Homeopathic medication is a useful approach.

EPILEPSY: Petit Mal and Grand Mal

Definition

Epileptic seizure: A brief disorder of cerebral function usually associated with a disturbance of consciousness and accompanied by excessive neuronal discharge.

Symptoms

Grand Mal

Prodromal phase: A warning phase lasting hours or days with a mood change.
Aura: An apprehension of brief duration that a seizure is about to occur.
Loss of consciousness: A sudden fall occurs.
Tonic stage: Loss of consciousness with muscular contraction, including contraction of the respiratory muscles, which creates a "cry" as the air is forced out through a partially closed glottis. This stage lasts 20 to 30 seconds.
Chronic stage: Tonic spasm is replaced by interrupted powerful jerks or spasms of face, mouth, jaw, body, and limbs. Foaming of the mouth may occur, along with incontinence of urine and biting of the tongue. This stage lasts 20 to 30 seconds.
Relaxation stage: The person lies flaccid and falls into a deep sleep lasting a few minutes to 1 hour or more. After regaining consciousness the person is often confused and may have a headache.

Petit Mal

A transient loss of consciousness with blank stare lasting 10 to 15 seconds. Some myoclonic jerks of the extremities may occur at this time. In rare cases

*Asterisks indicate the most frequently used therapeutic agents.

this is also accompanied by total loss of consciousness, falling to the ground, and immediate recovery of consciousness.

Partial or Focal Epilepsy

The commonest site of dysfunction is the temporal lobe. This form is manifested by hallucinations of smell, taste, sight, or hearing and "deja vu"-like feelings. There also may be experienced a dreamlike quality which may be accompanied with well-coordinated, seemingly purposeful motor actions of which no memory will be retained.

Jacksonian

Disturbance of function in one part of the body spreads to involve adjacent areas. An example is an involuntary twitch of a hand that spreads to the entire arm or whole side of the body. Consciousness may or may not be lost.

Etiologic Considerations

- Lymphatic lesion (Peyer's patches)
- Digestive disturbances
  Overdistended stomach due to excess intake of food
  Poor eliminations
- Spinal lesion
- Incoordination of cerebrospinal and autonomic nervous systems
- Nutritional or toxic causes
  Aluminum toxicity
  Copper toxicity
  Lead toxicity
  Mercury toxicity
  Chemical toxicity
  Pesticides
  Food additives
  Calcium deficiency
  Magnesium deficiency
  Manganese deficiency
  Selenium deficiency
  Trace element deficiency
  Zinc deficiency
  Vitamin A deficiency
  Vitamin B_6 deficiency

  Vitamin D deficiency
  Taurine deficiency

- Allergy
- Metabolic abnormalities
  Increased B_6 need
- Anoxia
  Heart block
  Anemia
  Vasoconstriction due to reflex from upper cervical vertebrae lesions
- Sensory triggers
  Flickering light
  TV-induced epilepsy
  Sounds
- Emotional triggers
- Head injuries
- Heredity
- Glandular imbalances
  Adrenals (hypoglycemia)
  Pancreas (hypoglycemia)
  Gonads
  Pineal
  Pituitary
  Liver
- Cerebral tumors
- Cerebrovascular disease
- Uremia
- Hypoglycemia (insulin-secreting adenoma)
- Sudden alcohol or drug withdrawal

Discussion

  The usual medical approach to epileptic seizures of unknown cause is the use of sedatives and anticonvulsants, with Dilantin the most frequently prescribed drug. Dilantin does not cure epilepsy, but does help control the frequency and intensity of seizures. Many cases are completely controlled. Most anticonvulsant drugs, however, tend to deplete the body's folic acid, thus creating folic acid deficiency. Hyperplasia of the gums can also occur.

Other side effects of anticonvulsant drugs include rashes, irreversibly enlarged lymph nodes, osteomalacia (rarefaction of bone), slurred speech, mental confusion, dizziness, insomnia, blood abnormalities, hyperglycemia, and possible liver damage. Obviously, no physician would prescribe such a strong drug unless he or she carefully monitored the patient for side effects, and unless it was essential. Unfortunately, I have observed some cases where its prescription has been seemingly more cavalier. I recall one patient in particular who experienced *one* seizure and was placed on Dilantin "for the rest of his life." Upon investigating his case it was discovered that he had been spraying with pesticides for 3 days prior to his seizure. Unfortunately, none of this ever came out in his initial case history, and Dilantin was prescribed. Certainly such cases are in the minority, but it does emphasize the importance of a complete case history prior to the administration of any drug medication.

The problem thus far in treating epilepsy through natural means has been an incomplete understanding of the multiple causes of the disorder. A clear picture of its causation has been sadly lacking. Fortunately, however, the more individualized holistic approach that naturopathic physicians employ has been successful in some cases in bringing about remarkable improvements.

The work of Edgar Cayce* has helped to present a fresh model to explain the complexity of this disorder. With his special sensitivity and ability to see hidden causes, some new insight into epilepsy has been presented. Cayce found the most frequent causative factor was an incoordination between the cerebrospinal and autonomic nervous system. This is caused by a lesion in what Cayce† calls the "lacteal ducts," which coincide loosely with Peyer's patches, lymphatic structures in the small intestine. This area, according to Cayce, but not yet substantiated by current medical knowledge, is a crucial center where both the cerebrospinal and autonomic nervous systems meet. A lesion, or a twisting of these meeting places, causes reflex lesions in the spine and brain, resulting in excessive abnormal neurological impulses. These reflex changes may also involve the endocrine system, causing disturbances.

Another common factor Cayce found was a digestive incoordination. Poor elimination can overload the lymphatic regions just past the duodenum and produce toxic substances which may affect the whole body and also contribute to the lacteal lesion as described above. Spinal lesions were also cited as a factor in many of the Cayce readings.‡

Evidence from other sources sheds further light on this perplexing disorder.§

---

*Cayce, Edgar, *Physician's Reference Notebook*, A.R.E. Press, Virginia Beach, Virginia, 1968, pp. 137–150.

†Ibid., pp. 137–150.

‡Ibid., pp. 138–150.

§Allen, R. B., "Nutritional Aspects of Epilepsy," *International Clinical Nutrition Review*, 3(3):3–10, 1983.

Some research points to vitamin B_6 deficiency as a possible factor in some cases of epilepsy. One study revealed a B_6 deficiency in certain baby formulas causing infantile epilepsy which was reversed by supplying vitamin B_6. Some infants have also been found to have an increased need for B_6 as the result of a metabolic abnormality. * Deficiencies of vitamin A, vitamin D, folic acid, zinc, and taurine (an amino acid) have also been linked with epilepsy in some patients. Other studies found that magnesium deficiency was a common cause with supplemental magnesium being curative. This was especially true in infants with excess calcium intake resulting in magnesium loss. †

It has been known for a long time that magnesium deficiency may cause muscle tremors and convulsive seizures. In 1976 magnesium was shown to be at lower levels in epileptics than in normal subjects. A magnesium supplement of 450 mg daily has successfully controlled seizures in a trial of 30 epileptic patients, restoring a proper physiological balance. ‡

Calcium deficiency also must be considered a possible cause. As recently as 1983 the *International Clinical Nutrition Review* reported cases of epilepsy successfully treated by restoring normal calcium levels. §

Toxic metals such as lead, copper, mercury, and aluminum have long been known to cause seizures. These toxicities are increasingly common in our modern society with aluminum cookware, auto exhaust, industrial pollution, and copper water pipes. Several other correlations have been found, pointing to nutritionally related causes of epilepsy.

Hypoglycemia has long been associated with convulsions. Serum glucose levels have been shown to fall just prior to seizures. It is estimated that between 50 to 90 percent of all epileptics have either constant or periodic episodes of low blood sugar, and 70 percent show abnormal glucose tolerance levels of the hypoglycemic type.

Allergy is another fairly well documented cause of epilepsy in some patients. Many case studies exist where exposure to chemicals, pesticides, food additives, or common foods such as peanuts or tea has been the sole cause of seizures for individual patients. In these cases drug therapy is not only clearly inappropriate, it is often detrimental.

Certainly, not all patients with epilepsy can be helped with natural therapies, but a careful investigation into each case may reveal possible avenues of therapy that may eventually help the patient reduce or in some cases even entirely eliminate the need for drug therapy.

*Crowil, G. F., and Roach, E. S., "Vitamin B_6 Dependent Seizures in Infants," *American Family Physician* 27 (3): 183–187.

†Pfeiffer, Carl, *Mental and Elemental Nutrients*, Keats Publishing, New Canaan, CT, 1975, pp. 278–279.

‡Allen, R. B., op. cit., pp. 3–10.

§Ibid.

Treatment

Diet

The diet should include low-fat (no fried foods, meat, or milk), low-carbohydrate foods, and no alcohol, salt, or sugar. This will promote regularity. The principles of a hypoglycemic diet regimen should then be followed for long-term care.

Physiotherapy

* Castor oil packs

   These packs should be used in series—3 days on, 1 day off, for at least 6 months. This is to help heal the intestinal lesions present in the majority of epileptic patients, according to Cayce.

   Use three to four thicknesses of undyed wool. Saturate this with hot castor oil and wring out lightly. (This is heated in a special pot used for this purpose only. You may reuse the same cloth twenty to forty times. Just store it in the pot and add more castor oil with each use.) This cloth is applied as hot as the body can comfortably bear, to the area on the right side of the abdomen, from the lower rib border to the iliac crest covering the liver to caecum and umbilicus. The pack is covered with oiled cloth or plastic and kept warm by a heating pad. If necessary, the bed may also be protected with plastic. The pack should stay on 1 to 3 hours. After finishing, wash the area with a weak solution of bicarbonate (1 tsp to 1 quart warm water). These packs should be done at the same time of day, in the evening. Take 2 tbs unrefined olive oil the evening of the third day of packs.

* Massage

   After the castor oil pack, a deep abdominal massage to help break up any adhesions is useful. Use a combination of peanut oil, olive oil, and tincture of myrrh.

* Spinal manipulation

   On the fourth day, after 3 days of castor oil packs, obtain a spinal treatment of C1, 2, 3, T9, 10, and sacrococcygeal areas, plus any specific lesions. These treatments are to be done about two times per week for 3 weeks, with 1 week of rest. Repeat the cycle over a 6-month period, minimum.

* Exercise
   Walking
   Swimming
   Calisthenics
   Keep active!

Therapeutic Agents

VITAMINS AND MINERALS

Vitamin A: 25,000 IU one to two times per day. *Use any dose of vitamin A over 50,000 IU per day with medical supervision only.* *

Vitamin B complex: 50 mg three times per day; essential to proper nervous system function. *

Intramuscular B complex, B_{12} plus folic acid: One to two times per week.

Vitamin B_6: 100 mg two times daily; anticonvulsant. *

Vitamin C: To bowel tolerance.

Folic acid: 1 mg two times per day. *

Vitamin E: 400 IU two times per day. *

Calcium: 800 to 1000 mg per day; sedative. *

Magnesium: 400 to 500 mg per day.

Trace minerals

Zinc: 25 mg two to three times per day.

Taurine: 1 to 3 g per day. *

OTHERS

Atomodine: 1 drop per day.

Pancreatic enzymes

EFA (essential fatty acids): 4 capsules three times per day.

Fletcher's Castoria as needed.

Lecithin: 4 capsules three times per day, or in granular form in drinks or on food. *

Octacosanol (wheat germ oil concentrate): 2500 to 5000 mcg per day. *

See also Hypoglycemia and Allergy.

BOTANICALS

Chamomile *(Anthemis nobilis)*

Catnip *(Nepeta cataria)*

Gota Kola

*Asterisks indicate the most frequently used therapeutic agents.

Hyssop *(Hyssopus officinalis)*: Petit mal.

Lobelia *(Lobelia inflata)*: Emetic doses at first signs.*

Passion flower *(Passiflora incarnata)**

Passion flower: Whole plant extract plus elixir of wild ginseng (Cayce product). Sedative, antispasmodic. Dose: 1 tsp four times per day and ½ hour before retiring. Decrease other medication slowly over 3 to 6 weeks with doctor's permission.*

Peony root *(Paeonia officinalis)*

Skullcap *(Scutellaria lateriflora)**

Valerian root tea *(Valeriana officinalis)*

USEFUL PRESCRIPTIONS

Antispasmodic tea:
    Black cohosh
    Lady's slipper
    Skullcap
    Valerian. Dose: 2 to 3 cups at first sign of attack.

Kloss antispasmodic tincture:
    Cayenne, ½ part
    Cohosh, 1 part
    Lobelia seed, 1 part
    Skullcap, 1 part
    Skunk cabbage, 1 part
    Dose: 8 to 15 drops, up to 1 tsp on tongue at first sign of attack.

FALLEN ARCHES (see Flat Feet)

FATIGUE

Definition and Symptoms

Abnormal tiredness and lack of energy. Weakness, mental and physical; lethargy; depression; inability to perform ordinary daily duties.

*Asterisks indicate the most frequently used therapeutic agents.

Etiologic Considerations

- Hypoglycemia
    Adrenal exhaustion and other results.

- Stress
    Nutritional and glandular reactions.

- Anemia
    Iron
    Vitamin B_{12}
    Folic
    Copper
    Vitamin C and others

- Toxicity
    Diet
    Pesticides
    Additives, etc.
    Drugs
    Smog
    Cigarettes, etc.

- Allergy

- Glandular imbalances
    Hypothyroidism
    Pituitary
    Adrenals
    Pancreas

- Poor eliminations or assimilation
    Constipation
    Enzyme deficiency, poor digestion and absorption of essential nutrients
    Poor skin function
    Liver, gallbladder disease

- Cardiovascular causes
    Low blood pressure
    High blood pressure
    Arterio- and atherosclerosis

- Improper diet
    Excess saturated fats
    Excess refined carbohydrates
    Junk foods (vitamin and mineral deficiency)
    Excess cow's milk (early infancy anemia)
    Overeating

    Skipped breakfast
    Coffee, alcohol, soda, sugar
    Excess animal protein
    Protein deficiency
- Lack of demanding exercise
- Excess sex or excess masturbation
- Birth control pill
- Overweight
- Overwork
- Lack of sleep
- Sedentary occupation
- Psychological
- Heavy metal poisoning
- Old age nutrition syndrome
    Lack of teeth, resulting in little fresh vegetable intake
- Degenerative disease
    Cancer
    Arthritis
    Most others
- Shallow breathing

Discussion

Probably the most common complaint of people today is fatigue. This is not a disease per se, but is a major symptom of many disturbances. Often, however, it must be dealt with generally as the single most obvious presenting disorder, without much else to aid in diagnosis. As you may understand from the long but still very incomplete list of possible causes, such a seemingly simple complaint can be very complex in its proper diagnosis and treatment.

A complete case history and good physical examination will usually reveal other clues to the origin of the fatigue. Although many etiologic factors are listed, in reality most of these in turn have a nutritional basis. Hypoglycemia, or low blood sugar, is one of the most frequent causes of a type of fatigue that is more obvious in the midmorning and afternoon in its early stages, becoming more continuous as the system becomes less able to cope with its repeated stress. The adrenal glands and pancreas become overburdened and eventually fail to function properly. The type of diet usually responsible for hypoglycemia, high in refined carbohydrates, is also deficient in the very vitamins and minerals essential for the health and well-being of these and others of the body's glands and organs.

Stress is also a common factor in fatigue. It may cause a form of hypoglycemia by depleting the adrenal glands which respond to any fear, anxiety, worry, or similar emotion, as if they were emergency conditions. A wide range of physiological actions are evoked to provide sufficient energy to meet this "danger." Eventually the adrenal glands become exhausted and, as vital energy reserves become overtaxed, fatigue results. Unlike true nutritional hypoglycemia, this type of fatigue does not necessarily occur between meals, but may be more related to an incident of intense stress or emotion. If this stress fatigue is coincident with a refined diet and especially if coffee or other caffeine-containing drinks such as black teas or soda are routinely consumed, the hypoglycemic state may take on a totally unpredictable character.

Caffeine is in reality a drug; a socially accepted drug, but a drug just the same. Unlike sugar, which at least draws part of its energy surge from its caloric nature, caffeine and caffeine-containing drinks such as unsweetened coffee or tea have no intrinsic energy value whatsoever. They do not give energy, but cause an endocrine emergency action to extract energy from the body's vital reserves in the liver and muscles. Caffeine causes glycogen stored in these tissues to be mobilized and converted to the body's fuel, glucose. Ultimately this extraction of energy leaves the energy reserves severely depleted, just as an unwise spender soon finds his or her pockets empty. The result is profound weakness and chronic fatigue. Caffeine drinks are probably the greatest curse to the body, after refined sugar. Habitual coffee or tea drinkers become literally addicted to their brew. So often we hear of people who just can't get going without their morning coffee, or who get a morning headache unless they drink coffee. What could be a clearer sign of dependency than this? Absolutely no progress will be made with chronic fatigue as long as coffee is a part of the diet.

Diet may influence the energy reserves in ways other than by the upsetting effects of low blood sugar. Many vitamin and mineral deficiencies are related to a lack of energy. The most widely accepted of these relate to the production of anemia. Deficiency of iron, B_{12}, folic acid, B complex, vitamin C, vitamin E, copper, and others may be involved. These deficiencies are fairly common as a result of devitalized food consumption; or may be related to conditions of blood loss such as profuse menstrual periods or bleeding ulcers.

Protein deficiency may be a cause of fatigue in some cases, while excess proteins may also be a factor. The habit of skipping breakfast or just having a sweet roll and coffee is associated with both low blood sugar and morning fatigue. Often, a change to a substantial high-protein breakfast will completely remove the morning "blahs." Excess protein, especially saturated animal fat proteins, cause a host of problems, including cardiovascular disease, liver and gallbladder disease and toxicity, all with symptoms of fatigue. Even excess vegetarian proteins may become a problem for a sedentary person. In general, the more demanding exercise a person does, the more protein he or she can eat and deal with effectively. Any excess clogs the system, causes toxicity, and lowers the body's vitality as it attempts to deal with the excessive amounts of unneeded and often toxic waste products of protein metabolism.

Another form of toxicity results from poor eliminations. Slow bowel transit time (loaded bowel syndrome, constipation) causes toxic residues in the colon to be reabsorbed, causing lethargy, depression, coated tongue, fatigue, and other signs of ill health. A high-fiber diet corrects this situation quite easily. One of the primary roles of the liver is detoxifying harmful or unwanted elements in the body. If the liver is overworked, general toxicity results. A congested liver due to excess toxins such as pesticides, food colorings, preservatives, etc., from foods, excess fatty foods, excess protein, chemical exposure, or drugs also will leave the person in a sluggish, toxic state.

Lack of demanding exercise and poor skin function cause poor circulation of blood and lymph. This results in stagnation and ultimately toxicity in various organ groups, causing lowered vitality and fatigue. It is paradoxical that exercise, which initially requires energy, produces such an abundance of vitality and more energy. Occupations that require little physical exertion are much more fatiguing than good, hard physical work. Exercise stimulates blood and lymph circulation, aids in tissue nutrition, stimulates the endocrine system, tones and cleanses the cardiovascular system, and generally acts to "grease" our entire body machine. Exercise also helps keep our energies directed and concentrated, preventing many emotional and mental disorders.

Food allergy is a frequently ignored cause of poor vitality, depression, listlessness, fatigue, and other similar symptoms. This may be caused by any food and may cause sudden acute symptoms almost to the point of prostration, or the more subtle chronic fatigue if the allergen is consumed on a regular basis.

Cardiovascular disease, arteriosclerosis, and atherosclerosis can reduce the efficiency of the blood circulation. If the blood flow to the brain is reduced due to narrowing of the vessels of blood supply, mental fatigue and lethargy may result. A similar effect occurs due to cervical arthritis, where the bony changes encroach on the vessels which pass through them and supply blood to the brain.

Other degenerative diseases such as cancer usually are first noticed by vague feelings of tiredness and lack of energy or vitality. All the other factors listed under Etiologic Considerations not previously mentioned may be involved in individual cases. As you can see, "simple fatigue" can be fairly complex and nothing to ignore.

Treatment

An attempt must be made to discover the basic cause of the fatigue and then treat specifically.

Diet

The hypoglycemic regimen using the blood-building foods found under Anemia is usually a safe choice. Some cases may benefit with periodic fruit or vegetable juice fasting and periods on a raw foods diet. No refined foods, coffee, or drugs are allowed. If this simple dietary approach does not prove effective, food allergy tests and a hair analysis may prove useful. If constipation is a problem, make sure the diet supplies adequate fiber.

Physiotherapy

- Meditation: 20 minutes, two times per day
- Deep breathing exercises
- Outdoor exercise daily (must induce perspiration)
- Aerobics
- Ice-cold foot baths
- Daily morning wet grass walks
- Alternate hot and cold showers
- Alternate hot and cold head baths or sprays (for brain fatigue)
- "Salt glow" skin rub (see Appendix I)
- Dry friction rub, skin brush (see Appendix I)
- Massage
- Saunas
- General spinal therapy
- Head stands, inversion therapy

Therapeutic Agents

VITAMINS AND MINERALS

Vitamin A: 25,000 IU one time per day. *Use any dose of vitamin A over 50,000 IU per day with medical supervision only.**

Vitamin B complex: 50 mg two to three times per day.*

Pantothenic acid

Vitamin B_{12}: oral, 250 mcg per day, plus 1 mg intramuscularly* per week.

Folic acid

Vitamin C: 1000 mg three times per day, or more.*

*Asterisks indicate the most frequently used therapeutic agents.

Vitamin E: 400 IU one to three times per day.*
Multivitamin, multimineral preparations
Chromium with hypoglycemia
Iron: due to iron deficiency anemia, 25 to 50 mg per day.
Calcium: 800 to 1000 mg per day.*
Magnesium: 400 to 500 mg per day.*

OTHERS
Bee pollen
Brewer's yeast (with hypoglycemia)*
Desiccated liver tablets*
Desiccated thyroid (with prescription)
Pancreatic enzymes
Kelp*
Raw adrenal tablets*
Raw heart tablets
Raw pancreas tablets
Raw pituitary tablets*
Raw thyroid tablets*
Spirulina

BOTANICALS
Ginseng (Panax spp.): general.
Oat (Avena sativa): mental.

FEVER

Definition

Elevation of the body temperature above normal. 98.6° F is considered average but this will vary from person to person and with time of day.

Symptoms

Skin is hot, dry or wet; the person suffers from malaise, general lassitude.

*Asterisks indicate the most frequently used therapeutic agents.

Etiologic Considerations

- Toxicity:
  Impurities in blood and lymphatic system
- Infection:
  Bacterial
  Viral
  Parasitic

Discussion

Body heat is normally generated at about 98.6° F. This temperature is produced by the body's internal work being performed day and night in its multitude of various tasks. The heart pumps, blood moves, muscles contract, air is expelled, food digested, hormones produced, etc.

Fever, or excessive body heat, is also produced by internal work performed by the body. In response to toxicity or infection the body institutes special defense mechanisms to help reestablish normality. These include an increase in the number of white blood cells and their transport to the area of need; antibody production; increased respiration to provide more oxygen; increased heart rate to pump blood, white blood cells, oxygen, and antibodies throughout the body; and formation of new blood vessels in areas of infection to allow closer and more effective contact of white blood cells, antibodies, and oxygen with foreign elements. These, along with many more activities, are all designed for defense. The best definition for fever is not a morbid or pathological disease state, but rather a state of hyperfunctional repair.

From this short explanation it becomes clear that fever is not the problem to be cured, but the *result* of the problem and *part* of the cure. Hippocrates once said "Give me fever and I will cure all disease," and by saying this he gives us insight into the true nature of fever.

Fever aids in eliminating toxins and helps destroy pathogenic bacteria. These bacteria usually have a very narrow optimum temperature range. Being pathogenic they live comfortably within the normal range of human temperature and can then actively reproduce. As the body's temperature rises to the upper limits of the bacteria's viable range, the generation time increases so that reproduction becomes slower and the body's defenses can combat them more effectively. At a critical point in the fever process, the body's defenses will engulf and destroy the bacteria faster than they can reproduce, resulting in a cure.

Recent research supports these views of fever. In a series of experiments on fever with fish, amphibians, birds, reptiles, and mammals, fever has been found to confer a clear advantage to the organism against any invading pathogens. Each of these groups of animals was found to respond in similar ways to fever.

When the onset of fever is first noticed the animals seek a warmer part of their environment. A fish will swim to a warm-water niche in its local habitat; a reptile will migrate to a sun-drenched sandhill, and a tree frog will climb to the uppermost branches to maximize its exposure to the warmth of the sun. Once a warm, comfortable location has been found, the animals become very inactive and cease to feed. Animals deprived of the ability to migrate toward warmth or kept active were slowed in their recovery and had a higher death rate.

Fever response in humans follows a similar course. The onset of fever is usually announced by an abrupt chill which occurs after the temperature has begun to rise. This is fever's most dramatic paradox. This chilly sensation usually causes the patient to seek warmth in bed, covered by several blankets, and even with a hot water bottle at the feet. Fever is also associated with a desire to rest and reduce all normal activities. As the fever progresses general weakness and muscular aches encourage this withdrawal and inactivity. Body movements become minimal. External stimuli become aggravating and the personality begins to disintegrate. The mind becomes dull and speech less articulate. The entire concentration is focused on the febrile condition. The appetite is characteristically depressed and even the most favorite dish is unappealing. As the temperature peaks and sweating begins, the second paradox of the febrile state is observed. In spite of the elevated fever, the aches and chills cease with the onset of sweating and a state of relative comfort supersedes.

This entire process of what is called *adaptive withdrawal* has been proven to be a definite survival advantage. When human subjects are given medication to lower their fever and eliminate the chills and muscular discomfort, discouraging the desire for warmth, rest, and abstinence from food, it has been found that their illness is lengthened and the prognosis diminished. In other words, subjects allowed to follow their normal instincts produced by the febrile state got better sooner and suffered less complications than those given fever-reducing medications.

Another study has conclusively found that antibiotics work far more effectively when the fever is *not* suppressed by aspirin. Once again, fever is a self-defense mechanism and is both a healing and cleansing process. Fever, *if properly managed* with natural means, does not cause brain damage. In fact, a real danger in fever is when it is artificially suppressed. Death can then result as toxins accumulate and attack susceptible organ groups.

The presence of fever by itself is not very informative. A normal high fever may be anywhere from around 104°F and 105°F and does not indicate how severe a disease really is. Children, however, develop notoriously high fevers in a very short time due to some fairly harmless bacteria and viruses, and if the fever is allowed to reach 106°F, brain damage *can* occur. In some isolated cases, however, severe complications or death have occurred after even relatively low fevers depending on the cause. Obviously, a doctor should be consulted for all severe or prolonged fevers.

As important a consideration as how *high* the temperature, is how *long* it has lasted, how the patient is coping, and whether the patient is *sweating*. A normal fever will run anywhere from 1 to 4 days. If it is prolonged it can indicate trouble. The patient's defense mechanisms may be weak and not up to the task on their own. If the fever is allowed to last too long, the body's energy reserves may be depleted, leaving it defenseless against the invader. If the patient is suspected of extremely low vitality, a more active approach to the problem is advisable. If the patient is not coping well with a very high fever, this also may be an indication for external intervention. And lastly, if the patient has a fever and is *not* sweating this *always* demands external intervention. Fever and sweating are two brothers that should never be separated. Sweating is needed to help expel toxins and keep the temperature regulated.

One very important footnote to the discussion on fever is that fevers in the newborn and infant should never be allowed to rise too high and never without medical supervision. The temperature control mechanisms in the newborn are still immature, and with a high fever will sometimes become uncontrollable. Infants' fevers climb very rapidly. If allowed to reach 106°F, brain damage can occur. There have been rare cases of brain damage and death reported as low as 103° to 104°. All moderate to high fevers in infants should be medically monitored.

For older children and adults I normally allow a fever to reach 104° to 105°F before advising simple hydrotherapeutic procedures to be used. Obviously, this will depend on the cause. Some fevers should be kept under control at a lower temperature. This certainly varies from case to case, and with children it depends very much on the condition of the child. I usually don't allow the fever to be lowered to less than 102°F in most circumstances.

Once an investigation is made so that you are sure that the cause of the fever is not serious and life-threatening, the following treatments may prove useful.

Treatment

Diet

All animals will fast when ill. Infants will refuse food and often even breast milk when they have a fever. Therefore we have before us the best example of the laws of nature at work. When you have a fever the best diet is the *liquid fast*. The old saying "feed a cold, starve a fever," although misunderstood, is at least correct when it comes to fever. The following liquids may be of benefit:

Water
Diluted fruit juices
Hot water and lemon juice
Hot teas (to sweat)

It is important not to allow infants to become dehydrated. If the infant refuses fluids, he or she must receive intravenous fluid and electrolyte replacement.

Physiotherapy

When advised:
- Cold compresses.

- Tepid (body heat 98.6°F), prolonged 30-minute bath.

- Baths followed by brisk towel rubs to increase skin function where patient's vitality is high.

- Trunk packs: These are advisable in most fevers. They work with the healing process and lower the body temperature by relieving internal congestion, increasing skin function with sweating, and increasing elimination. In this case a cold trunk pack draws blood from the congested interior to the surface, and then induces sweating as the pack heats up.

- Hot blanket baths, hot compresses, etc. (if goose skin). Use in conjunction with sweating teas.

- Hot Epsom salts bath (see Appendix I) followed by sweating in bed under many blankets.

Therapeutic Agents

VITAMINS AND MINERALS

Vitamin A: 5000 to 25,000 IU two to six times per day. *Use any dose of vitamin A over 50,000 IU per day with medical supervision only.**

Vitamin B complex

Vitamin C: 250 to 1000 mg per hour or as instant powder to drinks.*

OTHERS

Garlic: 2 capsules three to four times per day.*

Propolis: 10 to 15 drops tincture three to four times per day.*

Thymus: 2 tablets every 1 to 2 hours.*

TEAS

Catnip tea

Echinacea tea (blood purifier)

*Asterisks indicate the most frequently used therapeutic agents.

Elderflower tea

Hot pleurisy root tea (to induce sweating)

Lemon balm tea

Peppermint tea

Verbena tea

Yarrow tea

BOTANICALS

Boneset *(Eupatorium perfoliatum)*

Catnip *(Nepeta cataria)*

Coneflower *(Echinacea angustifolium)*

Elderflower *(Sambucus* spp.)

European vervain *(Verbena officinalis)*

Garlic *(Allium sativum)*

Lemon balm *(Melissa officinalis)*

Peppermint *(Mentha piperita)*

Pleurisy root *(Asclepias tuberosa)*: To induce sweating use hot infusion.

Yarrow *(Achillea millefolium)*

Therapeutic Suggestions

The key to the proper treatment of fevers in general (please refer to previous note on fever of infancy) is to allow the fever a wide range of action up to 104° to 105°F. Sweating must be encouraged and stimulated. The diet should be liquid only. The general situation and what symptoms accompany the fever (i.e., cough, body aches, excess mucus, etc.) influence if and what other medications are prescribed.

FIBROCYSTIC BREAST DISEASE (Cystic Mastitis)

Definition and Symptoms

Breast tenderness and cystic development which may recur with each menstrual cycle or become continuous. The breast becomes nodular, with freely movable cysts near the surface of the breast. Deeper cysts can occur.

Etiologic Considerations

- Hormonal imbalance
- Allergies
- Diet
    Methylxanthines (i.e., coffee, tea, cola, chocolate)
- Vitamin deficiency, especially vitamin E

Discussion

Although the cysts of cystic mastitis are benign there is a three- to seven-fold increase in the chance of cancer for those women with chronic fibrocystic disease. The condition usually progresses until menopause, when it is unlikely for new cysts to develop. There is an obvious correlation with the menstrual cycle. Approximately 20 to 50 percent of women are affected. Overstimulation of the breast by the female hormone estrogen is implicated. Until recently, little was known about the causes of this disorder. Within the past few years it has been observed that food and drinks containing methylxanthines, including coffee, tea, cola, and chocolate, are capable of aggravating this condition. Removing these substances from the diet is the most effective form of treatment for most women. Vitamin E supplementation has also been found to be very effective, in conjunction with these dietary changes.

Treatment

Although only foods containing methylxanthines have been implicated in this disorder, I usually suggest removing all negative health factors, to get the most complete cure. This includes eliminating not only coffee, tea, cola, and chocolate, but also cigarettes and alcohol, if possible. The diet should be composed of as many raw foods as possible, with emphasis on a more vegetarian protein-base diet, to avoid the hormones found in commercially raised meats.

The following supplements are useful:

Vitamins and Minerals

Vitamin A: 25,000 IU one to two times per day.

Vitamin B_1: 100 mg two times per day.

Vitamin B_6: 200 mg two to three times per day, especially if PMS symptoms coexist.*

Vitamin B complex: 50 mg one to two times per day.

Vitamin C: 1 to 3 g two to three times per day.

*Asterisks indicate the most frequently used therapeutic agents.

Vitamin E: 400 to 800 IU per day.*

Calcium: 1 g per day.

Arginine: 500 mg per day.

Kelp or other iodine source

Oil of evening primrose: 6 to 8 capsules per day.*

Flaxseed oil: 1 to 1½ tbs per day.

FLAT FEET (Pes Planus, Fallen Arches)

Definition

Collapse of the internal longitudinal and transverse arches of the foot. Eversion of the foot is associated in many cases.

Symptoms

A sensation of weakness and strain on the medial (inner) side of the foot. Pain and aching at night, which is increased on weight-bearing. The pain usually centers on the inner border, or at the metatarsal heads. Referred pain to the calf, knee, hip, or low back is common. Loss of "spring" in step, with awkwardness. Feet tire easily, numbness, cramping.

Etiologic Considerations

- Excess weight-bearing
  Carrying heavy weights
  Obesity
  Pregnancy
- Weak muscles
- Prolonged standing
- Improper foot wear
- Previous strain, sprain, or fracture
- Poor body mechanics—weight-bearing center incorrect
- Knock-knees
- External rotation of leg

*Asterisks indicate the most frequently used therapeutic agents.

- Congenital (abnormal talus bone)
- Heredity
- Shortening of Achilles tendon
- Arthritis, rickets, or calcium deficiency
- Muscle paralysis or weakness—due to disease such as polio or muscular dystrophy
- Improper walking habits
    Walking with foot everted
    Claw toe walking
- Spinal lesions

Discussion

The foot is a very complicated functional unit, composed of 26 articulating bones. It is supported by an internal longitudinal ligament (spring ligament), external longitudinal ligament, and anterior and posterior transverse ligaments. It is not the function of the ligaments, however, to withstand prolonged weight-bearing. It is the muscles that provide the foot with its real support.

In the weight-bearing position there is a natural tendency of the foot to evert (turn outward), which is counteracted by the muscles of the feet. If these muscles weaken and eversion becomes chronic, the weight distribution on the foot becomes severely altered. Instead of a balanced distribution of weight through all the ligaments of the foot, the whole weight is thrown onto the internal spring ligament, which is not designed to handle such stress.

In the normal foot, weight is first carried by the heel (calcaneus), passed down the outer border of the foot to the five metatarsal bones in the front of the foot, with a final push-off from the big toe. If the muscles become weak, the ligaments are overburdened and they begin to stretch. This leads to bone displacement and, finally, permanent bone changes. In specific medical terms, what occurs is a movement of the talus bone forward and medially (toward the midline). This can then be found displaced toward the inner side of the foot. The navicular bone is depressed and the heel (calcaneus) rotates posteriorly downward and everts, so that walking is done more on the inner border. With these actions, the entire foot can be seen to evert in the typical flat-footed position. The foot then widens as the transverse arch collapses and the forefoot abducts or moves away from the midline.

These foot changes may further affect muscular balance in the calf, leg, hip, and low back, causing tiredness, pain, rotation of the fibulae, and sacroiliac or lumbar spinal lesions.

The most detrimental influences causing flat feet are a combination of excess weight-bearing, weak muscles, calcium deficiency, and poor body mechanics.

The most obvious cause of excess weight-bearing is obesity. Occupations that require repeated or prolonged lifting also may be a factor. Muscles may become weakened by lack of general muscular tone, excess burden, nutritional deficiency (especially calcium deficiency), spinal lesions upsetting nutritional and nervous supply to muscles, trauma or previous strain, or poor spinal mechanics causing muscle imbalances and weakness.

Poor spinal mechanics may also be a factor in several other ways. Habitual walking with the foot everted places the weight burden on the weaker inner spring ligament, straining the arch and overburdening the muscles, which then weaken, allowing the ligaments to stretch. The big toe is then forced to push off in a position of adduction, creating the complication of hallux valgus, where the toe rotates and then crosses over its neighbor. The increased lumbar curve caused by wearing high heels throws the weight center forward onto the front part of the foot. The same situation occurs with the condition called visceroptosis, where the abdomen sags due to weak abdominal muscles, obesity, or spinal lesions, causing the center of gravity to alter, affecting the feet. The muscles between the toes (lumbricals and interossei) then weaken, due to the excess burden. The toes may also begin to "claw," favoring a collapse of the anterior transverse arch which is associated with the condition called metatarsalgia.

Treatment

Normally the arches only begin to form when the child has been walking for a year or so. This means that it is normal for a toddler to show some degree of flat feet and no cause for alarm. In some cases, however, arches do not form due to congenital causes and special shoes are required.

Three degrees of flat feet are recognized:

First-degree flat foot is a postural deformity with alteration in the muscles and ligaments but only minor displacement of bone or pain. Complete correction is possible with proper treatment.

Second-degree flat foot shows slight bone change and muscle damage. Complete correction is no longer possible, but stabilization and strengthening will relieve the symptoms of pain and weakness to a large degree.

Third-degree flat foot shows permanent bone changes with some arthritis and rigidity. No cure is possible.

As you can see, it is very important to treat flat feet in the earliest stages to prevent permanent joint deformity.

Diet

It is essential that the diet contain a large amount of readily absorbable minerals, especially calcium. Contrary to popular belief, dairy products are not the most desirable source of calcium. A far better source is raw green vegetables taken with a slightly acidic salad dressing containing apple cider vinegar or lemon juice. Salads or cooked vegetables should be eaten in large quantities with both lunch and supper. Dairy products, in most cases, should be reduced if a large portion of the diet has been concentrated on this source in the past. Less red meats and more fish or vegetarian proteins are also suggested.

Physiotherapy

The main part of therapy lies in physical therapies. These must be done daily for any real results.

EXERCISES—STANDING

- *Spring up:*   Stand on hard floor, rise gently onto toes and then "spring up." This should be done in the morning before shoes go on, and repeated fifteen to thirty times. Repeat again in evening.

- *Rise and sink:*   Stand on forefoot with hands over head and slowly rise onto toes. Lower arms in front of body and gradually sink down to the flat foot and heel. Repeat ten to twenty times two times per day.

- *Heel-to-toe-rock:*   Stand on the flat feet and rock heel to toe for 2 to 3 minutes two times per day.

- *Scrunch:*   With shoes on scrunch the toes up against the bottom of the shoe so that the foot arches. Do this six to ten times and repeat up to ten times per day.

- *Pick up:*   Pick up a ping pong ball or a large marble with the toes. Make this into a game.

- *Bean bag game:*   Make 3-in.-square or round bean bags. Pick up bags with toes and then toss them into a target such as a small wastebasket or hat.

- *Stand* with feet 2 to 3 in. apart. Contract gluteal muscles (seat) and rotate the hips outward while keeping the toes, outer foot, and heels firmly on the ground.

- *Stand* with the feet 2 in apart and attempt to force them apart, thus putting weight and stress on the outer portions of the foot, but do not move the feet. Slowly relax and repeat ten to twenty times.

- *Rise* onto the toes and slowly tilt the weight onto the outer borders of the foot. Repeat ten to twenty times two times per day.

- *Ostrich step:*   Walk in a straight line with weight on the outer borders of the foot and toes curled downward and inward. Raise each foot so that it is opposite the other knee before placing it down to the ground.

- *Knees* are held parallel and then slowly rolled outward so that the weight is placed on the outer borders of the foot.

- *Walk* on outer borders of foot.
- *Incline board walk:*   Nail two 8-to-10-ft-long × 8-to-12-in.-wide boards together at their long edges to make an equilateral triangle with the ground. Walk along the boards with one foot on each board. Repeat ten to twenty times two times per day.

Exercises—Sitting

- Heel raising and lowering.
- Sit with feet crossed resting on outer borders.
- Sit cross-legged.
- Press toes against ground but do not raise any part of foot off ground.
- Place thin book under toes and flex forefoot, keeping toes straight. This is a very important exercise.

Local Therapy

- Postural and muscular reeducation and exercises:
  With special work on Achilles tendon, calves, quadriceps, gluteals, paravertebral lumbar muscles, and abdominals.
- Deep muscle massage to plantar fascia, entire foot and lower limbs with:
  Peanut oil: ½ pint
  Witch hazel: 2 oz
  Rubbing alcohol: 4 oz
  Oil of sassafras: 3 to 10 drops
  Tincture of capsicum: 2 drops
  Mix well and repeat massage two times per day.
- Tannic acid foot and lower leg baths: Made by boiling old coffee grounds and water for 10 minutes. Apply hot and massage feet and lower legs while soaking. Time: 20 minutes per day.
- Alternate hot and cold foot baths.
- Spinal therapy (to specific lesions).
- Local manipulation: General joint mobilization. Treat talus which has rotated anteriorly and medially, navicular which is depressed, and calcaneus which is everted.
- Footwear: The front of the shoe should not compress toes and should have a straight inner border from heel to big toe. Soft, resilient arch supports are useful. In later stages of the disorder an *inner* wedge heel lift of 0.5 cm may be needed. This raises the inner border of the heel to counteract its tendency to evert.

Therapeutic Agents

VITAMINS AND MINERALS

> Vitamin A: 4000 to 25,000 IU two times per day. *Use any dose of vitamin A over 50,000 IU per day with medical supervision only.*
>
> Vitamin B: 25 to 50 mg two times per day.
>
> Vitamin C: 500 to 3000 mg per day or more.
>
> Multiminerals
>
> Trace minerals
>
> Calcium: 400 to 800 mg per day.
>
> Magnesium: 200 to 400 mg per day.
>
> Silica

BOTANICALS

> Horsetail (*Equisetum arvense*)

Therapeutic Suggestions

> Exercise, Exercise, Exercise!

FLATULENCE (Adult and Infant Colic)

Definition

Flatulence: Abnormal amounts of gas passing upward or downward, with or without intestinal discomfort.

Infant colic: Abdominal pain, distension, insomnia, extreme fretfulness, and hysteria.

Symptoms

Excess gas, abdominal distension, abdominal discomfort.

Etiologic Considerations

• Improper diet
   Excess acidity
   Poor food combinations

       Beans
       Hurried meals
       Frequent meals
       Allergies
       Liquids with meals

- Digestive enzyme deficiency
- Inadequate mastication
- Weakened digestion, poor eliminations
- Gallbladder/liver disorder
- Poor absorption
- Abnormal intestinal flora, yeast overgrowth
- Spinal (midthoracic)
- Visceroptosis: Poor spinal mechanics
- Diverticulitis
- Anemia
- Parasites
- Improper weaning

Discussion

Flatulence is not only uncomfortable and embarrassing, it is also a sign that some aspect of the digestive system is not functioning properly. What flatulence means, irrespective of its cause, is that food is not being completely digested, or is digested inadequately, for the particular part of the digestive system it is currently passing through to deal with it effectively. Digestive enzymes are essential in the digestive process to break down complex proteins, fats, and carbohydrates into small molecules for proper absorption. The result of food that is too complex passing out of the stomach and upper small intestine into the rest of the intestinal tract is fermentation, gas, and abdominal pain.

Diet is the most important consideration in all cases of chronic, excess gas formation. Certain foods such as beans* are well-known gas producers. They contain oligosaccharides (raffinose and stachyose) which have digestive enzyme-resistant chemical bonds between their sugar molecules causing food to be incompletely broken down and passed into the small intestine where fermentation

---

*If beans are soaked overnight and then cooked in fresh water, they usually lose their gas-forming characteristics. If this is not effective for you, cook beans after soaking for 15 minutes, then replace the water and cook until done. This is usually 100 percent effective.

and gas result. Many other foods will affect particular individuals in a similar way. These are usually easily determined and avoided. If this is the only cause, the problem is quickly solved.

More often, however, the problem is deeply ingrained. Food allergies or intolerances are a common cause of severe intestinal disorders with gas. Any food may cause a reaction, but the most frequent offenders are dairy products and gluten grains (see Celiac Disease). Generally unwise food combinations also may cause gas. The usual citrus/starch combination for breakfast is definitely a problem. These two require entirely different acid/alkaline levels for proper digestion and the two in the stomach at the same time simply become indigestible. Fruit and vegetables at the same meal or melons with anything else will have a similar effect. If these foods then pass into the intestine undigested, gas results.

The habit of drinking, especially milk, with meals is another bad nutritional habit. The liquids dilute digestive juices and hinder proper digestion. Excessively large meals also upset digestion by depleting the body's digestive enzyme capacity. Some food is then undigested or only partly digested, leading once again to fermentation and gas.

Meals taken at too-frequent intervals tend to upset the digestion of the meal taken previously, and also may cause enzyme depletion as above.

Hurried meals with inadequate chewing do not allow sufficient breaking down of vegetable cell walls. Cellulose, the main components of vegetable cell walls, is normally indigestible and unless food matter is thoroughly masticated, it may lead to gas formation and irritation in some people. Salivary digestive enzymes in the mouth, although of little use in partial breakdown of starches, have been overemphasized as a major digestive source. However, the process of chewing and tasting foods, along with the passage of sufficient salivary enzymes into the stomach, signals the secretion of other digestive enzymes absolutely essential to the digestive process.

Eating while under stress results in very poor digestion. Stress stimulates the sympathetic nervous system which governs danger responses and turns off the parasympathetic nervous system responsible for the secretion of digestive enzymes and intestinal motility.

Disorders of the liver and in particular the gallbladder upset fat digestion. Gallbladder disease is commonly associated with indigestion and gas.

Under normal circumstances the intestines are inhabited by friendly bacterial flora, absolutely essential for proper digestion. If the diet is high in vegetable matter and fiber, these bacteria do not cause any problems. If the diet is composed of sweets, refined carbohydrates, excess meat, and is low in fiber content, the amount and type of bacterial flora change, becoming less favorable to proper digestion and vitamin synthesis, and more favorable for gas production. Antibiotic use can totally upset this internal ecology, as can repeated enemas.

Poor eliminations and constipation may also be a cause of flatulence directly, or indirectly by causing diverticulitis with abnormal pain and gas.

Spinal lesions in the midthoracic region T4 to T10, or the condition of visceroptosis with poor abdominal tone, may cause abnormal secretion of digestive enzymes, reduced stomach or intestinal activity, or pressure on the intestinal tract, resulting in abnormal function.

Parasitic infections should always be considered as a possibility with any abnormal intestinal conditions. Some cases of infant colic are the result of *Candida* infections. This may be suspected in an infant whose mother had a yeast infection during her pregnancy, or if the infant has received antibiotic therapy for any reason. It is essential to reestablish normal bowel ecology as soon as possible. A preparation of lactobifidus powder added to the milk may be useful to correct this condition. If the infant is being breastfed, express a small amount and add the lactobifidus powder ($\frac{1}{8}$ to $\frac{1}{4}$ tsp) to the milk, two to three times daily. Other stronger medications should be avoided if possible.

Infant colic is included within this section on flatulence since some of the same considerations apply. The most common cause of colic in the totally breastfed infant is the mother's diet. Literally any food may cause the baby to suffer infant colic, gas, or diarrhea, but cabbage, onions, garlic, wheat, yeast, brussels sprouts, and broccoli are common offenders. Outside of the single irritating foods that may affect the infant at one time or another, I find the problem usually is a totally inappropriate diet of fried foods, junk food, and refined food in all manner of chaotic combinations. I remember one couple that came in red-eyed and extremely distressed since their 8-month-old daughter kept them up day and night with nearly constant screaming. Once the mother was placed on a "normal" diet the infant settled down within 2 weeks into a sweet, well-tempered child.

Colic that develops in a formula-fed infant obviously implicates the food given. The infant may be allergic to the milk, wheat, soy, or sugar in the formula. If breast milk is absolutely not available to the child, I find vitamin and mineral enriched goat's milk a better alternative to formula. Usually, however, the mother can breastfeed, or at least can with some effort, but has either been improperly educated about what is best for her child, or has some psychological hangup about breastfeeding. Even if the mother did not begin breastfeeding she can, with perseverance, develop a milk supply for her infant literally any time after birth and sometimes even years later by frequent attempts at breastfeeding over several months. If the infant does have colic and the mother could breastfeed, it is the best course of action in these formula-intolerance cases.

If colic has developed after weaning has begun, the obvious cause of the problem is one or several of the foods added to the diet. I am constantly amazed at what little understanding some parents have regarding the weaning process. I remember one couple vividly that came to me about their 3-month-old infant's colic. When asked what the child ate, I got the proud answer that he ate *everything* they ate! This was even more horrifying when you understand that their diet included fried eggs, bacon, pork, pastry, spaghetti, pizza, hamburgers, french fries, Coca-Cola, and so on.

When each new food is not slowly added and the infant carefully monitored for reactions such as colic, rashes, or any other unusual symptom, it can become very difficult to determine which food is the offender without totally reweaning the child. This is a difficult process for both parents and child, but is the only way to proceed if the diet has already become fairly complicated without care in weaning.

The two food groups, wheat and dairy products, are especially suspect and should be eliminated as a first step in all cases. Food allergies or intolerances to these two food groups are very common. In general, wheat and other grains are introduced far too early in the average infant's diet. Digestive capacity for concentrated starches only begins around 5 to 6 months in most infants. I usually advise grain to be introduced as one of the last foods and yeast bread added well after the first year of life. Fresh boiled goat's milk is usually less of a problem than cow's milk and this should be the choice if at all possible, to be introduced just before weaning is to commence. If these two simple rules were applied, there would be far fewer people with allergies in the world.

Treatment

Diet

General Rules

An old proverb states that nine-tenths of what we eat goes for our health, while the other one-tenth goes to the health of our doctor. In the case of indigestion and flatulence, this is clearly so.

- *Never eat until full. Meals must be unhurried.* It is wise to spend 10 to 15 minutes before each meal in quiet activity, and have a minute or two of silence before eating, to allow the nervous system to relax. Never eat when hurried or under stress, since the food will only cause you harm.

- *Each bite of food must be chewed thoroughly.* A person with a healthy stomach may gulp food with no obvious ill effect. The person with weak digestion must carefully chew each bite until almost liquid, to make the food more accessible to enzyme digestion.

- *Do not eat between meals.* Some people may benefit by eating between meals for conditions such as hypoglycemia, but usually it is better to allow complete digestion of each meal before eating again. I know some people who eat only one meal each day; however, it begins upon waking and only ends late at night. This will overburden the digestive system, leading to disease.

- *Do not drink with meals.* The dry feeding regimen is often sufficient in itself to correct many digestive complaints.
- *Never eat fried foods, hydrogenated fats, sugar, refined carbohydrates, or other junk food.*
- *Be careful in combining foods.*

The actual dietary regimen employed varies from patient to patient. With some it is enough to remove any allergic or irritating foods and follow the simple dietary rules above. Others need to be treated by treating the major causes affecting their case, such as constipation, gallbladder disease, etc. The following regimens are useful, depending on the patient:

3-to-14-day fruit juice or vegetable juice fast
10-day brown rice diet
Apple diet (no skin)
Raw foods diet
Constipation diet
Liver-cleansing diet and gallbladder flush

Physiotherapy

- Hot sitz bath (acute)
- Hot compresses (acute)
- Alternate hot and cold sitz bath (chronic)
- Enemas (acute and with cleansing diet regimens)
- Spinal manipulation
- Abdominal exercises

Therapeutic Agents

VITAMINS AND MINERALS

Dependent upon major cause, or none required. It is usually best to discontinue all pill supplements except those specifically recommended below for the flatulent condition, until full recovery has been attained.

OTHERS

Bran: Adds fiber and regulates bowel; not to be used in wheat sensitivity. May aggravate condition for first 7 to 10 days. Dose: 1 tsp with water before meals.

Charcoal tablets: 1 to 2 per hour in acute flatulence. *

*Asterisks indicate the most frequently used therapeutic agents.

Pancreatic enzyme tablets: 1 to 2 with meals.

Garlic: Some cases find this very effective; may aggravate others.

Glutamic acid hydrochloride

Hydrochloric acid: If hypoacid condition has been verified by test.*

Lactobacillus capsules: Not to be used if dairy sensitivity exists. Dose: 2 capsules three times per day.

Lemon juice and hot water.

Mucovata (Seroyal): Bulking agent.

BOTANICALS

American saffron (*Carthamus tinctorius*)
Adult: 1 cup infusion two to three times per day.
Infant colic: 1 tsp three times daily on empty stomach.

Anise (*Pimpinella anisum*): Tea.

Caraway (*Carum carvi*)

Cinnamon (*Cinnamomum zeylanicum*)

Cloves (*Eugenia caryophyllata*)

Comfrey (*Symphytum officinale*)

Coriander (*Coriandrum sativum*)

Cumin (*Cuminum cyminum*)

Dill (*Anethum graveolens*)

Fennel (*Foeniculum vulgare*)

Flaxseed (*Linum usitatissimum*)

Ginger (*Zingiber officinale*)

Goldenseal (*Hydrastis canadensis*): 25 drops in water three times per day as a bowel tonic.*

Parsley (*Petroselinum sativum*)

Peppermint (*Mentha piperita*)

Peppermint oil: 1 to 4 drops in hot water for flatulent colic.

Slippery elm (*Ulmus fulva*): 1 cup tea three to six times per day.

Thyme (*Thymus vulgaris*)

Wild yam root (*Dioscorea villosa*): Works rapidly in acute adult or infant

*Asterisks indicate the most frequently used therapeutic agents.

colic. Adult dose: 15 to 25 drops of tincture in water every ½ hour for 1 to 2 hours; then every 4 to 6 hours. Child dose: ¼ to ½ adult dose.

FLUORIDATION

Fluoride is now added to the water supply in many cities to prevent dental caries. It is also routinely prescribed by most pediatricians for infants and children in nonfluoridated areas. These practices follow the observation that certain areas with a high amount of naturally occurring fluoride in the form of calcium fluoride in the water supply show a significantly lower incidence of dental caries (tooth decay). The practice of fluoridation has been an intensely debated topic. Some people oppose fluoridation for health reasons. Many others feel the act of involuntary mass medication sets a very dangerous precedent. Still, enough evidence does seem to exist to shed considerable doubt on the safety of fluoridation.

Fluoride has always been considered a highly toxic element similar to lead or arsenic. At toxic levels symptoms of fluorosis appear. The most obvious of these symptoms is mottled teeth, a permanent change in the enamel of the teeth, first apparent as chalk-white patches with areas of yellow-brown staining. Later, pitting of the enamel may occur. When first estimating the amount of fluoride in preventing cavities, the toxic dose was also a consideration. Two parts per million (ppm) is considered toxic within 20 to 50 years, with 1.5 ppm considered the danger point. It was decided 1 ppm was the best therapeutic dose and also would prevent most cases of toxic fluorosis. At this dose it was expected that the "majority" of infants and children would be benefited by the increased protection against dental caries that fluoride reportedly gives.

There are, however, several other facts and factors not usually mentioned that are extremely important for us to know to properly evaluate fluoride and fluoridation. Fluoride is only effective in reducing cavities in infants and children. It has no anticaries effect on adult teeth. Some studies state the maximum benefit obtained for children is a 10 percent reduction in dental caries. Other sources claim a 30 to 50 percent protection.

The actual mode of action by which fluoride protects teeth is not certain. It is believed that fluoride strengthens enamel by joining with normally occurring hydroxyapatite in teeth to form fluoroapatite, which is considerably stronger and therefore protects against decay. It also makes enamel less soluble. Fluoride, however, does not affect only the teeth, but is also taken up by bones and is stored in the soft tissues, especially the aorta, ligaments, skin, bowels, kidneys, liver, and muscles. It is taken up more rapidly by immature bones and teeth and therefore children accumulate more than adults.

Several sources estimate that 10 to 20 percent of those who drink fluoridated water will get mottled teeth to some degree. Therefore, 10,000 to 20,000 in each 100,000 will be permanently disfigured by fluoridation. Normally a drug is not considered safe if more than 1 in 100,000 are harmed by it. Although mottling of teeth is fluoride's most obvious toxic effect, many studies implicate fluoride as a causative factor in other more serious conditions. Multiple studies link fluoridation with an increase in cancer. One such study found two times an increase in bone cancer in children in fluoridated areas. Another study of ten nonfluoridated and ten fluoridated cities of similar industrialization showed an increased cancer rate in the 10 to 20 years following fluoridation.

Comparison in England of Birmingham and Manchester shows an 850 percent increase in cancer in the 10-year period after the introduction of fluoridation in Birmingham. The Manchester area cancer rate, where fluoridation was not a factor, increased only 150 percent.

Cancer is not the only disease linked to fluoridation. Major U.S. studies show an increase in Down's syndrome in fluoridated areas (up to 38 percent more). Researchers in Japan also noticed that children with mottled teeth have a higher incidence of heart disease.

Other less dramatic but very important results of fluoridation follow as a direct result of fluoride metabolism in the body. Fluoride in the body combines with calcium to form insoluble calcium fluoride. This interferes with the dynamic exchange between the blood and bones of calcium. Normally the bones act as a calcium reserve to keep blood levels within normal limits. This is also a factor during pregnancy, especially if the mother is calcium-deficient.

Some researchers link fluoridation with congenital bone deformities. Fluoride also encourages crystals of fluoroapatite to form around joints and in soft tissues, characteristic of osteoarthritis. Calcification of arteries is also strongly associated with skeletal fluorosis.

Much of the problem of determining the usefulness of fluoride and fluoridation and its real toxic effects are the methods in which facts are evaluated. The only way we have to evaluate entire populations is statistical. Unfortunately it is impossible to control all variables of an entire city and equally impossible to establish any control populations for similar reasons. It has been said that "there are lies and there are statistical lies." It seems both sides of the fluoridation question have exploited these measures.

Another difficulty in evaluating fluoride's usefulness or danger is a matter of individual differences. Many reports are available showing cases where people drinking the optimal 1 ppm fluoridated water developed toxic fluorosis. We are dealing with the possibility of individual sensitivity to fluoride and also differences in individual consumption. Many people drink excessive amounts of water; others, especially in England, consume excessive amounts of tea. Ordinary tea contains 1 mg fluoride per 6 cups. One documented case was found where a woman in England, who consumed 6.3 to 9.3 mg of fluoride per day, suffered from a form of arthritis which was alleviated by curtailing her tea consumption.

Diet also is a factor. Refined diets have significantly more fluoride than whole grain unrefined diets. The average consumption on a refined diet is 1 mg in nonfluoridated and 1.7 to 3.4 mg in fluoridated areas. In areas or occupations that result in excessive sweating, fluoride consumption can increase drastically.

The point of all this is that it is impossible to guarantee the fluoride intake of any individual. Since fluoride only helps protect infants and children, it is unfair to subject the entire population to an involuntary mass medication that not only will not do good for the entire population, but is assured of doing at least some harm to a significant number.

Those at special risk are:

Calcium-deficient: Fluoride makes calcium reserves insoluble.

Vitamin C-deficient: C is essential for calcium absorption.

Elderly.

Those with impaired renal function.

Diabetics: Prone to kidney disease.

Arthritics: Disturbed calcium metabolism.

Fluoride-sensitive.

Thyroid disease: Fluoride is an iodine antagonist.

Women on the pill: Both pill and fluoride interfere with carbohydrate metabolism.

Pregnant women: Fluoride may bind minerals and trace elements needed for fetal development. (Associated with increase in Down's syndrome, congenital heart disease, anencephalus, stillbirth.)

Infants:
Causes abnormal bone development.
Delays dentition by depressing thyroid function.
Increase in heart damage.
Mottled teeth.

The most important aspect of the fluoride question, however, is that for dental caries (for which fluoride is employed as a preventative), it is entirely unnecessary. Every dentist knows that the true cause of dental disease is improper diet and lack of dental hygiene. A diet high in sugar, candies, refined carbohydrates, soda beverages, and too little fruit and vegetable fiber is the major cause in nearly all cases. (Some may be due to improper diet in the mother while pregnant or breastfeeding.) One study among many supporting this view showed that children given apples instead of sweets after meals got significantly less cavities and gum disease. It is far better to spend money on better food and desserts than on fluoridation, which is both expensive and dangerous.

Historical evidence gives us another example that high-fiber diets help prevent dental caries. Archeology shows that Egyptian mummies of aristocrats had extensive dental caries at a young age, but the peasants had very little. The main difference between the two was diet. Prehistoric humans, living on a diet of fruits, nuts, whole grains, and tuberous vegetables, also had little or no cavities. Once again, the relationship between sugar and refined carbohydrates and the presence of dental caries is well established. As one physician (Lendon Smith) humorously states, "Fluoridate sugar, not water."

For an in-depth look at fluoridation I suggest reading *Fluoridation, The Great Dilemma*, by George L. Waldbott.

(*Note:* Some children with weak enamel may benefit from fluoride use orally and topically. These should be *individually prescribed*.)

FROSTBITE

Definition

Freezing, or the effects of freezing, of an exposed body part. Usual areas involved are fingers, toes, cheeks, nose, and ears.

Symptoms

Tingling and redness, followed by paleness and numbness. Gangrene may occur.

Discussion

Frostbite can be a very dangerous condition, leading to loss of the affected area due to tissue damage and gangrene. Any frostbite damage should be seen by a physician at the earliest possible opportunity. Superficial frostbite, sometimes called frostnip, leaves the area firm, white, and cold. Peeling and blistering, which occurs 24 to 72 hours later, is usually the only complication, with occasional prolonged cold sensitivity of the area. In deep frostbite, the area is cold, hard, white, and painless while still frozen, and becomes blotchy red, swollen, and painful on rewarming. Depending on the severity, the complications may be few, or as bad as gangrene.

Treatment

The old technique of rubbing ice to the area to slowly rewarm the tissue is no longer recommended. The best technique now used is to rapidly rewarm the area by a warm bath whenever possible. The temperature range is between 100 to 110°F. Since the area will be numb and therefore without feeling, care must be taken not to burn the tissues. Due to tissue damage, care should be taken in drying not to injure the skin, and the area should not be used. If the feet are involved, it is suggested not to thaw them and then use the feet to walk. If considerable walking must be done, do not thaw the feet until at the destination, and then go to the hospital as soon as possible.

GALLBLADDER DISEASE: Gallstones and Cholecystitis

Definition

Gallstones (cholelithiasis): Concretions in the gallbladder.
Cholecystitis: Inflammation of the gallbladder.

Symptoms

Right upper quadrant abdominal discomfort (may be symptom-free for years); biliary colic (knifelike pain).

Dyspepsia (fatty foods cause gas, fullness, nausea, bloating, and/or belching).

Chronic constipation, headaches, irritation, quick temper, nervousness, pain between shoulder blades on right referred to right shoulder, possible fever and chills with positive Murphy's sign (acute).

(*Note:* In chronic cases the gallbladder is shrunken and scarred. Long-term complications of gallbladder disease include cancer.)

Etiologic Considerations

- Bile stasis: Dietary fats must empty the gallbladder frequently and forceably. Bile stasis allows the bile to become too concentrated. Incomplete emptying is a major cause of gallbladder disease plus stone formation.

- Bile blockage: 95 percent of all cholecystitis is caused by a stone in the neck of the gallbladder, in the cystic duct, or is due to inspissated bile (thickened bile). The gallbladder distends, becomes edematous, and inflamed. Secondary infection may then occur.

- Obesity: Overburdened gallbladder; sluggishness.

- Overeating and faulty diet: Fiber deficiency, fried foods, saturated fats, excess dairy products, excess sugar, refined carbohydrates.

- Food allergy

- Lack of exercise: Decreased bile secretion.

- Liver sluggishness and toxicity
- Female—pregnancy, many children: Associated with gallbladder disease.
- "The pill" doubles chances of gallstones.
- Stress

Discussion

Gallbladder disease and gallstones in particular are most common in the developed nations and are fairly rare in undeveloped nations. This places gallstones in the unique class of diseases called diseases of civilization. With this understanding it becomes clear that much unnecessary surgery can be prevented by simple changes in cultural, dietary, and social habits.

The surgical removal of the gallbladder (rarely necessary) robs the body of a useful organ and does nothing to correct the cause of gallstones or disease. To understand fully the real causes and treatment of these disorders, a little physiological background is useful.

Bile is secreted by the liver at the rate of about 2 L a day. It is then stored in the gallbladder in a concentrated form $(10 \times)$. Bile contains 90 percent water, mucus, bile pigments (bilirubin from hemoglobin breakdown—red blood cell pigment), cholesterol, bile salts (help emulsify fats), lecithin, and inorganic salts. Bile aids digestion and absorption of fat by increasing the solubility of fatty acids and emulsifying fats to make them more easily accessible to lipase, a fat-breaking enzyme from the pancreas. Bile salts are necessary for the absorption of fat-soluble vitamins. They help promote peristalsis and are mildly laxative. Bile is reabsorbed in the intestine, returns to the liver, and stimulates more bile secretion. Bile is initially secreted from the gallbladder due to the hormone cholecystokinin from the intestinal mucosa which is liberated when fatty foods enter the small intestine. This hormone causes the cystic duct and gallbladder to forceably contract and expel its bile contents. With these few facts, you can see that the gallbladder is essential for proper digestion of fat and fat-soluble vitamins, and aids in keeping the bowels regular.

Cholecystitis is almost always secondary to gallstones or thickened bile. Gallstones form due to a combination of factors, the most prominent being faulty diet and bile stasis. The typical American diet of high cholesterol and saturated fatty foods such as fried eggs, bacon, white toast, butter, and coffee with sugar and cream is a fine example of a diet carefully designed to cause gallstones, as well as other serious diseases. Saturated fats, such as excess eggs, milk, cheese, butter, meats, and hydrogenated margarine are all a major factor in causing gallstones. Ninety percent of gallstones are primarily cholesterol in composition. The problem with gallstone formation is not only excess cholesterol, but also a deficiency of many foods that normally keep cholesterol under control.

Refined carbohydrates and sugar upset cholesterol metabolism, and increase blood cholesterol levels. They also decrease bile flow. This effect is enhanced on a high-protein diet. When whole grains are refined, bran is stripped away. Bran has been found to therapeutically lower cholesterol levels. It influences the amount of chenodeoxycholic acid, a natural bile acid which lowers cholesterol and dissolves stones.

Vitamin E, also lost in carbohydrate refining, has been found to both prevent and dissolve gallstones. Vitamin E is commonly deficient in women on the Pill and during pregnancy. Lecithin, an element deficient in most modern diets, is a well-known fat emulsifier, and helps keep cholesterol in solution. Vitamin A helps keep the mucosal walls healthy and prevents excess dead cells from entering the gallbladder and bile. A diet rich in vitamin B complex helps empty the gallbladder more efficiently. Vitamin C helps convert cholesterol into bile acids and renders it harmless.

Unsaturated oils help stimulate the gallbladder to contract vigorously and thus cleanse itself on a regular basis. Raw, unrefined olive oil is the most efficient of all oils. This is the reason that Italians, who consume large amounts of olive oil in their diet, have a low incidence of gallstones. Olive oil has been used for therapy in gallbladder disease as far back as the Roman empire. (*Note:* A no-fat diet or very low fat diet will actually cause gallstones by decreasing bile flow and allowing the bile to become concentrated.)

Most gallstone patients are hearty eaters and high livers. While not all patients are "fat, flatulent, female, and over 40," certainly the majority are. Excess food puts an unnecessary burden on the digestive organs. Once the ingested food reaches a point of exceeding the body's enzymatic capacity, the rest remains undigested, or partially digested, causing bowel toxemia, gas, discomfort, and constipation (or diarrhea). A headache may soon follow. Smaller, more frequent meals increase bile flow, stimulate the gallbladder, and keep bile from getting too concentrated.

Exercise stimulates bile secretion by the liver. Too little exercise, therefore too little bile, causes a deficiency of bile digestion, especially if the foods eaten are of the wrong type.

Anger, fear, excitement, worry, and hate all cause bile to cease flowing, and therefore encourage stone formation.

Treatment

Therapy for gallstones and gallbladder disease is aimed at first flushing the gallbladder of its stones by use of specific time-tested dietary regimens and herbs. Many variations exist as to the type of foods and liquids consumed, and the relative proportions of the flushing agents. Several different examples will be given. Nearly all these regimens are based on the therapeutic effects of olive oil.

Prior to attempting these methods, an x-ray of the gallbladder is advised, to determine the size of the stones. If they are too large to be successfully passed and become lodged in the ducts, severe pain and possible surgery may be the result. For very large stones special methods are required to dissolve the stone so that it may be safely passed.

Diet

LIVER AND GALLBLADDER DIET

Stage 1: Begin treatment with a 3-to-5-to-7-day grapefruit mono diet:

Breakfast	Fresh grapefruit
Midmorning	Fresh grapefruit juice
Lunch	Fresh grapefruit
Midafternoon	Fresh grapefruit juice
Supper	Fresh grapefruit
Evening	Fresh grapefruit juice

Stage 2:

Breakfast Fresh grapefruit

Midmorning Fresh grapefruit juice, black cherry juice, parsley tea, carrot and watercress juice, raw beet juice, apple juice, or dandelion root tea.

Lunch A large, varied raw salad with nuts (other than peanuts) or soy-based protein with one or two whole wheat crisp breads with vegetarian margarine.

Midafternoon Same as midmorning.

Supper
1. Same as lunch; *or*
2. Any vegetarian meal (excluding the use of dairy products or eggs), with baked potato and two other green or root vegetables; *or*
3. Steamed vegetables and brown rice or other whole grain. Dessert: Any fresh, baked, or stewed fruit.

Evening Grapefruit juice
Olive oil plus lemon, garlic, and honey as salad dressing.

OLIVE OIL THERAPY

Olive Oil Flush 1:
8:00 A.M. ½ pint raw unrefined olive oil plus juice of 2 lemons.

9:00 A.M.   Repeat

10:00 A.M.   Repeat

1:00 P.M.   2 tsp Epsom salts in a glass of warm water.

Olive Oil Flush 2:
On empty stomach, drink 4 oz raw unrefined olive oil mixed with 4 oz lemon juice. Lie on right side with hips elevated for 2 hours.

Olive Oil Flush 3:
1 pint pure olive oil
8 to 9 lemons (juiced)
Drink plenty of apple juice or grapefruit juice for 24 to 72 hours before starting diet.
Begin at 7:00 P.M.: 4 tbs olive oil with 1 tsp lemon juice, separately or mixed. Repeat every 15 minutes until all the oil is gone.

Gallbladder and Liver Flush 4:*
Follow Stage 1 of the liver diet for 3 to 5 to 7 days, then continue Stage 2 for 7 to 14 days. Five days preceding the day of the olive oil therapy, take as much apple juice as can be consumed, in addition to your normally prescribed Stage 2 diet. On each of these 5 days also take 90 drops of orthophosphoric acid diluted in water. (After flush take 10 drops per day unless otherwise directed.) Three hours after lunch take 1 tbs Epsom salts in approximately 1 oz water (chase with citrus juice to avoid the bitter taste). Instead of supper, have citrus juice (grapefruit). At approximately 7 P.M. take a strong coffee enema in which 2 tbs Epsom salts are dissolved. Then do *either:*

Straight Flush:
Just before bed, take ½ cup of unrefined olive oil and ½ cup citrus juice. They may be blended or taken separately.

Royal Flush:
Eight 2-oz doses of olive oil taken over 2-to-4-hour period, approximately every 15 minutes. Citrus juice may be blended with it. (*Note:* Some people find olive oil difficult to get down. Sometimes sipping it through a straw so that the oil does not come in contact with the lips helps considerably.)

Therapeutic Agents in Diet

ACUTE CASES

    Apple juice*
    Beet extract tablets
    Beet root tops, beet juice*
    Beet tops, carrot, and lemon juice

*Asterisks indicate the most frequently used therapeutic agents.

Chamomile tea: To dissolve.
Dandelion tea and dandelion greens: Clears obstruction.*
Grapefruit juice*
Olive oil plus lemon*
Pear juice
Peppermint tea
Pineapple juice
Potassium broth
Radish
Watercress and nasturtium

CHRONIC CASES SUPPLEMENTS

Vitamin A (micellized): 10,000 to 25,000 IU two times per day. *Use any dose of vitamin A over 50,000 IU per day with medical supervision only.*

Vitamin B complex: 25 to 50 mg two to three times per day.*

Vitamin B$_6$: 50 to 100 mg one to two times per day.*

Vitamin C: 500 to 2000 mg three to six times per day.*

Vitamin E (micellized): 400 IU one to three times daily.*

OTHER

Alkaline foods*

Beet tablets*

Bran: 1 tsp with water two to three times per day.

Brewer's yeast

Choline, inositol, and methionine are useful lipotrophics and bile stimulants.*

Black radish plus olive oil (to dissolve): 2 tbs grated radish with 1 to 2 tbs olive oil, mixed. Eat ½ hour before breakfast for 40 days.*

Corn oil

EPA (Eicosapentaenoic acid): 5 to 10 g per day.*

Laxative foods

Lecithin as concentrated phosphatidyl choline: Take 1 to 2 capsules three to four times per day.

Olive oil: Include in diet daily.*

*Asterisks indicate the most frequently used therapeutic agents.

Orthophosphoric acid*

Smaller meals

Taurine: Thins bile (for prevention).

BOTANICALS

Celandine (*Chelidonium majus*): Reduces inflammation of bile ducts.

Chamomile (*Anthemis nobilis*)

Dandelion (*Taraxacum officinale*)*

Fringe tree (*Chionanthus virginicus*): Increases bile flow.

Oregon grape root (*Berberis aquifolium*): Stimulates bile.

Wild yam root (*Dioscorea villosa*): For colic.

Yellow dock (*Rumex crispus*): Stimulates bile.

(Note: Be sure to drink six to eight glasses of water to help prevent gallstone formation.)

GALLSTONES (see Gallbladder Disease)

GASTRIC ULCER (see Peptic Ulcer)

GASTRITIS (see Digestive Disorders)

GLAUCOMA

Definition

Elevated intraocular pressure with gradual vision loss. No early symptoms; later, colored halos around lights, eye ache, headache, tunnel vision, visual abnormalities, frequent changes of eyeglass prescriptions.

Etiologic Considerations

• Blockage of outflow of aqueous humor
• Increased production of aqueous humor
• Prolonged stress

*Asterisks indicate the most frequently used therapeutic agents.

Adrenal exhaustion
- Glandular imbalance
    Adrenals
    Thyroid
- Toxicity
- Allergy
- Arteriosclerosis
- Heredity
- Autonomic system disturbance
- Spinal lesion—cervical, upper thoracic
    Disturbed nervous and blood supply
- Cranial lesion
- Drugs
    Antispasmodics
    Steroids
- Coffee, caffeine, nicotine, and alcohol
- Blood vessel constriction
- Blood sugar abnormalities (diabetes-associated)
- Trauma

Discussion

The basic problem with glaucoma is an increase in fluid pressure within the eye which eventually damages the delicate optic nerve at the back of the eye. This nerve is the connecting link between what your eye sees and its interpretation by the brain. Intraocular pressure depends on an equilibrium between inflow of fluid called aqueous humor from an area called the ciliary body and its outflow from the tissues of the iridocorneal angle. If fluid production is too great, or more commonly, if fluid outflow is obstructed, pressure builds, causing tissue (nerve) damage. The higher the pressure above normal, the more serious and rapid is the damage. However, even lower pressure increases over a prolonged period of time may cause nerve damage and thus vision loss.

Once damage has occurred and vision partly lost, it can never be regained. Since early symptoms are not present, or are not very noticeable in most cases, an early diagnosis depends on routine eye pressure checks. Many optometrists offer this check as part of a normal eye examination.

The actual cause of glaucoma is not entirely clear. Some cases clearly show a hereditary predisposition. Blood sugar abnormalities, specifically diabetes, are also associated with glaucoma. Prolonged stress may precede glaucoma, as may a history of improper eye use such as reading in dim lights, watching excessive amounts of television or movies with poor lighting, or habitual use of sunglasses. Some physicians feel that there is a clear connection between glandular imbalances such as adrenal exhaustion or hypothyroidism. Others point to general toxic causes as a factor.

Whatever the actual cause, it seems likely that the way in which these tissues suffer damage is by reduced nutrition in the form of altered blood lymph, or hormonal or nervous supply. This may be due to hormonal or glandular imbalance, constitutional toxicity, spinal lesions, cranial lesions, habitual use of coffee, tea, alcohol, cigarettes, or any other factor such as allergy, which might disturb the body's normal functioning.

Treatment

Orthodox treatment for glaucoma consists of eye drops designed to reduce the fluid production in the eye, or to increase its outflow. Should these fail several types of surgery are now available, including new procedures using laser technology.

However, there is hope for a more complete and natural cure of glaucoma for some patients. The most well-documented treatment alternative in reducing intraocular pressure is megadoses of vitamin C. In studies where 5 to 7 g of vitamin C were given up to seven times a day, remarkable decreases in eye pressure were noted. The higher the initial pressure, the more dramatic the pressure reduction. However, even with mildly elevated pressures, significant reductions occurred.

Another well-recognized substance found in experimental studies to lower intraocular pressure is marijuana. This, at present, is a controlled drug, but available by prescription for this purpose from a sympathetic ophthalmologist.

Other less well-known approaches to glaucoma involve generalized constitutional treatment along with local physiotherapy and spinal manipulations. These therapies base their methods on correcting hormonal imbalances, circulatory and nervous supply deficiencies, and toxic causes.

Diet

The basic dietary changes are aimed at supplying adequate nutrition, encouraging internal cleansing, and establishing equilibrium. Periods on vegetable juice (carrot) and fruit juice fasting are recommended, followed by short, exclusively raw food diets. The interim diet emphasizes carrots, greens (lettuce, celery, sprouts, beet tops, etc.) and plenty of seafoods (fish, oysters, seaweeds, kelp, etc.). Potassium broth should be taken regularly or as a stock base for other soups. Gelatin should be included whenever possible in this regimen. These three stages (fast, raw foods, and interim diet) should be rotated at intervals, the length of each depending on the condition of the patient.

Absolutely no alcohol, coffee, black tea, cola, or cigarettes should be taken during the diet since these interfere with the normal blood circulation to the eyes and upset the hormonal stability in the system as a whole.

Physiotherapy

• Spinal manipulation: Specific lesions will usually be found in the upper cervical region (especially C1) with others in the general cervical and upper thoracic regions. Cranial lesions may also be found as a result of trauma. The endonasal technique (see Appendix I) may be useful. Precede all spinal therapy with moist heat.

• Atomodine fume baths: Put 1 tsp of Atomodine in 1 pint of boiled water. Make an improvised steam tent by placing pot under wooden chair and covering chair and body up to neck with a blanket. This will allow the Atomodine fumes to settle upon the body, helping to correct hormonal imbalances. Repeat two times per month.

• Sweat baths, saunas: One to two times per week.

• Massage: Follow each spinal therapy, sweat bath, and especially each Atomodine fume bath with massage from the midthoracic area up to the occiput, along the paravertebral muscles. This should be deep neuromuscular type massage with the following mixture:
    Olive oil: 2 oz
    Peanut oil: 2 oz
    Oil of sassafras: ¼ oz
    Liquefied lanolin: 1 tsp
Follow each massage session with alternate hot and cold showers, including alternate hot and cold head douches.

• Ice-cold baths: Fill a large basin with ice-cold water. Immerse both eyes in the container and rapidly blink eyes open and shut five to ten times. Rest and then repeat two to three times, two times each day.

• Alternate hot and cold eye compresses: Apply a hot, moist towel or folded washcloth to both eyes for 2 to 3 minutes; then apply an ice-cold cloth for 2 to 3 minutes. Repeat three times, ending with cold.

• Ice-cold eye compress: Apply ice-cold moist towel or folded washcloth for 2 to 3 minutes; rest 1 minute and reapply three to four times. Repeat two times per day.

- Bates eye exercise**
- Neck exercises

Avoid dark TV viewing, excessive movie attendance, reading in poor light, or wearing sunglasses excessively.

Therapeutic Agents

VITAMINS AND MINERALS

Vitamin A: 25,000 IU two times per day (micellized). *Use any dose of vitamin A over 50,000 IU per day with medical supervision only.**

Vitamin B_1: 100 mg two times per day.*

Vitamin B_2

Niacin*

Vitamin B_6 Diuretic

Vitamin B_{12}

Vitamin B complex: 50 mg two times per day.*

Vitamin C: 5 to 7 g seven times per day; average for 150-lb person 35,000 mg per day (extra B_6 and magnesium is required to prevent increased calcium excretion which is associated with the tendency to form kidney stones).*

Vitamin E: 400 to 800 IU per day.

Rutin: 20 to 30 mg three times per day.*

Bioflavonoids

Calcium: 800 to 1000 mg per day.*

Chromium

Magnesium: 400 to 500 mg per day.*

Potassium

OTHERS

Kelp or other iodine source (i.e., Atomodine or 636) (Cayce products)*

Spirulina: 1 tsp three times per day.*

---

*Asterisks indicate the most frequently used therapeutic agents.
**Found in *The Art of Seeing,* by Aldous Huxley, pp. 6–183.

(*Note:*   These nontoxic therapies may help control glaucoma or reduce pressure levels to prevent need for surgery. *In all cases remain under the care and supervision of your ophthalmologist, who can regularly check your intraocular pressure.*)

GOITER (see Thyroid Disorders)

GOUT

Definition

A recurrent form of arthritis affecting the peripheral joints. The metatarsophalangeal joint of the great toe is the most common site affected.

Symptoms

Acute joint pain, warmth, swelling, acute tenderness, and redness. The skin is tense and shiny red or purple.

First attacks usually occur at night with pain that is throbbing and excruciating. These first attacks are usually short-lived, but subsequent ones last longer, for weeks or even months. Gradual joint destruction may occur. Chalklike soft-tissue nodules may form in the earlobes, tendons, and cartilage.

Etiologic Considerations

• Excess meat consumption

• Excess refined carbohydrates and sugar: increases uric acid levels

• Overindulgence in alcoholic beverages

• Excess coffee

• Lack of fresh fruit and vegetables

• Acidosis

• Reduced renal clearance of uric acid

• Excess purine synthesis

• Obesity

- Hyperlipidemia, hypertriglyceridemia

- Hereditary: Enzyme deficiency causes excess production of uric acid, resulting in uric acid kidney stones and gout.

- Sedentary existence

- Stress causes increased uric acid levels.
  Executive syndrome
  Adrenal exhaustion

- Previous injury to area

- Previous oral antibiotics causing friendly intestinal bacteria deficiency

- Lead poisoning

- Adrenal exhaustion

- Drug-induced: Penicillin, insulin, diuretics.

- Intestinal toxemia

- Gout may be associated with psoriasis, thyroid and parathyroid disease, cardiovascular disease, kidney disease, obesity, and hypertension.

Discussion

Gout results from the deposition of sharp crystals of monosodium urate in tendons and joints. It also may be deposited in the intestine and kidney tissues, and may cause kidney disease and death. Hyperuricemia is associated with disease in affluent societies. It has been considered a disease of the wealthy. As such it has often been called "the rich man's disease." Throughout history the sufferer of gout has been depicted as a portly, middle-aged gentleman sitting in a huge leather chair with one foot resting painfully on a soft cushion as he consumes great quantities of meat and wine. This picture has arisen from the fact that many an acute attack of gout follows an evening of wining and dining. Certain nucleic acids (purines) in many foods increase the uric acid content of the blood. This occurs because uric acid is the ultimate oxidation product of the purine bases adenine and guanine. Organ meats and alcoholic beverages are the worst offenders. While meat actually contains purines and so helps raise uric acid levels directly, alcohol inhibits uric acid excretion by the kidneys, thus retaining uric acid in the body.

Other factors also influence the amount of uric acid in the body. A high-fat diet will increase the uric acid level. Also associated with raised uric acid levels is obesity. As weight increases, so does the uric acid level in the blood.

Another form of gout, which can be called "poor man's gout," results from consumption of an excessive amount of refined carbohydrates and sugar.

The dietary explanation of gout has come under some disrepute in recent years. Although it is not denied that a large portion of uric acid comes from dietary sources, it has become clear that this is not the only source. Endogenous uric acid, or uric acid made in the body through the breakdown of purine bases, is also a major source. This discovery has led many physicians to abandon the classic uric acid avoidance diets and employ new drugs that are aimed at lowering the uric acid levels artificially. On such therapy a person is enabled to continue moderate alcohol and meat intake.

I personally feel the drug dependence approach is short-sighted. A raised uric acid level and consequent gouty arthritis are valuable danger signals telling us that something is wrong with our manner of living. Once we understand this message we have the opportunity to reestablish proper equilibrium and prevent other diseases also associated with excess meat, fat, and alcohol intake.

Treatment

Diet

Noncitrus alkaline fasting is the best method for eliminating uric acid from the system and establishing equilibrium. These fasts need to be very short (3 to 4 days) in duration and repeated often over a period of at least 6 months, however, since uric acid levels rise sharply as keto acids increase in the blood due to fat breakdown. A highly alkaline urine helps keep uric acid in solution and a high fluid intake helps remove uric acid from the system. For these reasons noncitrus fruit juice, vegetable juice, or potassium broth are excellent liquids to use in the fast.

It is important to understand that gout has taken many years to develop and will also take some time to correct. Naturopathy does not offer quick and easy ways to remove symptoms. What it does offer is the possibility of a total cure. True treatment and cure is possible if the patient both understands and is willing to follow these simple methods. For those who truly wish to rid themselves of the pain and disfigurement gout causes, the road is long but very rewarding.

Liquid fast (any or all):

Noncitrus juice (may make worse at first)
Vegetable juice
Celery and parsley juice
Red cherry juice (neutralizes uric acid)
Carrot juice
Potassium broth

Diet between fast: Low uric acid, low purine, low fat, and no alcohol. In general, the diet should consist of 75 percent raw foods, with the greatest portion of these being nonstarchy vegetables. Vegetables to include in large quantities are celery, carrots, alfalfa sprouts, kale, cabbage, parsley, and any other green leafy vegetable (other than spinach). As far as fruit is concerned, bing cherries, bananas, and strawberries are especially useful.

If possible, this cleansing diet, devoid of any carbohydrates or protein, should be adhered to for 5-day intervals between the first two 3-to-4-day fasts. This will encourage elimination and weight reduction and help detoxify the system. Should this diet become too difficult, the next stage of the treatment should then be started. This consists of the addition of low-purine foods such as raw goat's milk with yoghurt, poached eggs, low-fat cheese, a few nuts, brown rice, millet, and corn bread. The bulk of the diet still remains as above (green vegetables).

The following chart will help give some basic guidelines for the long-term diet:

HIGH-PURINE DIET (AVOID): GROUP 1

Anchovies	Mussels
Meat broth	Porridge (oatmeal)
Meats	Roe
Heart	Sardines
Herring	Scallops
Kidney	Sweetbreads
Liver	Yeast
Mackerel	Spices
Meat extracts	Organ meats

MODERATE PURINE DIET: GROUP 2

Bran	Spinach
Fish	Beans
Fowl	Lentils
Shellfish	Mushrooms
Asparagus	Peas
Cauliflower	Whole wheat

LOW-PURINE DIET: GROUP 3

Rice	Green vegetables
Millet	Nuts

Goat's milk	Cornbread
Goat's yoghurt	Sea vegetables
Low-fat cheese	Fruit
Eggs	

A high fluid intake is essential, as well, to cleanse the system of uric acid. The best therapeutic procedure is to alternate the fast and low-purine diet every 7 to 14 days, fasting 3 to 5 days, and then going on the diet for 7 to 14 days.

Therapeutic Agents

VITAMINS AND MINERALS

Vitamin A: 25,000 to 75,000 IU. *Use any dose of vitamin A over 50,000 IU per day with medical supervision only.* *

Vitamin B complex: 50 to 100 mg one to three times per day.*

Folic acid: 25 mg three times per day.*

Pantothenic acid: 100 to 250 mg per day.*

Vitamin C: Up to 5000+ per day.*

Bioflavonoids: 1000 mg per day.

Vitamin E: 400 to 1200 per day.*

OTHERS

Lecithin: 2 to 4 capsules three times per day.

SOD (Superoxide dismutase): 2 to 3 tablets three to four times per day.

BOTANICALS

Burdock root (*Arctium lappa*)*

Colchicum (*Colchicum autumnale*): Use tincture: 5 to 15 drops three times per day during acute attack only.*

Celery (*Apium graveolens*): Use tincture of seeds, 10 to 30 drops two or three times per day. Eat stalk in very large amounts daily.*

White bryony (*Bryonia alba*): For pain made worse by motion; use as tincture or low-potency homeopathic dilution.*

*Asterisks indicate the most frequently used therapeutic agents.

Therapeutic Suggestion

See Arthritis for physiotherapy.

GUM DISEASE (see Teeth and Gum Disease)

HALITOSIS (Bad Breath)

Definition and Symptoms

Offensive mouth odor.

Etiologic Considerations

- Digestive disturbances
  Digestive enzyme deficiency, hydrochloric acid deficiency, food intolerance, improper diet or food combinations.
- Diet
  Overeating (exhaustion of digestive enzymatic capacity)
  Food allergy (milk, wheat, and others)
  Fiber deficiency
  Excess meat
  Excess refined carbohydrates
  Mucus-forming diet
- Gum or tooth disease (poor dental hygiene; improper diet)
  Pyorrhea
  Gingivitis
  Cavities
- Sinusitis
- Postnasal drip
- Tonsillitis
- Respiratory problems
- Constipation (poor eliminations)
- Smoking
- Anxiety (stomach derangement)
- Heavy metal poisoning (selenium and others)
- Liver disease

- Diabetes
- Dehydration
- Mouth breathing

Discussion

Foul breath is *always* a sign of some internal disorder and should never be treated only with palliative mouth washes. The first investigation should be of the teeth and gums. A visit to a good dental hygienist or dentist will reveal if tooth or gum disease is the cause. If the mouth is healthy, all other local problems should then be eliminated, including sinusitis, chronic nasal allergic symptoms, postnasal drip, tonsillitis, and chronic lung conditions. Should these problems be absent, the most probable cause of the offense is a digestive disturbance, usually due to improper diet. The most common problem involves poor eliminations and constipation. As the bowel contents are retained for prolonged periods within the body, toxins are reabsorbed, which cause coating of the tongue and foul breath. (See Constipation for further discussion and treatment.)

Another common factor is digestive enzyme deficiency. In a few cases an actual deficiency of hydrochloric acid or other digestive enzymes may be the primary cause. In most cases the enzymes were of normal character and amount, but have over a period of time become depleted in their production by dietary abuse.

Very large meals or too-frequent meals exceed the body's ability to produce digestive enzymes. This causes large portions of only partly digested foods to enter the small intestine, setting up fermentation which causes both flatulence and halitosis. Improper food combinations also create conditions impossible for proper digestion. Such foods as citrus fruits and complex carbohydrates (i.e., bread), a common combination at breakfast, is a common offender. Mixing fruits and vegetables or melons with just about anything else also will upset digestion.

Fiber deficiency and an excess consumption of refined carbohydrates along with too much milk or meat seems to be the worst dietary regimen as far as breath is concerned. Not only is this diet highly mucus-forming, but it favors tooth and gum disease, digestive weakness, constipation, and a host of other diseases, both related and unrelated to halitosis.

Certain individual foods may be the culprits in isolated cases. Many people simply cannot digest either milk or wheat. Others have special food intolerances or allergies that may upset digestion. These need to be diagnosed and eliminated. Useful tests include the cytotoxic food allergy test, RAST test, pulse test, or food elimination diets.

Stress and anxiety are often the main cause of bad breath. Prolonged stress will make normal digestion impossible by affecting both the nervous and endocrine systems.

Certain heavy metal poisoning may cause halitosis. Selenium has been known to give a garliclike odor to the breath.

Treatment

Dental Hygiene

If dental problems are the cause no treatments will be beneficial until the offending cause is treated. Pyorrhea must be treated with a proper high-fiber diet, herbs, Ipsab (Cayce product), or myrrh, *Hydrastis* (goldenseal) and glycothymoline mouth rinse, proper brushing, and dental flossing.

Diet

Proper digestion and elimination may be reestablished by a short 3-day apple mono diet or a longer brown rice mono diet. This is then followed by the constipation regimen, or simply by converting to a high-fiber diet with sufficient raw vegetables and fruit. Meals should be smaller than normal and taken dry, without drinks or soups. Don't drink liquids within the half hour before meals and not until an hour to an hour and a half following meals. This helps prevent digestive juices from becoming diluted and therefore less efficient. Although water is easily acidified by the stomach acid normally, a hydrochloric acid-deficient individual needs all the acid he or she can produce for digestion. Milk is particularly detrimental if taken with meals, since it requires such a great amount of acid to be acidified, leaving little or none left for the meal itself. This may be why kosher laws do not allow dairy products to be consumed with meat at the same meals. Hydrochloric acid is essential for proper protein digestion. Drinking water between meals, however, is very important to help cleanse the body. Cases of bad breath are improved by drinking six to eight glasses of water per day. In some cases more prolonged liquid fasting with enemas or colonics may be useful. Often the mono diet or fast will need to be repeated several times to gain complete results.

Physiotherapy

- Colonics
- Enemas
- Outdoor exercise
- Skin brushing (see Appendix I)
- Wet salt skin rubs (see Appendix I)

Therapeutic Agents

VITAMINS AND MINERALS

Vitamin A: 25,000 IU one to two times per day. *Use any dose of Vitamin A over 50,000 IU per day with medical supervision only.* *

Vitamin B$_6$

Vitamin B complex: 250 mg one to two times daily. *

Zinc: 15 to 50 mg two to three times per day. *

OTHERS

Bran: 1 tbs with water before all meals. *

Charcoal

Pancreatic enzymes with meals.

Fresh fruit, especially apples. *

Fresh vegetables, especially carrots and greens. *

Glycothymoline: 6 drops internally per day. *

Ipsab (Cayce product): Applied to gums where gum health is cause.

Lactobacillus: Normalizes bowel ecology; 2 capsules three times per day.

Laxatives (see Constipation regimen)

Liquid chlorophyll: As much as possible. *

BOTANICALS

Chew any of the following:
Anise seeds (*Pimpinella anisum*)
Cardamom seeds (*Elettaria cardamomum*)
Caraway seeds (*Carum carvi*)
Fennel seeds (*Foeniculum vulgare*)
Parsley (*Petroselinum sativum*)
Whole cloves (*Eugenia caryophyllata*): Suck.
Coneflower (*Echinacea angustifolia*)
Goldenseal and myrrh gargle for gum disorders.
Goldenseal (*Hydrastis canadensis*): For internal causes.
Peppermint tea (*Mentha piperita*): For digestion.

*Asterisks indicate the most frequently used therapeutic agents.

HEADACHE AND MIGRAINE

Definition

Headache: Pain in or around head.
Migraine: Recurrent attacks of headaches with visual and gastrointestinal disturbances.

Symptoms

Headache: Irregular attacks of pain in various parts of head or in the sinuses in the facial area.
Migraine: Recurrent pain with associated nausea, vomiting, and photophobia. The pain is usually confined to one side of head or eye. The patient is irritable and desires seclusion without direct light. Attacks may be preceded by flashes of light due to intracerebral vasoconstriction and followed by head pain due to dilation of extracerebral cranial arteries in the dura and scalp.

Etiologic Considerations

- Spinal
  Atlas (C1)
  Axis (C2)
  C1 to C7
  Cervical/thoracic junction (C6 to T2)

- Muscular spasm
  Suboccipital triangle, neck and shoulder tension, toxicity

- Arthritis
  Nerve compression (direct and indirect due to osteophytes or inflammatory disease)

- Stress
  Teeth grinding, anxiety, perfectionist, depression, insomnia

- Digestive problems
  Constipation, indigestion, intestinal toxicity, inflammation of stomach

- Diet
  Coffee (including coffee withdrawal), junk foods, tea, cocoa, salt, fats, excess carbohydrates and sugars

- Hypoglycemia

- Allergy

- Toxic

    Drugs, infections, kidney disease, liver disease, arthritis, food additives, gas appliances, paint fumes, nicotine excess, vitamin overdose, coffee excess, monosodium glutamate (Chinese restaurant syndrome due to excess MSG for sensitive individuals leading to headache, nausea, vomiting, and diarrhea)

- Liver disease

    Toxicity, congestion, gallbladder disease, blood toxicity

- Head injuries

- High blood pressure

- Circulation

    Cerebral hypoxia

- Disease of eye, ear, nose, throat, sinuses, teeth

- Anemia

- Water retention

    Menstruation, premenstrual tension, pregnancy, vitamin B_6 deficiency

- Birth control pill

- Menstrual disorders

- After spinal puncture

- Meningitis

- Tumor

- Eye strain

    Poorly fitting glasses, prolonged concentration, poor vision

Discussion

Headaches and migraines are frequently confused and the terms have been used by many almost synonymously. However, they are two very distinct entities and should always be accurately diagnosed. The case history usually is sufficient to establish a migraine with its recurrent one-sided nature and the associated visual and gastric disturbances. A migraine diagnosis is important since this condition is deep-seated and therefore may take longer to correct. Specific allergy is commonly found in migraine patients and tyramine-containing foods such as cheese, wine, citrus, and then to a lesser extent, avocados, plums, bananas, raspberries, and alcoholic beverages all have been known to initiate an attack. The exact mechanism by which tyramine, a breakdown product of the amino acid tyrosine, works is not proven. It is suspected that tyramine causes a release of norepinephrine, causing vasoconstriction of the blood vessels in the scalp and brain. This results in a reduced blood supply, which may be the cause of the visual symptoms that so often warn of a migraine. As the norepinephrine supply is exhausted, the blood vessels respond by dilating, according to the law of dual effect where every action has an equal and opposite reaction. The enlarged vessels are the postulated cause of the migraine pain. Other food allergies or sensitivities may be a factor. Chocolate is a common offender, but any food may be the cause. It is estimated that at least 25 percent of migraine cases are due to food sensitivity. Refer to Allergy for more detail on allergy diagnosis and treatment.

From the lengthy list of possible etiologic considerations, it becomes obvious that to first cure chronic headaches a thorough case history is important to help isolate the major cause. Often, several factors will coexist and all these must be dealt with to obtain permanent relief. The most frequently occurring causes are spinal lesions, intestinal disturbances, liver congestion, poor circulation, hypoglycemia, allergy, menstrual disorders, sinusitis, muscular tension, and arthritis.

In regard to stress, muscular tension, and cervical arthritis, I feel that these are generally progressive. The most common syndrome I see is the middle aged (usually female) patient with severe headaches due to stress and inability to relax. This slowly restricts cervical movements and circulation. Chronic muscle hypertonicity causes local toxicity (due to accumulated metabolites) and decreased disc space. The result is chronic headaches with or without other referred pains down to the hands. Over the years this lack of circulation and restricted movement becomes recognizable on x-rays as osteophytic lips and spurs, the classic findings in osteoarthritis. This is a perfect example of how improper emotions eventually affect the physical body, causing disease.

An interesting note about migraines and coffee consumption comes from the action of coffee, which constricts blood vessels and therefore helps relieve many headaches of vascular origin (a migraine headache is one type of vascular headache). Many people report chronic morning headaches until the first cup of coffee is consumed. This "coffee cure" has little real curative effect. In fact, due to the law of dual effect which governs all drug activity in the body, any agent which elicits a given action by the body will later cause an equal but opposite reaction. Therefore the vasoconstriction caused by caffeine is followed by vasodilation (the cause of vascular headaches) later on. This is one of the reasons a midmorning and midafternoon headache will recur in heavy coffee consumers.

Treatment

Treatment depends on predisposing causes. If liver congestion is a major factor, as it often is, a liver-cleansing fast and liver-cleansing herbs are indicated. Intestinal toxemia also calls for fasting and enemas. Hypoglycemia-related head aches require frequent high-protein meals and specific nutrients related to that disorder (refer to the specific headings that apply). In general, alkaline fasts repeated 3 to 7 days are usually very therapeutic, with an enema taken on days 1, 2, 3, 5, and 7.

Fasts

Apple juice (general)
Fruit juice (general)
Grapefruit juice (liver congestion)
Mucus-cleansing diets (see Appendix I): Sinusitis
Hot water and lemon juice (general, liver)
Fruit diet (less severe general)

Enemas

Coffee (to relieve acute migraine)

Emetics

The induction of vomiting will usually abort an early migraine and may help relieve a severe headache in many cases.
Lobelia is taken in emetic doses.

Hydrotherapy

Ice compress to base of head while lying in darkened room.
Ice to forehead with simultaneous hot foot bath is also effective to abort an attack.

Exercise

Vigorous daily exercise seems to help reduce frequency of attacks.

Therapeutic Agents

VITAMINS AND SUPPLEMENTS

Vitamin B complex: 25 to 200 mg one to two times per day.*

Vitamin B_{12}: 10 mg three times per day in acute conditions.

Niacin/niacinamide: 50 to 200 mg three times per day in acute conditions.*

Vitamin B_6*

*Asterisks indicate the most frequently used therapeutic agents.

Vitamin C complex

Calcium: 800 to 11,000 mg per day or 200 to 400 per hour in acute attacks.

Magnesium: 400 to 800 mg per day or 100 to 200 mg per hour in acute attacks.

OTHERS

Atomodine
Detox formula (Seroyal)
Garlic

BOTANICALS

Betony (*Betonica officinalis*): With vertigo.

Black cohosh (*Cimicifuga racemosa*): Relaxing nervine, antispasmodic, sedative, especially for headaches of menstrual origin.

Blue flag (*Iris versicolor*)*

Celandine (*Chelidonium majus*): Liver involvement.

Chamomile (*Anthemis nobilis*): Peppermint plus catnip tea for sick headache and nervous stomach.*

Culver's root (*Leptandra virginica*): With liver involvement.

Fringe tree (*Chionanthus virginicus*): For bilious headache.

Goldenseal (*Hydrastis canadensis*): For bilious headache.

Hops (*Humulus lupulus*): Hypnotic.*

Jamaica dogwood (*Piscidia erythrina*)

Lady's slipper (*Cypripedium pubescens*): Headaches of climacteric; hysterical headaches; reflex headaches from ovaries or uterus.

Lavender (*Lavandula officinalis*): To forehead.

Lobelia (*Lobelia inflata*)*

Mistletoe (*Viscum flavescens*): Headaches due to increased blood flow to brain, high blood pressure.

Pulsatilla, or pasque flower (*Anemone pulsatilla*): Nervous and gastric headache; neurotic headache with menstrual disorders.

Passion flower (*Passiflora incarnata*)*

Peppermint (*Mentha piperita*): Headaches of stomach origin.

---

*Asterisks indicate the most frequently used therapeutic agents.

Salicin willow (*Salix alba*)

Senna (*Cassia marilandica*)

Skullcap (*Scutellaria lateriflora*)*

Valerian (*Valeriana officinalis*)

Wintergreen (*Coaultheria procumbens*)

Yellow jessamine (*Gelsemium sempervirens*): Drink ½ to 1 cup infusion every ½ to 1 hour until headache is relieved.*

USEFUL PRESCRIPTIONS

1. Chamomile (*Anthemis nobilis*)
   Peppermint (*Mentha piperita*)
   Rosemary (*Rosemarinus officinalis*)
   Skullcap (*Scutellaria lateriflora*)
   Valerian (*Valeriana officinalis*)

2. Catnip (*Nepeta cataria*)
   Chamomile (*Anthemis nobilis*)
   Peppermint (*Mentha piperita*)

3. Chamomile (*Anthemis nobilis*)
   Senna (*Cassia marilandica*)

(*Note:* Severe headaches may be due to a serious medical disorder. An example is the headache of glaucoma which may, if left untreated, lead to vision loss or blindness in a very short period of time. Another example is the severe headache with vomiting that results from intracerebral hemorrhage which must be considered a medical emergency.)

HEARTBURN (see Digestive Disorders)

HEAT STROKE

Definition and Symptoms

An acute and dangerous reaction to excess heat exposure characterized by a high body temperature (105°F or more), reduced sweating, headache, numbness, tingling, confusion and delirium, rapid pulse, increased respiratory rate, and elevated blood pressure.

*Asterisks indicate the most frequently used therapeutic agents.

Etiologic Considerations

- Hot environment
- Inadequate ventilation
- Heavy insulating clothes
- Fluid loss
- Electrolyte loss

Treatment

Heat stroke is a serious emergency, and unless properly and vigorously treated, may result in convulsions, permanent brain damage, or death. If possible, wrap patient in an ice-cold wet sheet and transport to a hospital immediately, continually applying more ice-cold water. Take care not to lower temperature below 101°F. Take temperature at least every 10 minutes. If distant from a hospital, immerse in an ice-cold bath and use fans to aid cooling, or if ice bath is unavailable, use a cold stream or lake until medical attention can be obtained. Time is of the essence. Begin cooling treatments as soon as possible. Massage extremities to increase circulation while the patient is in the cold bath.

Heat exhaustion, a less severe condition, may occur over a period of days. Early symptoms include malaise, weakness, and tiredness. Dehydration may eventually lead to blood volume loss, poor heat regulation, and shock. Treatment in early stages is to drink large amounts of mineral-rich vegetable and fruit juices to replace water and electrolyte loss in perspiration. The worst drink in hot weather is water, since it does not replace electrolytes. Sea salt use is recommended in hot climates, as well as potassium-rich vegetable broths.

HEART DISEASE: Arteriosclerosis, Atherosclerosis, Angina, Coronary Heart Disease

Definition

Arteriosclerosis: A degenerative change in the arterial walls, affecting first the middle and later the inner layers, and resulting in loss of elasticity and possible calcification. Commonly referred to as hardening of the arteries.

Atherosclerosis: A degenerative change in the arterial walls which principally affects the larger arteries such as the aorta, coronary, and cerebral vessels. Systemic changes in other arteries also occur. The basic lesion is plaque formation on the inner walls of the vessels, causing narrowing and possible embolism when the plaque breaks loose into the circulation, with possibly disastrous results. The plaque is composed primarily of 70 to 80 percent tissue, cholesterol, and other fats.

Angina: Recurrent substernal pain lasting 1/2 to 1 minute, which may be precipitated by stress, exertion, a large meal, emotion, extreme cold, or other factors. Pain is characterized by the sensation of a viselike tight band drawn across the chest. Coronary atherosclerosis is the major cause. Average life expectancy after first onset of angina is 5 to 7 years.

Symptoms

Cold extremities, lethargy, dizziness, senility, difficulty thinking, high blood pressure, pain in legs on exertion, angina, blurred vision, enlarged heart, difficulty breathing, palpitations, heart attacks, embolism, death.

Etiologic Considerations

- Diet
    Excess saturated fats
    Excess use of overheated or oxidized vegetable oils
    Deficiency of fat emulsifiers
    Excess salt
    Excess refined carbohydrates and sugar: sugar increases triglycerides, platelet adhesiveness, uric acid levels, and blood pressure
    Vitamin and mineral deficiency
    Excess vitamin D (3000 mg or more per day is atherogenic)
    Coffee
    Alcohol

- Cigarettes
- Lack of exercise
- Stress
- Obesity
- Heavy metal poisoning
- Soft water
- Birth control pill
- Diabetes
- Hyperinsulinism: May cause atherosclerosis
- Family history
- Gout

- High blood pressure
- Elevated cholesterol, triglyceride, and uric acid levels
- Low HDL-to-cholesterol ratio
- Long-term ox bile supplementation

Discussion

Heart disease is the number one killer in civilized nations. Evidence clearly shows that the incidence of heart disease is directly related to our abnormal dietary habits. Wherever people live on a diet high in refined carbohydrates and animal fats, high blood pressure, arteriosclerosis, atherosclerosis, angina, and other degenerative heart changes occur most frequently.

A great deal of confusion presently exists about the role of animal fats in the causation of heart disease. Until a few years ago it was a commonly accepted assumption that excess consumption of saturated fats found in meat, eggs, and dairy products was the main cause of these disorders. This view, however, never could adequately explain why traditional Eskimos or other tribal people who eat a very large amount of animal fats do not show an increased incidence of heart disease. Still, most doctors stuck to their beliefs and reiterated the meat–heart maxim regularly. It may not be totally correct, but at least it is simple and easy to quote without having to go into too much time-consuming detail.

The problem with much past research has been the traditional tendency to try, whenever possible, to find a single, simple "something" that will explain a particular disease. However, this only rarely is possible. Heart disease, and most other degenerative diseases for that matter, is the result of a total lifestyle, not a simple dietary excess or deficiency.

In analyzing the true causes of degenerative heart disease, it is essential always to bear in mind that people are individuals and as such respond to various causative factors differently. Diet is definitely a major factor in degenerative heart disease. Saturated fats (those commonly found in animal products) are a problem, as has long been suspected, and the situation is getting worse, not better. Animal products contain a very high percentage of complicated fats said to cause a rise in blood cholesterol, which has been associated with formation of atherosclerotic plaques on arterial walls. Certainly the western diet contains a significantly larger amount of animal proteins and thus cholesterol than many other populations with less heart disease, and as such is definitely implicated.

The problem, however, is not only how much meat or dairy products we eat, but what kind. Domesticated animals have a much higher percentage of saturated fat than wild animals, due to a different diet, activity level, and the hormones used by various cattle and poultry industries to fatten their stock artificially. The meat or poultry we eat now is very different from that our grandparents ate, much to our detriment. Cow's milk, ignoring for the present the fact that this product was not designed by nature for humans, has also changed considerably over the past hundred years. We now break the fat molecules in milk up into easily absorbed particles by homogenization, and feed this food designed by nature for baby cows to our infants, resulting in cases of atherosclerosis by the age of 5! It is no wonder that heart disease, once a disease of middle age, is now being found in those in their late twenties.

The cholesterol story, however, is far from simple. Although multiple studies prove that an elevated blood cholesterol level is definitely associated with an increased risk of coronary heart disease, it cannot be said from these data that dietary cholesterol is the single most important factor causing this increased blood cholesterol. In fact, a modest increase in dietary cholesterol has been shown to give no significant rise in blood cholesterol levels. While it is true that excessive cholesterol in the diet will affect blood cholesterol levels, of far more importance to the total blood fat picture is the body's ability to form cholesterol within the body from other nonfat energy sources, such as protein.

In support of the old observation that vegetarians in general have lower cholesterol levels than those who eat meat, it has been found that certain amino acids (histidine, arginine, and lysine) found in highest concentrations in animal products are capable of being converted to cholesterol within the body.

While it is clear that the average vegetarian does have less incidence of coronary heart disease than the average meat eater, and while evidence does show clearly that elevated blood cholesterol levels, as found more frequently among meat eaters, are associated with an increased risk of coronary heart disease, this evidence alone still does not clearly state that increased blood cholesterol levels per se cause heart disease. The actual causes of the pathological changes found in the blood vessels of those with heart disease are not known. Several as yet unproven theories do exist but the final answer is not as yet agreed upon.

One of the most interesting and appealing of these theories is the so-called *monoclonal theory*. This model of the causation of atherosclerosis is based on the observation that plaque initially forms within the wall of the artery at the site of a bump or tumor growth, which originates from a single cell growing abnormally. This irregularity in the artery wall forms a site where cell debris, platelets, and cholesterol may collect and slowly narrow the artery wall, impairing blood supply to the heart. This is interesting in its implications since it suggests that some factor in the blood may cause a mutation of the artery wall cells, leading to tumor growth which is attacked by the body's defenses, thus explaining fibrous buildup in the area. Of specific interest to our discussion of cholesterol is that cholesterol can be acted upon by oxidation within the body into substances known to cause mutagenic reactions in the body.

Cholesterol is also a component of the platelet cell membrane and as the blood cholesterol level rises, so does platelet cholesterol. Along with this, the tendency for the platelet to stick to the cell wall also increases. Once the platelet adheres to the artery wall, it releases chemicals that cause a narrowing of the blood vessel and that also are capable of causing mutagenic cell reactions.

Over the past few years other extremely interesting research has helped clarify many of our previously unanswerable questions about the diet/heart disease link. One study examined some of the original research data which showed that cholesterol in high amounts fed to experimental animals led to a high percentage of developing coronary heart disease. This study has often been quoted to prove the causative link between cholesterol and coronary heart disease. In recent tests, however, using proven *pure* cholesterol, no such results were found. However, when cholesterol that was allowed to go *rancid* was used, coronary heart disease *did* result. The conclusion was that the harmful effects of rancid oil products were the primary factor, not simply cholesterol. This study has particular significance when we compare it with studies showing the usefulness of antioxidants (antirancidity factors) in the diet for both prevention and treatment of heart disease.

While the old cholesterol/heart disease connection is still valid as shown by the most recent 10-year study of human subjects, proving that decreased blood cholesterol levels definitely reduced the incidence of coronary heart disease, no mention is ever made that dietary consumption of cholesterol, while important, is the least important source of *blood* cholesterol. Most blood cholesterol is made within the body and this in turn depends on the amount and kind of protein eaten, the amount and kind of fat eaten, the levels of certain vitamins, minerals, and fatty acids, as well as stress, alcohol consumption, exercise level, and the interrelationship of all the rest of our previously noted causative factors. Once again, at the risk of being redundant, coronary heart disease is not caused by a single factor.

Saturated fats, although central to the increase of heart disease, do not work in isolation in the diet. Refined carbohydrates and specifically sugar are also known to increase fat levels in the blood. The combination of sugar or refined carbohydrates taken with saturated fats seems to cause the highest of all increases of cholesterol and triglycerides in the blood. This combination of foods is extremely common in the modern diet from early childhood on. Take, for example, the typical milkshake (sugar and milk) or a hamburger and Coke (meat, refined white flour bun, and sugar). While saturated fat consumption has increased only 10 percent in the past 100 years, the increase in refined carbohydrates and sugar has gone up to an incredible 700 *percent*. This increase in consumption of refined carbohydrates, especially sugar, is the single most important factor effecting a rise in blood triglycerides. There is a definite link between societies with an extremely high sucrose consumption and coronary heart disease.

Recent research indicates that *unsaturated* vegetable oils may also be related to some degenerative diseases. This may well be true when you consider the type of oils normally consumed in the United States (i.e., refined, heat-treated, and partly hydrogenated oils). Heat-treated unsaturated oils undergo a transformation from the chemical *cis* form to the more stable but abnormal *trans* form. The *trans* form, not normally found in these oils, if cold pressed or unheated, is more reactive with oxidants, producing rancidity by-products that, as we have seen, cause an elevation in the circulation of possible mutagenic substances which may initiate damage to the arterial walls. This may be a significant factor in the production of atherosclerotic plaque buildup, plaque being the local lesion found associated with coronary heart disease.

Partly hydrogenated, unsaturated oils (i.e., margarine) may also be a factor. Originally many people converted from butter to margarine to reduce their total dietary cholesterol intake. This seems logical; however, it turns out that the use of partly hydrogenated oils not only does not decrease blood cholesterol levels, it increases them! Hydrogenated oils are high in *trans* forms of fatty acids. This form inhibits a liver enzyme responsible for converting cholesterol into bile acids. Bile acids transport cholesterol out of the body. If cholesterol is not converted to bile, it accumulates in the blood, the exact opposite of the desired result.

Individual elements of the diet, even saturated fats and refined carbohydrates, do not function in isolation within the body. Many factors influence the way in which the body handles fats and are important in preventing and curing heart disease.

Fats, being water-insoluble, must be carried in the blood in the solutized form of a protein-fat molecule called a *lipoprotein*. It has been discovered that lipoproteins come in various sizes, compositions, and densities. The low-density lipoproteins (LDLs) are large, cholesterol-laden molecules. When found at high levels in the blood they are a risk factor associated with increased risk of coronary heart disease. High-density lipoproteins (HDLs), however, are smaller molecules with more protein and less cholesterol and triglycerides. When these are found in high levels in the blood there is a reduced risk of heart disease. The cholesterol-to-HDL ratio is very important as a diagnostic aid for risk of heart disease. The HDLs help transport cholesterol from the blood to the liver where it can be converted to bile, and thus removed from the body. With the discovery that these lipoproteins can be predictors of the risk of heart disease came a new area of research showing how individual foods, vitamins, or minerals affect the interrelationship of these factors—as well as cholesterol and triglycerides, giving us a guideline to their relative effectiveness. From this research the following facts have evolved:

• Vitamin C helps increase HDL levels and lowers LDL levels, thus protecting against coronary heart disease. It also dramatically reduces high elevations of blood cholesterol by activating the conversion of cholesterol into bile salts. At a dose level of 1 to 2 g per day, a 30 percent reduction in cholesterol levels of 400 or above can be expected. Less dramatic decreases occur with lower initial cholesterol levels. Vitamin C also lowers triglyceride levels.

- Vitamin B complex, lost in the refining process of starches and essential in the metabolism of carbohydrates, is known to help keep cholesterol from collecting in plaque.

- Vitamin E, also stripped away with the germ of grains and lost in the refining of oils, is essential for a healthy heart. It helps dissolve blood clots, dilates blood vessels, and conserves oxygen so that the heart can work less. As an antioxidant it prevents fatty acids from becoming toxic within the body.

- Lecithin, containing choline of the vitamin B complex group, is essential for the proper use of fat and cholesterol in the body. Lecithin in the diet significantly lowers blood cholesterol levels.

- Essential fatty acids as found in salmon, cod, and other cold-water fish oils rich in omega 3EFA decrease platelet adhesion, increase bleeding time, and reduce risk of heart disease. They reduce blood cholesterol and increase HDLs. This is the newly discovered preventive factor in the traditional Eskimo diet.

- Bran fiber reduces blood cholesterol and triglycerides, increases HDL, and lowers LDL. It also helps *prevent* recycling of bile from the bowel back to the liver, which signals a reduction of cholesterol conversion to bile, causing a blood cholesterol increase.

- *Lactobacillus* lowers cholesterol levels by normalizing bowel ecology, preventing excessive endogenous cholesterol production.

- Brewer's yeast and chromium 15 lower HDL levels and will actually cause regression of atherosclerotic plaque.

- Alfalfa meal (from ground seeds) contains a large portion of saponins which help prevent bile-like substances from recirculating to the liver, with an action similar to bran.

- Cultured milk products (yoghurt, kefir, and buttermilk): Daily use can lower blood cholesterol 5 to 6 percent.

- Garlic or onion extracts lower blood cholesterol and reduce platelet adhesiveness. They reduce triglycerides and increase HDLs.

- Soy protein lowers blood cholesterol.

Other lipotropic and dietary substances also are factors in keeping cholesterol and triglyceride levels down, and we can expect this list to grow rapidly with the expanding amount of nutritional research now being done in this area.

A second major cause of heart disease is lack of demanding exercise. Lifestyles have changed drastically over the past 100 years, and as general physical activity levels have decreased, heart disease has increased. Demanding physical exercise, the kind that really gets the blood flowing, helps clear the arteries of any early deposits, and prevents atherosclerosis and high blood pressure. In general, a very active person will develop heart disease later than his or her sedentary peer, or not at all. Activity alone, however, is no real protection. To be effective, the heart rate as well as the respiration must escalate to the point of breathlessness for at least 5 minutes each day.

Stress, coffee, cigarettes, alcohol, and obesity are all contributing factors to be considered in individual cases. Stress causes an increase in cholesterol, glucose levels, and triglycerides. It also causes an elevation of blood pressure. There is a well-known association between stress and coronary heart disease.

Caffeine potentiates the action of Adrenalin by blocking its breakdown. This results in the same physiologic responses as does stress. Heavy caffeine consumption results in a twofold greater risk of coronary heart disease. Cigarette smoking is now a well-documented risk factor in heart disease. Stress, coffee, and cigarettes all cause a vasoconstriction or narrowing of the arteries which is especially important in cases of angina where atherosclerosis is present.

Although all the answers to the heart disease question are not in, it is clear now, as it has been for quite some time, that the only true prevention and cure is to be found in a *total* lifestyle change. For those who are waiting for a simple answer, or one that comes in a little package or easy-to-swallow pill, I offer no hope.

Treatment

Coronary bypass operations have become commonplace as the "cure" for coronary atherosclerosis and severe angina. A segment of vein from the leg is grafted to bypass the narrowed artery segments in one or all three of the coronary arteries. Dramatic as this therapy is in relieving the immediate threat of imminent death due to heart failure, it neglects the fact that the disease is systemic in the first place, and affects the entire circulatory system, not just the heart. It also does nothing to prevent further degeneration of even the new transplanted arteries. At best it is an emergency repair job which does not in any way remove the cause. All of this would be acceptable if the cause were not known, or the cure impossible, both of which are not true. Even the most advanced cases, short of a terminally fatal heart attack or severe infarction, can be benefited by natural treatment.

Diet

The basic diet regimen should be similar to that found under Hypertension. Periods of vegetable juice fasting are interspersed with a high-fiber, unrefined carbohydrate, mostly vegetarian protein diet, emphasizing plenty of fruits, vegetables, vegetarian proteins, and high-fiber whole grains. All foods known to help lower cholesterol and triglycerides in the blood are stressed, including soybeans, tofu, beans, peas, cold-water fish, brewer's yeast, bran, onions, garlic, fresh wheat germ, sunflower seeds, seed sprouts, lecithin, and plenty of raw vegetables. Salt, alcohol, coffee, sugar, refined grains, hydrogenated fats such as those in margarine (or those found in commercial peanut butter), fried foods, meats, and all dairy products except yoghurt, kefir, or buttermilk, are strictly avoided in the early stages of the regimen.

Perseverance and rigid adherence to the diet are essential to obtain permanent results. Weight reduction is a primary aim for the obese. It is important to remember that degenerative heart disease usually takes 20 or more years of wrong living for the effects to become noticeable, and cannot logically be totally reversed overnight. Natural therapies are generally slow, but sure.

DIET FOR A HEALTHY HEART

The following diet may be of some use as a guideline.

Choose from the following:

Breakfast

1. Whole grain cereal. Use soy milk or buttermilk if desired. A little honey or sweetener is allowed, but not necessarily suggested.

2. Low-fat yoghurt, fresh wheat germ, brewer's yeast, and a little fruit, especially green apples.

3. Two poached eggs (poached eggs cause less rise in blood cholesterol than fried), plus whole grain bread (two to three times per week only).

4. Fresh fruit salad plus nuts and/or yoghurt.

Midmorning

1. Whole grain snack (i.e., crackers, muffins, bread, etc.)

2. Cereal-grain coffee, or herb tea

3. Vegetable juice

4. *Spirulina* in water

5. Miso soup

6. Yoghurt

7. Mixed nuts (unsalted)

Lunch

1. *Always* have a fresh, raw, mixed salad including seed sprouts, plus any of the following:

   100 percent whole grain (i.e., brown rice, wheat, oats, etc.)

   Vegetarian protein (i.e., tofu, soybeans or other beans, nuts, seeds, or low-fat fermented dairy products).

   Cold water fish (i.e., cod or salmon); other fish less frequently.

   Chicken or turkey without skin.*

Midafternoon   As midmorning

Supper

1. Cooked vegetables

2. Vegetarian protein

3. Whole grain

4. Cold water fish (cod, salmon, etc.); other fish less frequently.

5. Chicken or turkey without skin.*

Physiotherapy

• Aerobic Exercise: Obviously all exercise programs must be instituted slowly, with care, and under the supervision of a doctor in the case of heart disease. No surer way exists, however, to correct the problem. Whatever exercise you are initially able to do, it must be increased gradually over a period of time until true aerobic conditioning is possible, involving continuous vigorous exercise for 15 to 20 minutes or more each day. If you can now walk only 50 yards slowly before becoming tired or breathless or suffering angina pain, gradually increase the distance and the pace, with the aim of soon being able to jog and then run. The same procedure is applied to any other activity— bicycling, rowing, swimming—anything as long as it is steady and continuous, once again with a doctor's supervision.

• Alternate Hot/Cold Showers: These are excellent at stimulating the circulation, but must be done gradually, to prevent sudden shock that the heart cannot yet stand. Begin by taking alternate hot then lukewarm showers, alternating the hot/warm every 2 to 3 minutes. Slowly, over the next 2 to 6 months, depending on the severity of the initial condition and your general improvement in health through diet, exercises, and the rest of your new health program,

---

*On doctor's approval—one to two times per week.

increase the difference between the water temperatures to hot/cool and then to hot/ice-cold.

- Chelation therapy for arteriosclerosis
- Daily meditation
- Spinal manipulation: Lower cervical/upper thoracic, one to two times per week, especially where spinal lesions may be aggravating or causing angina due to imbalance in the deep vs. superficial circulation.
- Massage
- Colonics or enema series—where bowel loading is affecting angina. General toxemia may be a factor in all degenerative heart disorders.
- Liver flush: Often the liver is found to be congested in these conditions. See Liver Disease for details of liver flush.
- Skin brush and "salt glow": Stimulates circulation, encourages proper skin function, and aids in elimination.
- Hot compress: In acute angina apply hot moist compress to chest or midback, then massage the muscles deeply along the spine and follow with spinal manipulation.

Therapeutic Agents

VITAMINS AND MINERALS

Vitamin A: 10,000 to 25,000 IU per day.

Vitamin B complex: 25 to 50 mg one to three times per day.*

Vitamin B_3: Especially useful for angina. 400 to 500 mg of mixed niacin and niacinamide two to four times per day.

Vitamin B_6: Helps in production of EFA, and lowers cholesterol; antithrombic agent, antiaggregation of platelets.

Inositol*

Choline: High potency phosphatidyl choline as lecithin; 1 tsp three times per day.*

Folic acid: Vasodilator. 75 mg per day in some cases.

Vitamin C with bioflavonoids: 500 to 2000 mg three times per day; helps keep plaque from forming, lowers triglycerides, strengthens capillaries and increases HDL.*

*Asterisks indicate the most frequently used therapeutic agents.

Vitamin E: Inhibits platelet aggregation. Gradually increases dose of natural mixed tocopherols from 100 to 400 IU two to three times per day. Higher doses of up to 2400 IU have been used.

Essential fatty acids

Calcium cholate: 600 mg to 1 g per day: Decreases cholesterol levels.

Magnesium chelate or orotate: 300 mg to 2 g per day. More may be useful in some cases up to a ratio of 1:1 with calcium. Especially useful in ischemic heart disease after a myocardial infarction, or for those on diuretic therapy. Magnesium is a natural calcium blocker (calcium blockers are used in angina and cardiovascular disease).

Selenium: 100 to 200 mcg per day; helps improve vitamin E efficiency. Low selenium levels are a risk factor in heart disease.

L-carnitine: 1500 to 3000 mg per day. Increases HDL. Decreases total cholesterol, promotes transport of fatty acids into mitochondria, reduces triglycerides; useful in angina.

Chromium as brewer's yeast: 1 tsp three times per day. Chromium is commonly deficient in heart disease patients. Decreases LDL, cholesterol, increases HDL, causes regression of atherosclerotic plaque.

Copper: Depends on hair tissue levels and zinc-to-copper ratio. Copper deficiency has been linked to increased serum cholesterol and decreased HDL.

OTHERS

Alfalfa: Decreases blood cholesterol.*

Atomodine: With angina take 1 drop twice daily for 5 days; stop 5 days and repeat five times.*

Bran: 1 tbs three times per day.*

Brewer's yeast: High in vitamin B complex, selenium, and chromium.

Bromelain: Acts as fibrinolytic agent to aid in dissolution of thrombi. Anti-inflammatory agent.*

Citric acid: A nutritional chelating (binding) agent.*

Desiccated thyroid: In hypothyroid-related heart disease.*

Chlorophyll*

Cod-liver oil: 1 tsp three times per day.*

*Asterisks indicate the most frequently used therapeutic agents.

Citrus fruits*

EPA (eicosapentaenoic acid): 5 g per day as preventative, 5 to 20 g per day as therapy.*

Garlic: Decreases cholesterol and blood viscosity; 2 capsules three times per day.*

Grape juice*

Heart Forte (Seroyal)*

Low-fat fermented milk products: Yoghurt, buttermilk, and kefir lower blood cholesterol levels.*

Pectin: Lowers cholesterol.*

Phosphatidylcholine: The most concentrated form of lecithin.*

Primrose oil: Decreases platelet aggregation.

Specta cardia (naturopathic formulations)*

Wheat germ oil

BOTANICALS

Angelica (Angelica archangelica)

Black cohosh (Cimicifuga racemosa) plus yellow jasmine (Gelsemium sempervirens) for angina.

Cactus (Cactus grandiflorus) for angina with irregular heartbeat.

Dandelion (Taraxacum officinale)

Hawthorn (Crataegus oxyacantha): Angina; infusion of berries (1 tsp to 1 cup water, plus honey) two to three times per day.*

Hawthorn and walnut

Mistletoe (Viscum album)

HEAVY METAL POISONING

Definition

Excess exposure and absorption of heavy metals in toxic clinical or subclinical doses.

*Asterisks indicate the most frequently used therapeutic agents.

Symptoms

These are dependent upon the type of metal and degree of exposure.

Lead: Cumulative doses may cause:

Constipation	Nausea
Vomiting	Diarrhea
Learning difficulties	Difficulty in concentration
Mental retardation	Confusion
Emotional instability	Restlessness
Hyperactivity	Insomnia
Vertigo	Muscle aches
Gout, arthritis	Fatigue
Kidney damage	Pituitary damage
Birth defects	Impotence, sterility
Ataxia	Tremors
Muscle weakness	Degeneration of motor neurons
Loss of appetite, anorexia	Schizophrenic-like behavior
Seizures	Growth problems in long bones
Cirrhosis of liver (jaundice)	Cataracts
Metallic taste	Headaches
Thyroid dysfunction	Impotence, sterility

Lead colic: Painter's colic with severe wandering pain in the abdomen and acute muscle spasm.

Anemia

Lead line on gum margin

Peripheral neuritis: Paralysis of muscles (i.e., painter's wrist drop).

Lead encephalopathy includes convulsions, drowsiness, excitability, vomiting, incoordination, insanity, and coma.

Cadmium:

Emphysema	Kidney damage, nephritis
Hypertension	Arteriosclerosis

Abdominal cramps, colic   Nausea, vomiting
Diarrhea   Liver disease
Acne, slow healing (zinc deficiency)   Anemia

Mercury:

Tremors   Chromosome damage
Birth defects   Insanity
Kidney damage   Abdominal pain
Nausea   Vomiting
Loss of hearing or vision   Mental retardation
Sore gums, gingivitis   Tooth loss
Vertigo   Headaches
Nervousness   Skin eruptions
Fatigue

Aluminum:

Digestive disorders   Seizures
Colic, gas   Motor and behavioral dysfunction
Gastritis   Skin rash
Brain degeneration,   Headache
senile dementia
Alzheimer's disease

Copper:

Mental disorders   Schizophrenia
Anemia   Copper deposits in kidney, liver,
Arthritis   brain, eyes
Hypertension   Insomnia
Nausea, vomiting   Autism
Hyperactivity   Stuttering

Rheumatoid arthritis (high copper levels)

Postpartum psychosis

Inflammation and enlargement of liver

Myocardial infarction

Toxemia of pregnancy

Wilson's disease

Cystic fibrosis
(high copper levels)

Etiologic Considerations

- Lead:
    Auto exhaust
    Industry:
        Smelters
        Paint factories
- Water:
    Lead pipes (soft water is the worst)
    Industrial pollution
    Pesticides runoff
    Water catchment: Lead-headed nails; especially severe if acid rain occurs (industrial or volcanic origin)
- Paint:
    "Painter's colic"
    Roof paint (water catchment systems)
    Pica: Children eating lead-based wall paint or paint on cribs due to lead's sweet taste (sugar of lead)
- Cigarettes: Lead arsenate used on tobacco as insecticide
- Insecticides/fungicides
- Newspaper ink: Burning newspaper "logs" increases lead in air; typesetters
- Soldered cans
- Gardens near main roads
- Children playing near main roads
- Jogging on main roads
- Commercial baby milk
- Industrial materials
    Nails
    Solder
    Plating
    Plaster

    Putty
    Lead
- Shellfish, oysters
- Gasoline: Lead tetraethyl forms lead oxide in engine exhaust.
- Bullets
- Lead weights: Melting down and casting without proper ventilation, including soldering.
- Auto body workers
- Organ meats, dog food
- Dolomite
- Cosmetics
- Paper clips
- Cooking utensils
- Enamel and cloisonné work
- Lead paint on goblets, lead crystal
- Hair colorings
- Wines
- Ceramic glasses: Improperly fired lead-glazed ceramics when used with acidic foods such as citrus, tomatoes, etc.
- Old pewter
- Machine shops
- Snuff in lead foil
- Leaded toothpaste tubes
- Cadmium:
      Cigarettes
      Fertilizers
      Water pipes (impure galvanized pipes)
      Soft drink dispensers
      Coal burning
      Zinc deficiency
      Old dental amalgams—were one part cadmium, two parts mercury. These are no longer used.
      Zinc smelters
      Low melting point alloys
      Refined foods (low zinc/cadmium ratio)

"Silver solder"—the type of "do-it-yourself" solder available in most hardware stores gives off cadmium when overheated.
Catchment from galvanized roofs
Hardware; cadmium-plated nuts, bolts, and wood screws have dangerous potential when heated above 626°F or if sanded or power buffed. Gives off onion/garlic odor.

- Mercury:

  Dental fillings

  Pesticides/fungicides

  Pollution

  Canned tuna/salmon

  Adhesives

  Fabric softeners

  Drugs

  Large fish

  Coal burning

  Cosmetics

  Water-based paints

  Chemical fertilizers

  Calomel laxatives

- Aluminum:

  Deodorants

  Cookware

  Emulsifier in cheese processing

  Baking powder

  Construction materials

  Antacids

  Foil

  Salt (anticaking ingredients)

  Beer and soda cans

  Catchment water

- Copper:

  Copper water pipes and copper water heaters (especially where water is acidic)

  Meats (copper sulfate given as growth enhancer)

  Soybeans (high copper)

  Frozen greens, canned greens (copper added to produce ultragreen color)

  Zinc deficiency

  Alcoholic beverages from copper brewery equipment

  Instant gas hot water heaters

  Hormone pills

  Soft water

  Pesticides, insecticides, fungicides

  Copper jewelry

  Copper cooking pots, especially if acid foods are cooked

Discussion

From the above list of possible harmful effects of heavy metal toxicity, it is obvious that these substances can pose a serious health risk. Knowledge of these dangers has come slowly and with much suffering. The entire Roman Empire routinely dosed itself with toxic lead by drinking out of lead goblets, lining its aqueducts with lead, or even adding it to wine in the form of lead acetate, called "sugar of lead," to enhance its flavor and sweet taste. Finally, in the seventeenth century the serious condition of "painter's colic" was recognized as being lead-related. Later, laws were enacted to prevent rum from being made in lead-containing pots. In the eighteenth and nineteenth centuries lead poisoning was epidemic in the upper classes, who habitually drank an excess of lead-containing port wine.

Exposure of workers to toxic metals has been the major source of knowledge about their harmful effects. Industrial toxicology now recognizes that toxic exposure to lead, cadmium, mercury, aluminum, copper, and other less common metals may cause serious disease and even be fatal. With this awareness came the establishment of permissible levels or threshold limit values to monitor workers and their environments. Blood and urine tests have been used primarily to diagnose a suspected toxicity, but for the most part estimation of probable heavy metal levels is the major preventive measure. Even among the orthodoxy there is dissatisfaction with these inexact methods and the heavy reliance on threshold limit values which do not take into consideration individual differences between heavy metal susceptibility (biochemical individuality), other sources of contamination off the job, the effect of a closed environment, or the fact that some heavy metals (i.e., lead) are *cumulative* in their effects.

The real question, however, has been at which point do these toxic substances cause even a slight deviation from health? The assumption is usually that some toxic metal absorption is harmless; however, many now feel that even *slight* amounts may cause abnormal physical and mental responses. Threshold limits are clearly designed to protect the *majority* of workers from *clinical disease*. It is the subclinical symptoms of heavy metal poisoning, however, that may be the greatest threat to the health and well-being of the industrial worker.

With the rise of industrialization, heavy metal pollution of the air, water, and the food chain became an increasing problem. Now environmental exposure is clearly unavoidable. Studies of snow layers in Greenland, far from industrialization, clearly show this increase, which progresses yearly. By the 1950s routine tests of "symptomless" U.S. children showed hundreds of thousands with toxic lead levels.

In reviewing once again the sources of metal pollution, the fantastic variety of ways we poison ourselves will become obvious. Cigarettes, auto exhaust, newspapers, canned foods, frozen foods, aluminum cookware, insecticides, fungicides, food additives, water piping, cosmetics, hair dyes, antacids, and even deodorants!

Prevention and Treatment

In this day and age prevention of heavy metal poisoning is not easy, but it is absolutely essential to health and well-being. The most obvious preventive measure is to avoid consuming food or water likely to be contaminated. All canned food or frozen green foods are suspect. Lead-containing solder is often used in canned foods and copper sulfate is used frequently in treating canned or frozen green vegetables to help give an ultragreen color to enhance marketing. Any food exposed to insecticides, pesticides, or fungicides may have high levels of lead, cadmium, mercury, copper, or other toxic chemicals and should be strictly avoided. The safest vegetables are organically grown. Make sure, however, never to grow food within 25 to 50 feet of a major road, to avoid lead toxicity. The further the better!

Cooking utensils with copper or aluminum cooking surfaces should be discarded. Use only tempered glass, stainless steel, or non-lead-glazed earthenware. Since heavy metals tend to concentrate within the ocean food chain, passing from bacteria to algae, then to small fish and later big fish, it is important to avoid frequent consumption of large fish such as tuna, marlin, and swordfish. In many areas swordfish is not allowed to be sold due to high heavy metal levels.

The source of fish, especially clams and other shellfish, is equally important. Avoid any shellfish caught near industrial towns. The best fish are freshwater lake or river fish from unpolluted waters, and small ocean reef fish.

Commercial meats are generally unfit for regular human consumption for many reasons, including heavy metal poisoning. Wild game may also have excessive amounts of heavy metals unless far from civilized areas.

Water supplies are difficult to change for most people. Those living in very old houses should check the plumbing to ensure that lead is no longer used anywhere in the system. The most potent dose of heavy metals from water comes in the morning after the water has been in the pipes for prolonged periods. The best prevention is to allow the water to run 1 to 2 minutes to drain away the pipes' reserve before you use it. Water filters also may be used.

Although it is considered the duty of the employer to prevent occupational heavy metal poisoning, many seem truly unaware of any health risk. I conducted informal spot checks on local auto body repair shops and did not find a single shop that required workers to wear air filter masks while on the job. Day after day, year after year, these workers are exposed to an incredible amount of heavy metals in the grinding, sanding, and painting process, completely oblivious to the dangers to which they are being subjected. Other occupations are equally exposed and just as unprotected. Any worker involved in such an industry should make the problem known to his or her employer or union. A routine yearly hair analysis should be provided for in all industrial contracts, as a preventive measure.

The human fetal brain concentrates heavy metals very rapidly. It is essential that pregnant mothers especially make all efforts to avoid these poisons. Children also are very susceptible. Playgrounds near major roads are possible sources of lead poisoning. Even soft drinks from beverage dispensers may cause toxic metal poisoning. Any child with behavior disorders or learning difficulties should be given a hair analysis to exclude toxic metals before being subjected to other treatments. This applies to adults as well.

Detoxification

Once heavy metal toxicity is diagnosed or suspect, the following regimen and nutritional supplements will help slowly reverse the process, provided the cause has been eliminated. It is important that the elimination take place in a controlled and gentle manner, since toxins will be released from body stores in muscles, organs, and bones, creating elevated blood levels for a short period of time. This can be extremely serious if the elimination process is too pronounced, causing exaggeration of the patient's symptoms, or even stimulating uncontrolled psychotic behavior.

Diet

Short periods of citrus fruit or apple mono diets are useful in the elimination process. Each case will determine the length of the initial mono diet. The more severe the toxicity, the shorter will be this first elimination. The usual period for the first mono diet is 3 to 7 days. This fairly rapid detoxification is followed with a mostly raw foods regimen with the exception of cooked beans as protein. A typical diet outline is as follows:

On Rising	Hot water and lemon juice
Breakfast	Fresh grapefruit or just-ripe green apples
Midmorning	Carrot juice
Lunch	Raw green salad with cooked beans
Midafternoon	Carrot juice
Supper	As lunch, or cooked vegetarian meal with plenty of ultra-green vegetables, seaweeds, and beans
Evening	Raw apple or carrot juice

1 tbs raw bran is to be taken with all meals. *Spirulina* should be added whenever possible. All water should be distilled. No alcohol or cigarettes are allowed, and all foods should be organically grown, if at all possible.

This diet may last 1 to 2 weeks and then alternated with the mono diets previously mentioned. The second mono diet series may be much longer than the first, since we now need to extract deeper stores of heavy metals. Some cases may benefit from a prolonged citrus fruit juice fast at this time.

Another 1 to 2 weeks on the mostly raw foods diet with cooked beans is then followed by a further fast or mono diet. By this time all symptoms will have disappeared and the patient must be educated on how to avoid all toxic heavy metals and placed on a mostly vegetarian diet, allowing fish three times per week, if desired. No other meat is allowed for at least 3 months or longer. Periodic fast, mono diets, or mostly raw food diets should be undertaken for at least 3 days two times per month.

Therapeutic Detoxifying Supplements

VITAMINS AND MINERALS

Vitamin A: 25,000 IU two times per day for 1 month, then one time per day. *Use any dose of vitamin A over 50,000 IU per day with medical supervision only.*

Vitamin C plus bioflavonoids: 1000 mg six times per day or more in acute toxicity, to bowel tolerance. High dose of C plus calcium. Vitamin C is a detoxifier and chelator (binding agent) of toxic metals. Given intravenously in high dose (30 g) for acute toxicity.*

Vitamin D: 400 IU two times per day.

Vitamin E: 400 IU two to three times per day.

Vitamin B complex: 50 mg two times per day.*

Vitamin B_6: 50 to 100 mg per day. This helps protect against kidney stone formation on a high C supplement regimen.*

Calcium orotate, calcium lactate, or bone meal (600 to 1500 mg per day): 2 tablets three to four times per day. Calcium decreases gastrointestinal absorption of some heavy metals and aids in their elimination. Milk as a calcium source is associated with *increased* lead levels and is not advised.*

Zinc: 15 to 30 mg two to three times per day.*

Magnesium orotate: 300 mg.*

Potassium iodide: 1000 mcg per day for 1 to 2 months.*

Selenium*

*Asterisks indicate the most frequently used therapeutic agents.

OTHERS

> Bran: 1 tbs three times per day.*
>
> Citric acid*
>
> Chlorophyll as supplement and in deep green vegetables.*
>
> Distilled water*
>
> Garlic*
>
> Kelp: 2 tablets three times per day.*
>
> Lecithin: 4 capsules three times per day or 1 to 2 tbs granules.
>
> Pectin: Found in just-ripe apples and white inner lining of citrus peels. It absorbs heavy metals and prevents absorption from gastrointestinal tract. It is a chelating (or binding) agent.*
>
> Sodium alginate: 250 mg four to eight times per day; helps chelate and eliminate toxic metals. Algin is found in sea vegetables such as kelp.*
>
> Sulfhydryl amino acids (L-lysine, L-cysteine, dimethionine): As found in legumes and as supplement form in many detoxification tablets.*

(Note: Once heavy metal poisoning has reached the stage of severe confusion, seizures, and disorientation (all signs of encephalopathy), the condition is a medical emergency and is best treated in hospital with chelating agents. Due to the chance of brain damage these severe symptoms should not be treated at home.)

HEMORRHOIDS (Piles)

Definition

Varicose veins of the hemorrhoidal plexus, external or internal.

Symptoms

Burning, itching, and pain with bowel movement; blood loss with bowel movement; dilated, painful, enlarged, and often protruding swellings in the anal region.

Etiologic Considerations

• Diet
> Refined foods (fiber deficiency)
> Overeating

*Asterisks indicate the most frequently used therapeutic agents.

- Constipation
  Straining at stool
- Laxative habit
- Poor abdominal tone
  Visceroptosis
- Lack of exercise
- Sedentary existence
- B_6 deficiency
- Pregnancy
- Improper heavy lifting
  Without breathing, increasing intraabdominal pressure
- Toxicity

Discussion

Hemorrhoids are extremely rare in countries where whole unrefined cereal grains are a major part of the diet. Again, this places hemorrhoids in the class of "diseases of civilization." The western diet, with its refined carbohydrates such as white bread, white rice, and macaroni, is one of drastically reduced total fiber intake. Associated with this low-fiber diet is a nation with chronic constipation, addicted to the habitual use of laxatives.

The major mechanical cause of hemorrhoids is increased intraabdominal pressure. This can occur during heavy lifting when the breath is held, and this factor has been mentioned frequently as a cause of hemorrhoids. More common, however, is the increased intraabdominal pressure created by straining to pass hard fecal matter during a bowel movement, which is the primary cause. With a lack of fiber in the diet, the stool becomes dehydrated, hard, and extremely difficult to pass. Laxatives are then resorted to, which act in several ways to ease bowel movements. Some act as irritants, while others are lubricants, softeners, or fiber additives. Of these only the fiber additives could be considered relatively harmless, as this approach is designed to *add* fiber removed from the diet by consumption of refined food. Most other laxatives, however, set up a vicious cycle of bowel movement followed by constipation, needing further laxatives. The powerful bowel movements so created leave the bowel in a flaccid state, further weakening future peristaltic action. I have seen patients literally addicted to both laxatives and enemas which, when used habitually, also cause bowel weakness and reduce peristaltic action (see Constipation).

Obesity with visceroptosis (sagging abdominal region) caused by weak abdominal muscles and lack of exercise will also predispose to hemorrhoids. This usually coincides with improper dietary habits as well.

Treatment

The prevention of hemorrhoids is much easier than their cure. Once the small blood vessels have been grossly dilated and fibrotic scar tissue has formed, it can be very difficult to totally remove the local damage. Surgical removal of hemorrhoids only gets rid of the immediate symptom and does nothing to prevent a recurrence. Surgery also creates more scar tissue. In spite of this, some hemorrhoids will need to be removed surgically if natural therapies fail to eliminate them. After this, prevention of further hemorrhoids should be the main priority.

The obvious dietary solution is to add fiber to the diet *naturally* through unrefined whole grains, fruit, raw and conservatively cooked vegetables, and nuts. While the addition of fiber alone in the form of bran will help most people have shorter transit times, larger stools, and will reduce constipation, this approach is not advised as the sole dietary change. Rather than eating refined foods and adding fiber later, it is much better to eat unrefined foods with all their protein, vitamins, minerals, and fiber intact. It is true, however, that bran is very useful in many stubborn cases of constipation and hemorrhoids. The dietary therapy for hemorrhoids is the same as for constipation.

Exercises

• Slant board exercises.

• All abdominal strengthening exercises.

• Stand with hands at side at attention. While inhaling, raise the hands over the head and rise on the toes. Stretch as far as possible, then breathe normally and lean as far forward as possible without falling. Retain this position for 3 to 5 minutes. Repeat two times daily.

Hydrotherapy

• Heat for pain relief:
    Hot compress
    Hot sitz bath

• Alternate hot and cold, to cure:
    Alternate hot and cold sitz baths
    Alternate hot and cold compresses
    Alternate hot and cold perianal sprays

- Icc-cold: In acute cases; also to help replace prolapsed internal hemorrhoids.
  Cold compresses
  Cold sprays
  Cold sitz baths
- Ice: In acute cases:
  Ice compresses
  Icicle suppository [These may be made artificially by placing a small copper tube in a halved potato (to act as a stand and prevent water draining away)]:
  Fill with water and put in freezer. When frozen, put under warm water to loosen icicle. Insert in the rectum for 30 seconds at first, later increasing to 1 to 2 minutes; repeat 1 to 2 times per day.
- Compresses and poultices:
  Witch hazel: Continuous day and night. Recommended in all cases.*
  Lemon juice compress, or inject juice of lemon and ½ pint cold water into rectum and retain 10 minutes, followed by cold sitz bath.

Therapeutic Agents

VITAMINS AND MINERALS

Vitamin A: 25,000 IU two times per day. *Use any dose of vitamin A over 50,000 IU per day with medical supervision only.* *

Vitamin B complex: 25 to 50 mg one to three times per day.*

Vitamin B_6: 25 mg three times per day.

Bioflavonoids*

Vitamin C: 1000 to 2000 mg two to three times per day.*

Vitamin E: 400 IU three times per day.*

OTHERS

Blackstrap molasses*

Bran: 1 to 2 tbs with meals.*

Increase fluids

Lemon*

Olive oil: 1 tbs prior to meals.*

Raw carrot cure

BOTANICALS

Aloe (*Aloe vera*) plus goldenseal (*Hydrastis*): Topical.

Bloodroot tea (*Sanguinaria canadensis*)

*Asterisks indicate the most frequently used therapeutic agents.

Calendula (*Calendula officinalis*) lotion: Topical use.

Goldenseal (*Hydrastis canadensis*)

May-apple or American mandrake (*Podophyllum peltatum*) (highly toxic; see p. 62): For complete prolapse.

Mullein tea (*Verbascum thapsus*)

Peony root (*Paeonia officinalis*): 1 cup infusion two times per day.

Psyllium seeds (*Plantago psyllium*)

Rhatany (*Krameria triandra*)

Stone root (*Collinsonia canadensis*): 2 capsules three times per day.*

Wintergreen (*Gaultheria procumbens*): For painful hemorrhoids.

SUPPOSITORIES

Goldenseal: Insert one nightly.*

Stone root (*Collinsonia canadensis*)

Stramonium: For extremely painful hemorrhoids.

Witch hazel, stone root, and Peruvian balsam.*

HEPATITIS

Definition

Inflammation of the liver due to infection or toxic substances. Infectious agents include viruses, bacteria, and parasites. Toxic agents include antibiotics, drugs, industrial solvents, anesthetics, carbon tetrachloride, and others.

Symptoms

Begins similar to influenza with weakness, lassitude, drowsiness, nausea, fever, and headache. Jaundice may or may not develop, with or without dark urine, gray stools, and skin irritation. The liver is tender and enlarged. Appetite is poor. Possible depression. Liver may develop necrosis or cirrhosis. Severe cases may be fatal.

Etiologic Considerations

• Infection
    Virus, bacteria, parasites

*Asterisks indicate the most frequently used therapeutic agents.

- Infectious hepatitis
  2-to-4-week incubation period. May be prevented by immune serum globulin injections. Contracted via blood, feces, contaminated food, water, and
  shellfish.

- Serum hepatitis (Australian antigen)
  4-to-23-week incubation period.
  Parenteral transmission.

- Toxic hepatitis (via inhalation, ingestion, skin absorption)
  Drugs (a large number)
  Chemicals (carbon tetrachloride)
  Insecticides
  Solvents
  Metallic compounds and others

- Hepatitis symptoms may be simulated by parasitic amebiasis, abscess of liver

- Improper diet
  Downgraded liver function
  Reduced vitality

- Bile obstruction
  Alcohol

Discussion

As a general rule, disease occurs only when resistance is low. Certainly, with
hepatitis, contamination by the infective agent is a major consideration. In both
infectious and serum hepatitis, feces and blood are considered infectious. Both
types may be spread by the fecal and oral route, with poor sanitation a factor.
However, a healthy system will resist such invasions more efficiently than would
otherwise be the case in downgraded health. Improper diet will leave the liver
more susceptible to infection by clogging it with unnecessary chemicals or toxins
which must be detoxified, and by supplying it with deficient nutrients. Gallbladder malfunction and liver toxemia are also major causes of degraded liver
vitality.

Treatment

The treatment of acute hepatitis and chronic hepatitis is somewhat different
than in other liver diseases. Although short liver-cleansing diets may be useful
in isolated cases, a high-protein diet rich in nutrients favors recovery. The type
of protein foods used are important and should be primarily lacto-vegetarian.

Yeast, wheat germ, egg yolks, low-fat yoghurt, acidophilus low-fat milk, tofu, soybeans, and *Spirulina* are good sources. The diet should also contain high-chlorophyll foods such as raw and cooked green vegetables. Of special importance in treating acute hepatitis are vitamin C injections (25 to 50 g of sodium ascorbate intravenously per day) with calcium gluconate (1 g per 10 g of vitamin C). Also useful are vitamin B complex and B_{12} injections intramuscularly in addition to multiple oral nutritional supports. Lecithin is of special significance and should be consumed as food and as a food supplement.

Diet

High protein, lacto-vegetarian, low-fat: Wheat germ, yeast, lecithin, egg yolks, low-fat goat's milk, eggnogs, and lecithin

Low-fat acidophilus milk and curds

Low-fat yoghurt

Hot water and lemon

Tofu, soy products

Beets plus beet tops

All greens, *Spirulina*

Papaya

Plenty of fluids

This diet may cause ammonia buildup if liver damage is severe. This must be monitored. *Lactobacillus* helps prevent this buildup from becoming aggravated by excess protein consumption. *(Note: Absolutely no saturated fats or alcohol can be consumed.)*

Therapeutic Agents

VITAMINS AND MINERALS

Vitamin A: 10,000 to 25,000 IU emulsified, two to six times per day. *Use any dose of vitamin A over 50,000 IU per day with medical supervision only.* *

Folic acid: 5 mg three times per day.*

Vitamin B complex, oral: 50 mg three times per day, plus intramuscularly.*

Vitamin B_{12}: 1 mg intramuscularly one to three times per week.*

*Asterisks indicate the most frequently used therapeutic agents.

Vitamin C: 1000 mg per hour in acute cases, 25 to 50 g sodium ascorbate intravenously (with 1 g calcium gluconate to 10 g vitamin C daily). *

Vitamin E: 400 to 1200 IU per day, prevents hemorrhaging and scar formation. Improves circulation. *

Essential fatty acids

PHYSIOTHERAPY, HYDROTHERAPY, AND SPINAL MANIPULATION

- Coffee enemas (see Appendix I): One to two times daily.
- Trunk packs (abdominal): Leave on for 1 to 3 hours or overnight.
- Alternate hot and cold compresses over liver area.
- Rest and sunlight baths.
- Spinal manipulation: Thoracic and lumbar.

OTHERS

Chlorophyll
Pancreatic enzymes
Crude liver intramuscular injections daily
Disodium phosphate
Garlic
Radish tablets
Raw liver tablets
Raw spleen tablets
Raw thymus tablets
Spirulina: 1 tsp three to four times daily*

BOTANICALS

Blue flag (Iris versicolor)

Celandine (Chelidonium majus): Dose: Tincture 1 to 10 drops three to four times per day. *

Culver's root (Leptandra virginica): Dose: Tincture 10 to 60 drops three to four times per day. *

Dandelion (Taraxacum officinale)

Fringe tree (Chionanthus virginicus): Dose: Tincture 5 to 30 drops three to four times per day. *

Goldenseal (Hydrastis canadensis)

Oregon grape root (Berberis aquifolium)*

---

*Asterisks indicate the most frequently used therapeutic agents.

HERPES GENITALIS AND COLD SORES

Definition

Cold sores, canker sores, fever blisters: A recurrent, contagious viral infection caused primarily by herpes Type 1 virus.

Herpes genitalis, venereal herpes, genital herpes: A recurrent, contagious viral infection usually caused by herpes Type 2 virus.

Symptoms

Recurrent fluid-filled blisters that rupture, leaving red, inflamed, painful lesions. These are preceded by a slightly irritating tingling. Once the lesion appears, pain is pronounced. Lesions may affect the lips, tongue, nose, face, genitals, thighs, or elsewhere. The first attack is most severe. Lesions tend to dry and crust over in 10 to 14 days. Repeated attacks in same area may cause scarring.

Etiologic Considerations

- Herpesvirus Type 1 and Type 2
- Stress (physical or emotional)
- Overwork
- Acid diet
- L-arginine excess
- Fevers
- Vitamin deficiency
- Citrus
- Some drugs
- Sunburn
- Menstruation
- Friction
- Sexual contact

Discussion

Genital herpes infections now affect over 35 percent of the population in the United States, with over one-half million new cases reported each year. Of these victims, 80 percent are 20 to 39 years of age, with most of the reported cases being Caucasian. Traditionally, the distinction between herpes Type 1 and Type 2 was that Type 1 infections occurred primarily on the upper half of the body (cold sores) and Type 2 on the lower half (genital herpes). This distinction is no longer considered very valuable, as either type may infect any part of the body. Many consider herpes a worse disorder than gonorrhea or syphilis. At least with these other venereal infections cure is possible. The orthodox medical field, however, can offer little hope presently for the herpes patient.

Although the herpes infection itself is moderately painful, the real concern is not with the lesions themselves. The most painfully difficult aspect of having genital herpes is the fear of giving the disease to someone else. Severe depression, self-reproach, hate, and anger often follow the initial attack, which may deepen into a major psychological problem in some cases. Great difficulties arise for the single herpes sufferer on whether, or when, to tell a prospective bed partner about the infection.

Herpes tends to cause recurrent attacks with intervals without symptoms. The virus is thought to live in the dorsal root ganglia of the dermatome affected and migrate to the lesion site under certain conditions. Gradually, most victims learn which factors lead to an outbreak for them. Commonly observed factors are physical or emotional stress, overwork, anxiety, fevers, friction, or menstruation. Although most herpes infections, either cold sores or genital, are passed from person to person by the intimate contact of a kiss or sexual activity, there is some evidence that herpes can live outside the body long enough for indirect infection to occur. Tests have shown that herpes can live up to 4 hours on toilet seats.

Outside of the lesion itself and psychological trauma, herpes has been implicated as a cause or factor in cervical cancer in women, and in severe infections of the newborn. If the mother has an active lesion during delivery, this represents a serious risk to the newborn since the infant's immune system is still too weak to prevent a systemic spread of herpes, which may cause blindness, nerve damage, and may even be fatal. In these cases many obstetricians recommend Caesarean section as a preventative.

Treatment

To my knowledge, no natural therapy has been successful in eliminating herpes completely. What I have seen in my practice, however, are patients who once had frequent attacks, even lasting 3 weeks out of every 4, who now have only very rare incidents, short-lived and fairly mild.

Diet

The nutritional approach to herpes is based partly on the observation that an amino acid, L-arginine, must be supplied in the environment for herpes to grow. L-lysine, another amino acid, has been found to decrease absorption of L-arginine and to increase the speed of its metabolic breakdown in the body. The key then is to decrease L-arginine-containing foods, increase L-lysine foods, or to simply take an excess of L-lysine as a nutritional supplement. High L-arginine foods are peanuts, peanut butter, cashews, pecans, almonds, seeds and chocolate, with peas and untoasted cereal grains being moderate sources. Foods with a better arginine-lysine relationship are brewer's yeast, dairy products, potatoes, meat, and eggs. In clinical practice we encourage these minor changes in diet, but advise L-lysine as a supplement, with the patient taking 500 mg each day when symptom-free, and 500 mg three to four times per day when a lesion is present. When L-lysine is taken it reduces the pain of an acute lesion, shortens its duration, lengthens the remission state, and decreases frequency of occurrence.

In general, the diet must be alkaline in reaction, avoiding sweets, refined carbohydrates, alcohol, and, for some people, citrus. All food must be unrefined and in as natural a state as possible. Fermented foods such as plain yoghurt, kefir, or acidophilus milk should be taken daily, along with 1 to 2 glasses of potassium broth. Foods such as brewer's yeast also should be eaten daily in food as well as in supplement form.

Physiotherapy

- Ultrasound direct to lesion when acute, or to spinal area related to dermatome affected. Repeat daily for 2 weeks, then three to four times per week for 2 to 3 weeks.

- Meditation: Learning to deal with stress is essential to prevent outbreaks.

- Acupuncture

- Ice applications topically

Therapeutic Agents

VITAMINS AND MINERALS

Vitamin A: 25,000 to 50,000 IU daily; also topical.*

Vitamin B complex: 50 mg three times per day.*

*Asterisks indicate the most frequently used therapeutic agents.

Vitamin B_1: 100 mg plus vitamin B_{12}—1000 mcg intramuscularly one to three times per week initially, then one to two times per month.*

Vitamin B_1: 200 to 300 mg per day.*

Vitamin B_6

Vitamin B_{12}: 25 mcg two times per day.*

Folic acid

N,N-Dimethylglycine

Pantothenic acid

Vitamin C complex: 1000 to 6000 mg per day (or to bowel tolerance). Increases natural interferon production.*

Vitamin E: 400 IU one to two times per day; also as topical application to cold sore or genital herpes.*

Zinc: 30 mg two to three times per day.

OTHER

Atomodine: Apply locally followed by glycothymoline.*

Lactobacillus, acidophilus, and *bulgaricus:* 4 capsules four to six times daily in acute cases; 2 capsules three times daily for maintenance. This must be *fresh* and *refrigerated* to be effective.*

L-Lysine:* 500 mg per day for prevention. 500 mg three times per day during an attack.

Thymus tablets: 2, three to six times per day.*

BOTANICALS

Butternut (*Juglans cinerea*): Local application, use decoction of root.

Comfrey (*Symphytum officinale*): Root powder; local.

Goldenseal (*Hydrastis canadensis*): Powder; local.

Green kukui nut: Apply sap to lesion three to four times per day.*

Oregon grape root (*Berberis aquifolium*): 1 oz herb to 1 pint water; 1 cup two to three times per day.*

*Asterisks indicate the most frequently used therapeutic agents.

HIATAL HERNIA

Definition

Protrusion of the stomach above the diaphragm through the esophageal hiatus, leading to a reflux regurgitation of acid pepsin through the incompetent gastroesophageal sphincter.

Symptoms

Heartburn, pain, difficulty with swallowing, inflammation, ulceration, gastrointestinal bleeding, pain from reflux on reclining, fibrositis, and possible stricture of esophagus.

Etiologic Considerations

- Increased intraabdominal pressure
  Constipation
  Obesity
  Pregnancy
  Heavy lifting
  Tight, restricting abdominal clothing (girdles, belts, tight jeans, etc.)
- Overeating
- Fiber deficiency
- Poor abdominal tone
- Slow stomach transit time
- Digestive deficiency
- Refined carbohydrates
- Weak diaphragm (especially in older age groups)
- Poor spinal mechanics
  "Dowager's hump" (kyphosis)
- Cigarette smoking
  Nicotine relaxes sphincter
- Spicy foods, acid foods, coffee

Discussion

Hiatal hernia is another of our "civilized diseases," being uncommon in underdeveloped nations. Looking at the etiologic considerations, it is easy to see why.

The most widely accepted causative factor is increased intraabdominal pressure. Western diets, with an abundance of low-fiber refined foods, favor constipation. The result is straining at stool with an increased intraabdominal pressure, literally forcing the stomach through the diaphragm.

Obesity, so common in developed nations, is another major factor associated with hiatal hernia. Restricting abdominal clothing such as girdles, tight belts, and skin-tight jeans is another factor fairly unique to "civilized" nations.

Of all the factors influencing formation of hiatal hernia, it is diet that has the most central effect. As previously mentioned, the western low-fiber diet will favor constipation. However, this is not diet's only role. Refined carbohydrates, stripped of their protective protein and fiber coverings, act to stimulate gastric acid production, without the ability to buffer that acid (see Peptic Ulcer). This causes an excess of acid in the stomach and sets up conditions necessary for gastric reflux into the esophagus, leading to heartburn. In fact, several authorities feel gastric reflux due to acid is the *primary* condition with a hiatal hernia, following *secondarily* from injury to the tissues by the acid.

Another aspect of refined carbohydrates is that due to the lack of fiber an overabundance of carbohydrates may be consumed, leading to obesity. Overeating is a major causative factor in hiatal hernias. Excessively large meals tend to slow stomach transit time. As the food sits for prolonged periods in the stomach, the esophageal sphincter relaxes and allows gastric acids to enter the esophagus.

Another factor slowing stomach transit time is meals containing large amounts of fats and fried foods. This may be the reason hiatal hernias are so often associated with gallstones. Consumption of foods that increase gastric acidity such as sweets, coffee, tea, alcohol, and spicy foods all predispose to hiatal hernias as well.

Treatment

Obviously, the treatment must first reverse the causes.

Diet

If constipation is present, the treatment for habitual constipation should be followed. The diet is changed to a high-fiber one of smaller meals. The bulk of the diet should be composed of raw fruits; raw and conservatively cooked vegetables; whole grains such as brown rice, millet, bulgar, barley, oats, rye, and wheat; nuts; beans; sprouts; and some animal proteins if desired, but little or no red meat. Periods of fasting or the apple mono diet should be alternated with this general high-fiber diet. Bran should be taken with all meals.

Weight loss is a major aim with obese patients. All sweets, coffee, tea, alcohol, fried foods, and spices are forbidden. Patients are told not to drink with meals and to eat only when hungry.

Physiotherapy

- Spinal manipulation: Improper spinal mechanics are corrected with spinal manipulation and back exercises to correct thoracic kyphosis.

- Abdominal exercises: Good abdominal tone is essential for proper bowel eliminations and diaphragm function. These must be done vigorously daily. Without proper abdominal tone, healing will not be possible with this condition.

Therapeutic Agents

VITAMINS AND MINERALS

Vitamin A: 10,000 to 25,000 IU one to three times per day. *Use any dose of vitamin A over 50,000 IU per day with medical supervision only.*

Vitamin B: 250 to 500 mg per day.

Vitamin B complex: 25 to 50 mg two to three times per day, if well tolerated.

Pantothenic acid: 250 to 500 mg per day.

Vitamin C: May require buffered forms. Dose depends on how well it is tolerated.*

Bioflavonoids

Vitamin E: 200 to 400 IU three times per day.

Manganese: 50 mg per day.

Choline: 1 to 2 g per day.

OTHERS

Kelp or other iodine source

Lecithin

Sodium alginate

Bran: 1 tbs with water before all meals.

Mucovata (Seroyal): Bulking agent.

BOTANICALS

Comfrey (*Symphytum officinale*)*
Goldenseal (*Hydrastis canadensis*)*
Marshmallow (*Athaea officinalis*)
Slippery elm (*Ulmus fulva*): Demulcent.*

*Asterisks indicate the most frequently used therapeutic agents.

Therapeutic Suggestion

The return to a high-fiber diet is the major therapy. Supplements may aggravate condition in early stages; use intramuscularly or liquid form where possible. Bran may aggravate condition at first, but it is essential (unless wheat allergy exists). Slippery elm will help soothe the mucosa and is useful even in early stages.

HICCUP (Hiccough, Singultus)

Definition and Symptoms

Repeated involuntary, spasmodic contractions of the diaphragm, which are then followed by a sudden closure of the glottis.

Discussion

This usually self-limiting condition is the result of irritation of the afferent or efferent nerves or the medullary centers controlling the muscles of respiration. Most episodes last only short periods of time; however, I occasionally hear of hiccups lasting for several days. Cases lasting for years have even been reported. You can imagine how irritating a prolonged case of hiccups would be. Unfortunately, simple techniques for stopping such a prolonged case do not work since the cause in these situations is usually pathologic. This may include such serious conditions as a tumor in the medulla oblongata, disorders of the stomach or esophagus, pancreatitis, hepatitis, or hepatic metastases. Fortunately, common cases of hiccups are not of this serious nature and are easily relieved. Most cases are caused by overeating or overdrinking, which will distend the stomach and irritate the diaphragm.

Treatment

A high blood carbon dioxide level is known to inhibit hiccups. Breath holding and/or rebreathing into a paper bag are the most commonly used techniques. Should these fail it is not difficult to gather tried and true pet techniques from literally anyone you care to ask. The following list reflects years of *un*scientific, *un*tested, and *un*proven clinical trial methods, which I'm sure will, if not cure the condition, at least entertain you.

A female patient of mine swears that this technique is 100 percent successful: She recommends taking ten (not nine or eleven) sips of water in rapid succession. Others are:

Lie on left side for 10 to 15 minutes.

Chew and swallow ice for 10 to 15 minutes.

Drink a glass of water from the opposite side of the glass.

Apply pressure with the flat hand just below the breastbone.

Hold breath while extending head as far back as possible.

Eat some sugar.

Apply ice to neck.

Take a hot bath.

Stand on your head.

Take a roller coaster ride.

Induce vomiting.

Have your stomach pumped.

Have someone apply traction to your tongue!

Apply strong digital pressure over the phrenic nerves behind the sternocla-
vicular joints (I use this one).

C5 mobilization, percussion, and manipulation (I also use this one).

Good (hic) luck!

HIVES (Urticaria)

Definition

Local wheals and erythema of the dermis.

Symptoms

Pruritus (itching), elevated wheals, swollen eyes, possible general and occasionally fatal anaphylactic response (edema of airways causes respiratory distress
similar to severe asthma); self-limiting, 1 to 7 days, except in cases of severe
hypersensitivity when death may result.

Etiologic Considerations

- Chlorine in drinking water
- Stress (histamine release)
- Imbalance between deep and superficial circulation
- Toxemia
- Food allergy: Shellfish, milk, eggs, wheat, pork, onions, some fruits
- Spinal lesion

- Allergy: Adrenal exhaustion; liver congestion
- Hydrochloric acid deficiency
- Lymph stasis
- Food additives: Food dyes, preservatives
- Disordered stomach and bowels; skin: Improper eliminations
- Drug allergy
- Acid condition
- Insect stings
- Chronic infection
- Drug sensitivity (may be hidden, such as penicillin in milk); aspirin
- Coffee, alcohol, tobacco may cause or aggravate condition.

Discussion

I believe the most common cause of hives is an imbalance between the deep and superficial circulations, accompanied or caused by poor eliminations. Toxins are then thrown into the superficial circulation and cause a typical histamine "wheal" response. Although allergy is the accepted exciting factor, I believe that instead of looking externally for the cause, it usually may be found within, in the intestinal tract. It is also possible to get hives from sensitivity to various foods or various external agents. We then must deal with the reasons for the hypersensitivity such as adrenal exhaustion, stress, diet deficiency, improper weaning, food additives, or pesticides. Many cases follow the use of a particular drug.

Lymph stasis and poor circulation may be caused by lack of exercise, poor skin function, poor eliminations, toxemia, general atony or even spinal lesions. Several interesting cases come to mind where all treatments failed to give relief until spinal manipulation was successfully tried.

With severe anaphylactic reactions causing respiratory distress, immediate hospital care is required.

Treatment

Prolonged fasting is the best method to eliminate recurrent hives. This will allow the intestine to heal, eliminate toxins, and reestablish proper eliminations. The following fluids are useful:

Distilled water
Carrot and green vegetable juice
Burdock seed tea

This diet should be continued as long as possible, or repeated at frequent intervals until the hives do not return. Enemas or other eliminants should be used during the fast. If constipation is a problem, follow the regimen under Constipation.

The diet between fasts should reduce sugars, fruits, and carbohydrates to a minimum. Eat an abundance of green vegetables, avoid saturated fats, or fried foods. Organically grown food is advised.

Physiotherapy

• Oatmeal or bran bath to relieve itching: 2 lb of either placed in muslin bag and set in hot (104° to 106°F) bath.

• Cream of tartar and water paste applied to hives.

• Trunk packs to induce sweating.

• Sodium bicarbonate bath for itching.

• Ultraviolet light.

Therapeutic Agents

VITAMINS AND MINERALS

Vitamin A: 25,000 IU two to three times per day for 2 months. *Use any dose of vitamin A over 50,000 IU per day with medical supervision only.*

Vitamin B complex: 50 mg two to three times per day. Helps prevent production of histamine from the amino acid histidine needed for adrenal function and natural cortisone production.

Vitamin B_6: 50 to 100 mg two times per day.

Vitamin B_{12}: 1 mg intramuscularly daily in acute stage.

Vitamin C: Essential for adrenal function; anti-inflammatory. 1000 IU three to four times per day or more. Ascorbates are best.

Calcium: 2000 to 3000 mg per day in acute, and 1 g intravenous with 5 g vitamin C.*

OTHERS

Raw adrenal tablets: Helps normalize cortisone production which is an anti-inflammatory and antihistamine.

Hydrochloric acid: 5 to 60 grains with meals.

Wheat germ oil: Rub on hives.

Marshmallow soap.

*Asterisks indicate the most frequently used therapeutic agents.

BOTANICALS

> *Apis mellifera** (Tincture)
> Burdock seed tea (*Arctium lappa*)*
> Catnip tea (*Nepeta cataria*)*
> Chickweed ointment (*Stellaria media*)
> Elder leaf ointment (*Sambucus*)
> Nettle juice (*Urtica dioica*): 1 tsp three times per day*
> Sassafras tea (*Sassafras albidum*)*

PRESCRIPTIONS

> Infusion:
> 1 part nettle
> 1 part yarrow
> 2 parts dandelion
> ½ part goldenseal

HYPERACTIVITY (Hyperkinesis, Hyperkinetic Impulse Disorder, Minimal Brain Damage)

Definition and Symptoms

A behavioral disorder of children and sometimes adults, manifested by impulsive activity, low stress tolerance, emotional instability, anger, anxiety, aggressiveness, destructive behavior, hyperresponsive actions, slow learning, short attention span, and sometimes a lack of coordination.

Etiologic Considerations

- Food additives, flavorings, colors, preservatives
- Pesticides, insecticides, fungicides
- Caffeine foods and drinks; soda, tea, coffee, chocolate
- Refined foods, junk foods
- Canned foods
- Food allergy
- Celiac disease
- Salicylate sensitivity (Feingold concept)
- Heavy metal toxicity
- Vitamin and mineral deficiencies and dependencies

*Asterisks indicate the most frequently used therapeutic agents.

- Hypoglycemia
- Fluorescent lights (lack of full-spectrum lighting)
- History of birth trauma, prenatal hemorrhage, toxemia, low birth weight, prematurity, difficult labor, or lack of oxygen at birth
- Monosodium glutamate (MSG)
- Environmental
- Parasitic infestation
- Glandular imbalance
- True psychological causes
- Drugs

Discussion

Hyperactivity of a child can totally destroy the hopes of a reasonably normal life for every member of the affected family. Each time such a child is brought into my office, I find the mother's physical and psychological condition even more upsetting than the child's. These parents suffer incredible tension, profound helplessness, frustration, and guilt, trying to deal with their own pent-up emotions which arise in response to their child's behavior. It is a rare mother indeed who does not break down into tears during the initial consultation. Hyperactivity transforms what was hoped to be the beautiful experience of parenthood into an endless nightmare.

Orthodox treatments have included drugs to sedate and tranquilize the child. This may remove some of the more obvious symptoms temporarily, but does nothing to deal with the cause. The mother frequently is told that nothing more can be done, and given the hope that, at least for some hyperactive children, the problem seems to resolve itself by the midteens.

The cause of hyperactivity is unknown. Abnormal conditions of pregnancy, labor, or the immediate postpartum period may account for some cases. This, however, accounts for only a small number of cases where the condition of minimal brain damage may in fact be the sole cause.

Recently, the Feingold diet has become popularized. This blends the age-old arguments of naturopaths and organic food enthusiasts against the use of refined, devitalized foods poisoned by additives, food colorings, preservatives, flavorings and pesticides; and the more original discovery by Dr. Ben F. Feingold that a significant number of hyperactive children have a salicylate sensitivity. Salicylates are not only found in aspirin, but also in many common foods such as almonds, apples, apricots, cherries, cranberries, cucumbers, grapes, nectarines, oranges, tangerines, peaches, peppers, plums, prunes, raisins, and tomatoes.

Further useful research has come out of the orthomolecular psychiatry approach. Many physicians have found that a significant number of hyperactive individuals are suffering from vitamin dependencies. In such a situation, the patient may require more of an individual nutrient than an otherwise normal person. This research is very similar to that done with schizophrenia and I refer you to that section of this book for more detail.

Both of these approaches have done a real service in presenting at least a part of the nutritional concept to the public attention. Unfortunately, they are both incomplete, failing to present the entire range of possible causative factors in any given case. It is of course no new discovery that diet and nutrition are the single most influential factors in the cause of hyperactivity. The really big surprise would have been that it were otherwise! Naturopaths have been successfully treating hyperactivity with simple diet changes since the turn of the century. The fact that some children are hypersensitive to the blatantly poisonous substances used in the agriculture or food processing industries should be accepted as common sense. Even if every Tom, Dick, or Harry, or in this case Billy, Bobby, Jennie, or Joey, does not show the ill effects of such poison in the form of hyperactivity, other manifestations may result. This is one of the great human mysteries, that each is unique.

Going one step beyond this, it is not too surprising that some people would respond unfavorably to a group of foods containing a naturally occurring substance such as the salicylates. There certainly is evidence that other food groups can cause or aggravate specific conditions, such as the nightshade group (potatoes, tomatoes) in its relation to some cases of arthritis. I must admit that personally I have never taken salicylates into account in the treatment of hyperactive children, but still have had excellent results.

Hypoglycemia is another factor commonly found associated with behavioral disorders, including hyperactivity. Low blood sugar is an increasingly common problem as a result of the objectively bizarre diet most people now consume. From bottled baby food onwards we are literally bombarded with highly refined, devitalized foods and incredible amounts of sugar. Even a casual observer must surely be appalled at the typical junk food diet—or perhaps common sense has left us. Not only does the hypoglycemic state itself create glandular and behavior disorders, but some individuals develop such a severe sugar sensitivity that even minute amounts cause allergylike reactions sometimes manifested as emotional instability or hyperactivity.

Food allergy or sensitivity is another dietary factor often related to hyperactivity. Milk and wheat are the two most common factors, along with sugar, as mentioned above. Any food, however, may be suspect. Celiac disease has been a recognized problem in many cases of behavioral disorders.

Heavy metal toxicity is now becoming more recognized as a cause of behavioral disorders. In children this often accompanies a typical devitalized diet, high in canned and frozen foods. Sometimes the cause may be found in the water supply or some other chronic exposure (see Heavy Metal Poisoning for sources of contaminants).

More subtle factors such as environmental lighting may be important with some individuals. Once again, just because some people might be able to live in a dark, smoggy city in a small box with artificial light does not mean that all could do so unharmed. A wonderful book on the effects of natural and artificial light on humans and other living things is *Health and Light* by John N. Ott.

Treatment

Diet

The most obvious, and for many the most difficult change in diet must be the conversion to *100 percent* organically grown, unrefined foods, with absolutely no additives, colorings, preservatives, pesticides, or any other chemical adulterations. This includes avoiding sugar, salt, most soy sauce, yeast, canned foods, frozen foods, most commercially baked goods, most restaurant foods, etc. You must be absolutely *sure* of the contents of every item consumed. This rarely is an easy process unless you happen to live in an area where organic foods are readily available, or can have your own garden. Unlike other conditions where organic foods are highly recommended, they are an absolute necessity in hyperactivity. Even a small amount of the offending chemicals can trigger an attack of behavioral problems lasting up to 5 days. If you only allow one minor slip every 5 days, and it happens to be the primary irritant, the child will experience a continuous reaction. In other words, no improvement will be seen.

Specific allergy tests may be very revealing. Unfortunately, no food or chemical allergy test is perfect and none has as yet been devised that tests for all types of allergic reactions. Still, the RAST, cytotoxic, and pulse tests should be used to find any specific factors that may be present. Don't be confused if one test shows a specific allergy and others do not confirm this. Each tests for a specific type of reaction and they often do not overlap.

The basic diet is similar to the hypoglycemia regimen with the exclusion of wheat, gluten grains (see Celiac Disease), dairy products, and yeast. These foods are so commonly dietary problems that they are eliminated routinely until all symptoms are gone. They may be carefully reintroduced later to see if a recurrence takes place. The first to be reintroduced is dairy foods in the form of goat's yoghurt. Next comes organically grown wheat in any unyeasted preparation. Last of all, yeast is tried.

A hair analysis is performed to determine any excess heavy metal toxicities and to trace the source. A general heavy metal detoxification program is then instituted if significant levels are found (see Heavy Metal Poisoning).

Once the body has been normalized by proper diet and the child has returned to normal, it is essential to maintain the program for at least 6 months. At this time it is often possible to become more flexible with the diet, but any return to the old habits will certainly result in a return of the old behavioral patterns.

Physiotherapy

* Saunas: One to two times per week.

* Daily exercise: Whatever the activity, it must induce sweating.

* Throw out your TV.

* Spinal manipulation: One time per week.

* Massage: One or two times per week. Massage along spine with cocoa butter.

Therapeutic Agents

VITAMINS AND MINERALS

Vitamin A: 10,000 to 25,000 IU one to two times per day. *Use any dose of vitamin A over 50,000 IU per day with medical supervision only.*

Vitamin B complex: 25 to 50 mg two to three times per day, plus intramuscular injection. *

Vitamin B_3: 1 to 6 g per day. *

Vitamin B_6: 100 to 400 mg per day. *

Pantothenic acid: 200 to 500 mg per day.

Vitamin B_{12}

N,N-Dimethylglycine

Vitamin C: 1 to 6 g per day. *

Vitamin E

Essential fatty acids: GLA (gamma-linoleic acid). *

Calcium: 800 to 1500 mg per day. *

Magnesium: 400 to 800 mg per day.

Zinc: 15 to 30 mg two to three times per day. *

---

*Asterisks indicate the most frequently used therapeutic agents.

Chromium: 200 mcg per day for glucose intolerance.

Trace minerals

Oil of evening primrose

OTHERS

Raw brain tablets*

Raw pancreas tablets

Raw adrenal tablets*

Tranquil Forte (Seroyal)*

Glutamine*

BOTANICALS

Chamomile (*Anthemis nobilis*)

Passion flower (*Passiflora incarnata*)*

Refer also to Allergy.

HYPERTENSION (Essential)

Definition

Increased blood pressure that cannot be ascribed to a single cause. Average blood pressure is 120/80 for men and slightly lower for females. A reading of 140/90 is considered suspicious. Higher readings are considered clinical hypertension. The lower figure (diastolic) is usually considered the most important, as this is the pressure the arteries are under, even at rest.

Symptoms

Headache, dizziness, nervousness, irritability, energy loss, fatigue, insomnia, and intermittent increase in blood pressure, later becoming permanent. Late symptoms are hypertensive heart disease with enlarged heart and possible left ventricular failure, myocardial infarction, possible senility, cerebral hemorrhage, paralysis, and death.

Etiologic Considerations

Although there are several factors that may raise blood pressure, such as increased cardiac output, an increase in the viscosity of the blood, or increased peripheral resistance, in most cases of hypertension we find that increased peripheral resistance is the primary cause, with little or no change in the other two factors. This increased peripheral resistance or narrowing of the blood vessels occurs chiefly in the arterioles (small arteries) and may be anatomical or functional. The initial cause may be vasoconstriction (narrowing), added to by stress or spinal lesions. This sets up a vicious cycle of narrowing and resultant hypertension, which in turn causes further vascular narrowing, etc. The renal arteries may play a key role in the process and seem to be the most sensitive to change due to increased blood pressure.

Another postulated cause of hypertension is narrowing of the blood vessels due to cholesterol and other fatty molecules. Recent research implicates both saturated fats with their high cholesterol and even some unsaturated vegetable oils in this process. It is not as yet clear, however, if it is the unsaturated oils themselves or the artificially processed unsaturated oils that may cause this effect. To my knowledge, no research has been done to differentiate the effects of refined unsaturated oils from the effects of unrefined cold pressed unsaturated oils. The refined oils are a questionable health risk since many changes occur in the natural oil as it is processed at high temperatures. Certainly, hydrogenated oils such as margarine are a definite risk factor. The fatty acids found in this preparation have been altered from the *cis* form to the entirely unnatural *trans* form, which has no known metabolic function. It also interferes with essential fatty acid metabolism. One of the known symptoms of essential fatty acid deficiency, in fact, is high blood pressure. * Cold pressed unsaturated oils, however, should still retain their vitamin E content, as well as their normal essential fatty acid content, which keeps them from going rancid. Both of these factors are essential for good health, and have been used therapeutically to help reverse and control high blood pressure. Further research on this is needed.

Drugs given to treat high blood pressure either reduce cardiac output, reduce peripheral resistance, or are diuretic in action to reduce total blood volume. The common approach is to begin with very mild diuretics and mild hypotensive drugs and increase the dose as required, or change to more powerful drugs, when the milder ones are no longer effective. An important factor to understand here is that in most cases the progression from mild hypertensive drugs having few side effects to stronger hypotensive drugs having significant side effects is the rule, rather than the exception. In my practice, I frequently see the situation where a person has been treated for hypertension with drugs that have lost their effectiveness. These patients have been lulled into a false sense of security, feeling that their blood pressure is under control with diuretics and other drugs, only to find on examination a reading of 160/100 or 110! On questioning, this was

*Horrobin, David, *Clinical Uses of Essential Fatty Acids*, Eden Press, London, 1982, pp. 1–37

the very figure that had prompted drug therapy in the first place, several years before.

The most revealing and upsetting fact of all is that in my experience over 85 percent of all cases of high blood pressure are both treatable and preventable *without* drugs and most physicians know it. The problem is that both the prevention and treatment of hypertension require lifestyle changes which are both difficult and time-consuming to accomplish.

The evidence supporting lifestyle causes of hypertension is readily available. Certainly, *excess weight* is a known factor, as is *excess consumption of animal fats* (vegetarians have long been known to have both lower blood pressures and less incidence of hypertension), *fiber deficiency* due to consumption of excess refined carbohydrates, *stress, lack of demanding exercise*, and *excess salt intake*.

The common argument I receive from physicians is that patients are simply unwilling to change. They show as evidence that even if patients are told to cut out salt, increase their exercise, and lose weight, very few ever do more than reduce their salt intake without making other lifestyle changes. I concede that many patients are unwilling or incapable of change; however, from my experience I have found a growing number who are ready for change, and most willing to do so if educated properly.

It is true that this education process takes considerable time and effort on the part of both doctor and patient, but rewards are high. The end result is a patient carefully weaned off high blood pressure medication and nearly ecstatic with a feeling of self-control of his or her health—and a physician satisfied that yet another human being has begun to understand the true causes of high blood pressure.

Treatment

The first and most important stage of treatment begins by exploring in detail with the patient all the common causes of hypertension, and showing which of these factors relate to the patient's condition.

Diet

In most cases diet remains the single most important factor in the causation of high blood pressure. The ordinary western diet of fried eggs, white toast, bacon, and fried potatoes for breakfast, a meat sandwich for lunch, and meat again for supper (all usually highly salted), not to mention excess dairy products (saturated fats again), coffee, sugar, tobacco, and alcohol, is a prescription for physical disease, especially high blood pressure. (*Note:* There is no one aspect of the western diet that causes high blood pressure, but rather the multitude of improper foods and eating habits.)

I find the best procedure is to have the patient make a list for 3 days of every bit of food, solid or liquid, that enters his or her mouth. We can then gently and carefully analyze the diet in the light of a few clinical facts. The first is that most people who are overweight and have hypertension can usually lower their blood pressure significantly simply by losing weight. The other is that it has been shown over and over that most people with hypertension can lower their blood pressure by eating *less* meat and *more* vegetables. In fact, the most effective way to lower blood pressure safely, rapidly, and permanently, is an entirely vegetarian diet.

Obviously, not all people are able or willing to become totally vegetarian. This is where the skill of the physician comes into play. It is the physician's job whenever possible to convince the patient that a regimen of total vegetarianism for from 3 to 6 months is in his or her best health interests, and that such a diet can and should be not only bearable, but enjoyable. It should be emphasized, however, that once blood pressure is under control, moderate meat eating, especially fish and fowl, can once again be resumed, but this is by no means suggested.

It is always essential for the physician to keep firmly in mind the type of diet optimally beneficial, tempering this with what the patient can achieve. It is, however, important not to be so lenient that results are not achieved. I find the best approach is a period of 4 to 8 weeks of a very strict whole food vegetarian diet, so that both patient and physician can see a true change. This encourages both and makes the long road ahead more achievable.

Below you will find a sample diet regimen for high blood pressure. There is nothing magical about the diet. All that is being stressed is a diet composed of a very large proportion of raw and cooked vegetables, fresh fruits, whole grains, and vegetarian proteins. Salt is restricted totally from the diet. This one change alone will help reduce the average blood pressure considerably. The early stages restrict carbohydrates for weight reduction, if needed; and also protein to achieve a true elimination effect. Brief fasting periods are very useful for rapid blood pressure reductions and then finally eliminating the last of the blood pressure drugs. These diets are alternated as deemed suitable by the physician and are followed by a good general diet, either vegetarian or including light meat eating (fish or poultry), with plenty of fruit, vegetables, and unrefined whole grains.

HIGH BLOOD PRESSURE DIET REGIMEN

Stage 1:

On Rising	A glass of red grape juice or other fruit juice.
Breakfast Day 1	Any ripe fresh fruit (e.g., apples, grapes, grapefruit, pears, papaya, mango, etc.), excluding bananas.

Day 2	Fresh fruit (with or without goat's yoghurt) or stewed fruit or baked apple with a little honey or malt if desired. Wheat germ and soybean lecithin granules are desirable and may be added.
Midmorning	Vegetable juice such as carrot or carrot and other juices, mixed.
Lunch	A large, varied raw salad with plenty of green vegetables such as lettuce, onions, cabbage, green peppers, parsley, celery, carrots, and a few walnuts or other nuts or nut-meats (excluding peanuts); fresh fruit for dessert if desired.
Midafternoon	As midmorning
Supper Day 1	Same as lunch
Day 2	Steamed green leafy vegetables and root vegetables (other than potatoes, including onions, always). Fresh fruit for dessert, if desired.
On Retiring	Same as midmorning
Drinks	Grape juice, apple juice, spring water, or dandelion coffee between meals when thirsty; drink moderately.

If you are taking any drugs prescribed by a doctor for your condition, you must not on any account stop taking them when you begin this diet. As you progress with the dietetic treatment and your health improves, the dosage may gradually be decreased, but *only* with the consent of your doctor.

Stage 2:
Three-day fast on fruit juice (one glass sipped slowly at 4-hour intervals). Grapefruit or apple juice is recommended; however, most fruit juices will do fine. Make sure never to mix juices at any given meal. It is best to restrict oneself to one juice type per day.
Or:
Four-day mono diet of grapes and grape juice. Eat ½ to ¾ lb of red grapes at 4-hour intervals, with red grape juice to drink when thirsty, between meals.
Or:
Four-day apple mono diet of apples and apple juice.

Stage 3:

On Rising	A glass of red grape juice or other fruit juice.
Breakfast Day 1	Any fresh or stewed fruit with lecithin granules, wheat germ, and a little honey if desired.

Day 2   Plain yoghurt (goat's, if possible) with fresh or
                               stewed fruit, lecithin granules, wheat germ, and
                               a little honey if desired.

Midmorning   Vegetable juice

Lunch   A large, varied raw salad with nuts and one or
                               two crispbreads with nut spread, cottage cheese,
                               or vegetarian margarine. Fresh fruit for dessert
                               (especially grapes) if desired.

Supper   Any vegetarian meal (though restricting eggs or
                               cheese to two times per week each. These foods
                               are not encouraged due to their high fat content).
                               Tofu, soybeans, and whole grains or brown rice
                               and buckwheat are especially beneficial. A baked
                               potato may be eaten (including the skin) and two
                               other vegetables. A fresh or stewed apple with
                               soaked and simmered raisins and a little honey
                               for dessert, if desired.

Drinks   Grape juice, apple juice, vegetable juices, dan-
                               delion coffee, or herb teas when thirsty, and in
                               moderation.

General Considerations   1. No salt!

                               2. Eat smaller meals than usual and get as much
                                  rest from stress as possible.

                               3. No alcohol, coffee, or tea, and no smoking.

                               4. Foods especially useful are:
                                     Buckwheat
                                     Onions
                                     Garlic
                                     Brewer's yeast
                                     Miso
                                     Wheat germ
                                     Lecithin granules
                                     Soybeans
                                     Tofu
                                     The pulp of citrus fruits (inside of skin and
                                     outside of fruit)

Other specialized diets useful in some cases are:

Brown rice diet
Lemon juice fast
Vegetable juice fast
Fresh juice fast

In addition to the dietary regimen, certain foods, food supplements, and herbs are useful in speeding up the process, as found under Therapeutic Agents.

Exercise

Lack of demanding exercise usually associated with a sedentary occupation is a second major factor in causing hypertension. A person needs a minimum of 5 minutes per day of the type of exercise that leaves you breathless. This helps clear artery walls of adhering fatty molecules and prevents narrowing of blood vessels. Obviously, a person who already has hypertension needs careful supervision in increasing his or her daily exercise safely until this minimum has been reached. Any type of exercise is acceptable but must be done regularly.

Relaxation Exercises or Meditation

Stress is also considered a major factor in some cases of hypertension. For patients with tension problems, it is useless to simply say "avoid stress." Usually these people will be overstressed under any circumstances, showing a basic tendency of character rather than a simple reaction to a single life situation. For these people progressive relaxation exercises or meditation will be essential. I usually advise patients to find a class of this type that appeals to them and then practice consistently twice daily. The type of exercise or meditation is of little matter, as long as the result leads to physical relaxation, and hopefully better self-awareness. One very useful relaxation exercise I advise frequently is called the "draining exercise." This was given to me by a very special man who really knew how to relax to the very foundation of his soul.

Sit in a comfortable chair with eyes closed and take a few deep breaths, relaxing as much as possible. Quiet your mind and feelings to the best of your ability and let yourself go, once again to the best of your present ability. Next, imagine that you are filled with tension in a *liquid* form, from the top of your head to the tips of your fingers and toes. Further imagine that your body is like a bathtub filled with this liquid tension, and that all ten fingertips and toe tips are the plugs where this liquid may be drained away. In your imagination I want you to pull these plugs from the fingers and toes and let this fluid tension drain out of your body. First, draw your attention to your scalp and head and visualize and feel this liquid tension lowering out of your scalp into your face and neck. As it passes out of your head feel the muscles of your face relax. At the same time you are aware of a constant draining away of tension out of your fingers and toes. Next, feel the tension lowering into your neck and shoulders and into your upper arms and chest. You will begin to notice your breathing becoming more relaxed and regular as the tension drains through your solar plexus and down into your elbows and lower arms. Next, feel this liquid tension flow into your wrist and hands, as well as your abdomen and lower back. As the liquid drains further into your hands and fingers, feel the tingling as it escapes from your body out of the fingertips.

Continue to allow this tension to flow constantly out of the fingers as it continues to drain into your lower abdomen and pelvic region, deep into your sexual organs, and then down to the thighs. Next, it flows to the knees and calves and on into the ankles. Feel the tingling sensation as this liquid tension drains into the feet and out your toes. Maintain this sensation of feeling the liquid tension now draining out of both your fingers and toes for 3 to 5 minutes, or longer. Then take three or four deep, relaxing, cleansing breaths. The object is that with each of these cleansing breaths, you take in new, pure energy to replace the old tension energy you have just drained away.

At this time, if you are a religious person, be open to prayer and let yourself be filled with that grace that may now flow into your empty, open vessel. If not of such a temperament, many other avenues are open that will help unlock your feelings. One technique is to visualize some real or imagined scene of beauty, trying actually to feel the refreshing air on your face, or smell the sea breeze or flowers. In time you will be able to retreat into this peaceful scene and learn to find rest and relaxation.

If you do this "draining exercise" twice daily, early in the morning and before bed, you will soon find that this peace and relaxation becomes a part of you. At first you may find it difficult to let your mind go, or your feelings. Do not criticize yourself for this but gently redirect your mind to the draining exercise each time it wanders. Your reward for perseverance will be an entirely new approach to life, filled with the freedom and joy of a child's. And more to the point, it will lower your blood pressure.

Physiotherapy

Hot showers or baths are discontinued and replaced by warm showers, alternating with cool showers. These alternating warm and cool showers should be 3 minutes each, repeated two to three times. Later, as the cardiovascular system strengthens, the temperatures may be more extreme, with hot and ice-cold water being used. This should be followed by drying with a rough towel to redden the skin, thereby increasing superficial circulation.

Therapeutic Agents

VITAMINS AND MINERALS

Vitamin B complex: 50 mg three times per day.*

Vitamin C complex (with bioflavonoids): 1000 mg three times per day.*

Vitamin E: Begin with 100 IU two times per day and increase slowly over 1 to 2 weeks to 400 IU two times per day. In some cases 1200 IU daily is required. A rapid increase in vitamin E intake has been known to raise some blood pressures while a slower increase will lower them.*

Niacin/Niacinamide: 100 to 400 mg one to two times per day.*

Calcium: 800 to 1200 mg per day.

Magnesium: 400 to 800 mg per day.

OTHERS

Chlorophyll

Essential fatty acids: GLA (gamma-linoleic acid).

Garlic: 2 capsules three times per day.*

Lecithin: 1 to 2 tbs three times per day (emulsifies fats).*

Rutin: 2 tablets with meals.*

Taurine: 50 to 100 mg per kilogram of body weight in three divided doses per day.

Wheat germ oil*

BOTANICALS

Foxglove (*Digitalis purpurea*): Congestive heart failure.

Garlic (*Allium sativum*)

Hawthorn berries (*Crataegus oxyacantha*): Cardiac depressant, hypotensive; helps dissolve deposits on arteries.

Indian snakeroot (*Rauwolfia serpentina*): Hypotensive, contains reserpine. May cause severe depression. Take only under medical supervision.

Lime flowers (*Tilia americana*): Arteriosclerotic hypertension.

Mistletoe (*Viscum album*)

Watercress (*Nasturtium officinale*)

Green hellebore (*Veratrum viride*): Very poisonous. Take only under medical supervision. 2 to 10 drops to lower blood pressure and pulse rate.

See also Heart Disease.

*Asterisks indicate the most frequently used therapeutic agents.

Therapeutic Suggestion

Reduction of drug therapy must be done slowly and sanely. I usually advise 6 to 12 weeks of strict application of all therapeutic suggestions before reducing drugs. At this point, if I am convinced that the patient has been applying the therapies correctly, we cut drug medication in half and put the patient on a 3-day strict juice fast of either citrus juices, vegetable juices, or grape juice. This further lowers the blood pressure.

After several more weeks medication may again be cut in half while the patient fasts, then the drugs are taken on alternate days for a week or two before stopping entirely, again during a short fast.

Botanical medication to lower high blood pressure should be used only until the rest of the naturopathic program has had a chance to reverse the cause (refer also to Heart Disease).

HYPOGLYCEMIA AND HYPERINSULINISM

Definition

A defect of carbohydrate metabolism where the blood glucose level (BGL) reaches levels lower than normal. In some cases, symptoms are better associated with elevated insulin levels.

Symptoms

Nervousness, irritability, emotional problems, fatigue, depression, craving for sweets, inability to concentrate, cold sweating, shakes, palpitations, tingling of skin and scalp, dizziness, trembling, fainting, blurred vision, cold extremities, nausea, midmorning tiredness and mid- to late afternoon tiredness, anxiety, indecisiveness, crying spells, allergies, convulsions, hyperactivity. Symptoms are usually episodic, being related to the time and content of the previous meal. Symptoms are usually improved by eating.

Etiologic Considerations

- Refined carbohydrates (i.e., excess sugar, candy, fruit juice, vegetable juice, dried fruit, or refined grains).

- Adrenal exhaustion: May be primary or secondary due to diet or stress.

- Stress: Depletes vitamin B complex, vitamin C, and adrenals.

- Sucrose sensitivity
- Large meals
- Alcoholism
- Excess coffee and/or nicotine
- Pregnancy
- Liver damage, hypothyroidism, pancreatic tumor, pituitary insufficiency

Discussion

Hypoglycemia is probably one of the most widespread disorders in America and the civilized nations today. It is not a disease as such but a symptom that may result from a wide range of hormonal abnormalities reflecting irregular function of many glands and organs. Unfortunately, it often goes undiagnosed and its multitude of symptoms are frequently labeled as emotional or psychological in origin.

To understand hypoglycemia a little physiological background is essential. The body needs a steady supply of readily available energy to function. It derives this energy from food primarily in the form of carbohydrates which are converted, in the process of digestion, into their simplest common denominator, glucose. Glucose is essential for all bodily activity, and is especially necessary for the function of the nervous system and brain, which responds drastically to abnormal variations of the BGL.

Normally the BGL is kept within a very narrow range of variation by various hormones which respond rapidly to even slight changes. Insulin from the pancreas is released when glucose enters the blood from digested food. This lowers the BGL to the normal range. The sugar is then stored in the liver and muscles in the form of glycogen, or converted to fat for later use. Cortisol and growth hormone counterbalance this insulin action. If any of these hormones are secreted too rapidly or too slowly an imbalance of the BGL can occur.

If the blood glucose level rises above normal, or if glucose is delivered to the blood too rapidly, as it is following a meal of simple refined carbohydrates, the body deals with this excess in two ways. It initiates a *sudden* burst of insulin to counteract what the body perceives as a very dangerous imbalance. It also begins to convert the excess glucose in certain "glucose-insensitive cells" found in the eye, kidney, myelinated nerves, and red blood cells, first into fructose and then sorbitol. This is important since both fructose and sorbitol are relatively insoluble within the cell and tend to crystallize out, leading to cataract formation in the eye, basement membrane thickening in the kidney, damage to nerves, and altered oxygen-carrying capacity in red blood cells. This sorbitol pathway is initiated each time the blood glucose levels rise rapidly on the glucose rollercoaster ride that hypoglycemics travel daily.

In some cases of hypoglycemia insulin is often secreted in excess and thus lowers the BGL too far and too rapidly. This is what is often called hyperinsulinism. In functional hypoglycemia the insulin response may be normal, but the insulin antagonism may be out of balance, once again leading to a low BGL. The most commonly involved glands are the adrenal glands. Most commonly, both the pancreas and adrenal glands are malfunctioning. The liver is also usually involved in this imbalance. Some cases of hyperinsulinism show normal insulin levels but a reduced sensitivity to insulin. This results in a prediabetes type of glucose metabolism where sugar levels remain elevated for a prolonged period and then fall rapidly below normal.

The causes of the endocrine imbalances of hypoglycemia are usually easy to find. As I mentioned previously, in my opinion hypoglycemia is rampant in the civilized nations. The two most significant factors are diet and stress. The average American diet is literally a prescription for hypoglycemia, with its common foods such as white bread, sugar, soda, and coffee. Sugar and refined carbohydrates are absorbed very rapidly into the bloodstream since they require little digestion due to the stripping of their protein and fiber in the refining process. This rapid increase in the BGL causes the pancreas to become hypersensitive to sugar. In time the pancreas learns to secrete very large amounts of insulin in response to a rise in BGL. This causes a rapid *lowering* of the BGL, in this case far lower than normal. During this low period the symptoms of hypoglycemia become manifest. This is primarily due to a deficiency of glucose supply to the brain and the resulting adrenal "shock" response. The adrenal glands recognize the low sugar level as an acute danger and institute an appropriate response. In time the adrenal glands become overstressed by these recurrent emergencies and lose their ability to cope adequately with the situation.

Most people fail to recognize that excess table sugar is not the only "refined carbohydrate" that may cause this disinsulinism leading to hypoglycemia. Excess honey, fruit, fruit juice, dried fruit, or even vegetable juice will cause a rapid rise in blood glucose levels, causing pancreatic hypersensitivity.

Stress also plays a major role via the adrenals since stress also is recognized by the adrenals as an emergency situation and triggers similar responses, thus once again overburdening the adrenals. To further aggravate the complexity of the situation, you should also understand that stress depletes vitamin B complex and vitamin C, both of which are necessary for proper adrenal function, in addition to which vitamin B complex is an essential nutrient in the metabolism of carbohydrates. In turn, the carbohydrates have *already* been stripped of vitamin B complex in the refining process and therefore need extra vitamin B complex for utilization! And we are not off the merry-go-round yet! Coffee stimulates the adrenal glands, which act to mobilize the body's energy reserves in both the liver and muscles. This removes the body's fail-safe mechanism to further keep the BGL in balance, and further abuses the adrenal glands.

The importance of the diagnosis and proper treatment of hypoglycemia should not be underestimated. In the past, and even to some practitioners presently, hypoglycemia has been considered a non-disease. Some doctors claim that the label "hypoglycemia" is too often used for any emotional problem that enters the practitioner's office. Hypoglycemia can be diagnosed clinically using the 5-hour blood glucose tolerance test. Some cases show normal blood glucose levels but elevated insulin levels, which are associated with hypoglycemic symptoms.

Recently, new medical research is supporting the view that the effects of even mild hypoglycemia may be far-reaching.* Hypoglycemia has now been clearly associated with a significant proportion of physical, mental, and emotional disorders, including hyperactivity, schizophrenia, anti-social behavior, criminal personalities, drug addiction, impotency, alcoholism, epilepsy, asthma, allergies, ulcers, and arthritis.

As much attention should be placed on preventing and treating hypoglycemia as has been the case with diabetes. These two disorders are often manifestations of a similar endocrine imbalance, due to the same causes.

Back in the 1960s the seriousness of hypoglycemia was often dismissed. Often a physician, upon discovering hypoglycemia, would recommend a candy bar whenever the patient felt weak. This caused a rapid rise in blood sugar which later resulted in an even more precipitous drop. This "candy bar" therapy for hypoglycemia was clearly a case of a short-term solution that ultimately caused the problem it was meant to solve.

The only effective treatment is the removal of the initial causes and the reestablishment of normal hormonal controlling mechanisms. Unfortunately, once the pancreas has been hypersensitive to sugar over a long period of time, complete recovery is not always possible. In experiments with rats who were fed refined carbohydrates until clinical hypoglycemia developed, it was found that the hypoglycemia could be corrected and kept under control with a change in diet, but once the old diet was reverted to, the hypoglycemia returned fairly rapidly.

Obviously, the longer a person has hypoglycemia and the more severe the condition, the less probable is a complete cure. All that can be expected in these cases is that with a change in lifestyle and diet, no hypoglycemic symptoms will be present. These people, however, do remain hypersensitive to sugar and can react with hypoglycemic symptoms should they revert to their old diet and stress patterns.

*"Hypoglycemia emulating emotional, social and clinical disorders," *Orthomolecular Psychology*, 10(2):77–92, 1981.

Treatment

Diet

The body is very similar in its proper energy needs to a good wood-burning stove—with a supply of high-fiber fuel it will burn evenly and at the right consumption rate. If, however, the body is supplied with refined carbohydrates, stripped of both fiber and protein, the situation becomes similar to paper burning in the stove at a very high heat for a very short period of time.

The traditional low-carbohydrate diet, or high-protein diet, so often advised for hypoglycemia, is not the answer. What is needed is a high-fiber carbohydrate diet with adequate protein. Instead of three large meals per day, the diet should consist of six smaller meals, or three smaller meals and three snacks between meals. The basic concept of the diet is that all foods should be unrefined and slow to digest.

Dried fruit, fruit, fruit juices, and vegetable juice are all considered rapidly absorbable and should be consumed in moderation. When fruit is eaten, it should be taken with some protein such as a handful of nuts, cottage cheese, or yoghurt. Fruit juice, if taken at all, should be diluted 80 percent with water, taken in small quantities, preferably near the time other food is eaten. The rest of the diet is composed of vegetables, whole grains, and protein.

The following diet is an example of the type used in this condition. Choose from the following suggestions:

Breakfast

1. Granola (unsweetened)

2. Cooked whole grain cereal, especially oatmeal.

3. 1 to 2 soft-boiled or poached eggs, 1 to 2 slices whole grain bread. Yoghurt, plus wheat germ and brewer's yeast for dessert, if desired.

4. Yoghurt and wheat germ, kefir, acidophilus milk, buttermilk, or raw unpasteurized cow's or goat's milk. Add brewer's yeast wherever possible.

5. Fresh fruit with yoghurt and wheat germ.* Sweet fruits are to be eaten only rarely and in moderation. Grapes are too sweet for this diet. Recommended fruits are papaya, apple, grapefruit, orange, banana, or fresh berries. Nuts may be added. ½ tsp honey may be used if desired, but no more.

Midmorning   Choose from:

*With doctor's consent.

1. Almond milk: 12 almonds blended with water, a little juice, brewer's yeast, and lecithin.

2. Unsweetened herb tea.

3. ¼ to ⅓ handful raw nuts (almonds, brazils, hazels, sunflower, etc.).

4. Whole grain crackers, biscuit, bread, or other source of unrefined carbohydrate.

5. 1 tsp *Spirulina* in warm water.

Lunch

Fresh raw salad, always as the main part of the meal. (Use olive oil and lemon and herb dressing, avocado dressing, or yoghurt dressing on salad, or other nonsweetened natural dressing.) Then choose from:

1. 1 slice 100 percent whole meal bread and cottage cheese or other protein

2. ⅓ avocado plus lemon

3. Whole grain brown rice, millet, or buckwheat

4. A little cheese

5. Fish, fowl, or lean meat

6. 100 percent whole meal sandwich

Dessert: If desired, a little yoghurt plus wheat germ and brewer's yeast

Midafternoon

As midmorning

Supper

Choose from:

1. 2 to 3 cooked (never boiled or fried) vegetables

2. Whole grain (rice, millet, buckwheat, etc.)

3. A vegetarian savory meal with cheese, eggs, or vegetarian protein

4. Lean meat or fowl two to three times per week only

5. Fish

6. 100 percent whole meal bread with butter or cottage cheese

7. Baked potato (be sure to eat skin)

Desserts:

1. Yoghurt and wheat germ plus brewer's yeast if desired

2. Fresh fruit, especially papaya

Evening

1. Raw goat's milk, cow's milk, or kefir drink, with ½ tbs brewer's yeast; nuts may be added in a blender

2. Almond milk

3. 100 percent whole grain snacks

If hungry at any time your best choice is a slow-burning fuel food made of 100 percent carbohydrate sources.

Never eat

1. Sugar (white or brown) or anything that contains sugar. Honey is permitted only in absolute moderation (1 tsp per day) and best avoided altogether when possible.

2. White flour and its products

3. Refined grains, rice, macaroni, etc. Use whole grains, whole wheat macaroni, etc., instead.

Very important to avoid

4. Alcohol

5. Coffee

6. Cigarettes

7. Dried fruits, dates, figs, plums, grapes. Eat bananas in moderation only.

Foods of special usefulness

Whole grains (especially oats and oat flour)

Nuts

Raw milk products (if no sign of allergy exists)

Avocado

Brewer's yeast

Jerusalem artichokes

Note: When eating fruit, eat in moderation and slowly. Always eat with some protein. When drinking fruit or vegetable juices, drink no more than 2 to 3 oz at a time. It may be best to avoid juices altogether. Eat only when relaxed. Avoid stress whenever possible.

Therapeutic Agents

VITAMINS AND MINERALS

Vitamin B complex: 50 mg three times daily.*

Vitamin B$_3$ (niacinamide): Very useful for nervous hypoglycemics, stress-induced hypoglycemia, or adrenal exhaustion cases. 500 mg time-release capsules, two or three times per day, can be as effective as Valium for these patients. If nausea occurs, reduce dose. (Hepatitis has been reported to occur at very high doses of Vitamin B$_3$ intake in susceptible subjects. Nausea is an early warning sign and should be heeded.)*

Vitamin C: 500 to 1000 mg three to four times daily.*

Vitamin E: 400 IU per day.*

GTF (Glucose tolerance factor composed of chromium, nicotinic acid, and glutamic acid): This is essential for carbohydrate metabolism. GTF is essential for proper insulin function. (GTF is found in yeast or separately in pill form.) 1 tsp brewer's yeast three times daily.*

Chromium. Dose depends on type and amount of brewer's yeast (GTF) taken. 200 mcg per day is the usual dose.*

Zinc

Spirulina: 1 tsp three times daily.*

Lecithin: 1 tsp three times daily (a good source of choline).*

Raw adrenal: 1 tablet one to three times daily.*

Raw pancreas: 1 to 2 tablets two to three times daily.*

Bran: 1 tsp two to three times daily. Fiber helps regulate absorption of carbohydrate from the intestine.

(Note: For further information on this disorder, an excellent book to read is *Hypoglycemia: A Better Approach*, by Paavo Airola.)

IMMUNE DEFICIENCY

The immune defense system is designed to protect against infection. Its actions are mediated by antibodies (immunoglobulins) and the cells of the lymphocytic system (cellular immunity). A deficiency, either genetic or acquired,

*Asterisks indicate the most frequently used therapeutic agents.

of either system will increase susceptibility to infections in general and some diseases. Since the discovery of the first immune deficiency disease in the early 1950s, over twenty distinct types have been reported, most of which are hereditary. The immune system, however, is very susceptible to acquired malfunction from a number of directions. One very controversial cause of immune malfunction is the procedure of vaccinations and immunizations against common childhood and epidemic diseases. The thymus gland seems to be the site most severely affected, altering the function and activity of this all-important kingpin of the immune system.

While severe infectious diseases may be the result of immune deficiencies, they may also be the preceding cause. For example, it is common for allergies, a frequent result of immune malfunction, to follow a severe case of mononucleosis, hepatitis, rheumatic fever, or other acute viral or bacterial disease which may reduce the production by the thymus gland of T-helper cells necessary to moderate the allergic response. Toxic exposure to chemicals or radiation may have similar results. Prolonged stress also depresses the immune system.

The most common source of immune deficiencies, in my opinion, however, is single or multiple nutritional deficiencies. The immune system can only be as healthy as its organized cells and tissues. Various nutritional deficiencies have been associated with immune malfunction. As the immune system becomes weakened, the body becomes susceptible to any opportunistic virus or bacteria which can take hold with sometimes devastating results.

Literally any infectious disease may be considered an immune deficiency. If the immune system is functioning adequately, no such infection could take place. This includes the range of infectious diseases from colds to pneumonia, or diseases of unknown origin such as multiple sclerosis, multiple dystrophy, and AIDS (acquired immune deficiency syndrome).

Treatment

Each case of immune deficiency has to be considered individually. Classic forms of immune deficiency will obviously need to be treated by an immunologist. Other less severe cases may benefit by the following treatment. The tissues affected most will need local therapy, and will give clues to specific nutrients needed. Following is a list of nutrients found useful in enhancing immune function:

Thymus: 2 to 4 tablets, three to six times per day.

Vitamin A: 50,000 to 1,000,000 IU per day. *Use any dose of vitamin A over 50,000 IU per day with medical supervision only.*

Vitamin B complex: 50 mg one to three times per day.

Vitamin B_6: 250 to 500 mg per day.

Vitamin B_{12}: 1 mg intramuscularly one to seven times per week.

Folic acid: 400 mcg to 10 mg per day.

Pantothenic acid: 250 to 500 mg per day.

Vitamin C: Up to bowel tolerance; 30 to 100 g intravenously may be helpful.

Vitamin E: 400 to 800 IU per day. However, very high doses tend to temporarily depress the immune system.

Iron: Dose depending on need and response.

Magnesium: 400 to 800 mg per day.

Selenium: 200 mcg per day.

Arginine: 3 to 5 g per day.

Zinc: 25 to 50 mg two to three times per day.

Copper: 1 to 3 mg per day.

Essential fatty acids (GLA, oil of evening primrose, EPA).

Protein

IMPETIGO (see Staphylococcal Infections)

IMPOTENCE (Male)

Definition and Symptoms

Inability to attain or maintain an erection during sexual intercourse.

Etiologic Considerations

- Physical abnormalities
- Psychological
  Fear of failure
  Inhibitions
  Feelings of inadequacy
  Psychological trauma
- Endocrine imbalance
- Systemic disease
  Diabetes

Disseminated sclerosis
Tabes dorsalis

- Stress
- General debility
- Nutritional deficiency
- Heavy metal poisoning
- Drugs (i.e., Inderal and reserpine)

Discussion

Two main types of impotence exist. *Primary impotence* implies that the problem has existed since birth (males achieve erections at very early ages). In this case a normal erection does not occur and normal sexual relations have never occurred. *Secondary impotence* is a loss of the ability to gain or maintain a normal erection adequate for sexual relations. Primary impotence shows a greater percentage of abnormal physical problems; however, it does not exclude early psychological trauma or other factors. Secondary impotence points to factors other than physical abnormalities of birth and development. Lack of a morning erection points to organic causes.

The psychological factors influencing normal sexual function in the male are well recognized. Few men have never experienced a lost erection due to an inopportune comment at the wrong moment, stress, fear, anger, insecurity, or some other similar emotion such as fear of failure or various inhibitions. Many men experience these problems in the early periods of their sexual activity, finding that an erection occurs easily and spontaneously prior to actual sexual activity, but melts away as soon as intercourse is attempted. These cases are usually caused by fear of failure, insecurity, or similar psychological factors that ordinarily accompany attempts at performing "skilled" tasks by the inexperienced. The only difference in this case is that the tool used is extremely fickle, being unduly influenced by pre-performance butterflies. The individual's reaction to this fairly normal early failure is extremely important in the development of normal sexual performance. Depending on the level of general psychological adjustment, the individual may conclude quite rightly that the whole embarrassing scenario was simply due to the "jitters" and will be short-lived. The next opportunity with a willing partner probably will prove successful. Others less secure, however, may fear the worst from the outset and assume that they are, or will prove to be, impotent. This fear builds upon normal feelings of insecurity to become a self-fulfilling prophecy.

Similar psychological factors may affect the older, more sexually experienced man. Even one failure due to any number of interrelated factors can set up self-doubt. These initial factors may be psychological or they may be due to any one of several little-recognized physical factors. Many prescription drugs have impotence as a side effect. If the individual is presently taking one of these drugs and is not aware, or has been inadequately informed of this possibility, he may wrongly interpret this lack of performance as psychological or senile impotence, which in turn creates psychological stresses that may cause a self-perpetuating condition, even if the drug is withdrawn.

Nutritional factors such as extreme vitamin deficiencies or heavy metal poisoning may affect sexual performance, with similar secondary psychological reactions as observed above.

Treatment

Diet

All therapy should be preceded by a hair analysis to exclude toxic metal causes. If this proves to be a factor, a heavy metal detoxification program should be started. A general detoxification and rejuvenation regimen is required even in the absence of metal toxicity, since toxicity may be caused by many substances. The best program for impotence is an initial fast on fruit and vegetable juices, followed by a raw foods lacto-vegetarian diet similar to that described under Parkinson's Disease. This will encourage toxic elimination and supply essential nutrients often missing in the average diet. Foods to stress are whole grains, green vegetables, fruits, seeds (especially sunflower and pumpkin), nuts, fermented dairy products, free-range fertile eggs, cold pressed oils, sprouted seeds and beans, brewer's yeast, wheat germ, fish, kelp, and other seaweeds. Exclude meat and fowl from the diet totally, unless these are obtained wild or are free from feminizing hormones routinely used as fattening agents. Avoid alcohol, cigarettes, and drugs.

Physiotherapy

* Alternate hot and cold sitz baths: This is the most effective measure in rejuvenating the sexual organs. Repeat one or two times per day, if possible.

* Ice-cold plunges: These are an excellent tonic for the body generally and pelvic region specifically, if the plunge is confined below the waist. Precede ice plunge with a sauna where possible.

* Spinal manipulation: I have seen quite dramatic results with regular spinal therapy in these cases. Repeat one to two times per week for 8 to 12 weeks.

Therapeutic Agents

VITAMINS AND MINERALS

Vitamin A: 25,000 IU per day.*

Vitamin B complex: 25 to 50 mg two to three times per day.*

Vitamin B_6: 100 mg per day.*

Vitamin C

Vitamin E: 400 IU two to three times per day.*

EFA: GLA, EPA, and oil of evening primrose.*

Zinc: 30 to 45 mg two to three times per day.*

OTHERS

Kelp: two to three times per day.

Raw pituitary tablets*

Raw thyroid tablets

Wheat germ oil

BOTANICALS

Ginseng (*Panax* spp.)

INCONTINENCE (Female): Urinary Stress Incontinence

Definition and Symptoms

The involuntary loss of urine in very small amounts, accompanying coughing, sneezing, laughing, walking, running, lifting, or any sudden shock or strain.

Etiologic Considerations

• Repeated births

• Failure to do prenatal and postnatal exercises

• Poor pelvic floor tone

• Damage to supports, sphincter mechanisms, and pelvic floor

• Visceroptosis

*Asterisks indicate the most frequently used therapeutic agents.

- Poor abdominal tone
- Overweight
- Obstetrical trauma
  Tears
  Instrumental delivery (forceps)
  Large baby
  Prolonged labor
  Improper management of labor (failure to empty bladder before second stage)
- Increased intraabdominal pressure

Discussion

Stress incontinence is the commonest variety of urinary incontinence in females after the childbearing years. It may first be noticed after a prolonged labor where much stretching of the pelvic floor has taken place. In a young and healthy woman this will usually heal, but may return insidiously in later years, especially if postnatal exercises were ignored, or if excess weight becomes a factor. Stress incontinence can occur in the nullipara, or woman never having had a baby, but it is much less frequent. Weak abdominal tone, visceroptosis (a drooping of the entire abdominal contents which puts pressure on the pelvic organs), obesity, and lack of pelvic muscle tone are the major causative factors involved in these cases.

To understand what causes stress incontinence, some knowledge of anatomy is essential. Normally the pelvic contents, in this case the uterus, bladder, and urethra, are maintained in place by ligaments and supported by what is called the pelvic floor. This consists of a group of muscles extending from the pubis to the tailbone. This sheet of muscle is pierced by three openings—the anus, vagina, and urethra. Circular muscle layers surround these openings to form two main sphincters, one controlling the anus, another governing the vaginal and urethral openings. Placed just between the anus and vagina is a firm, fibrous area called the perineal body. A strong pelvic floor keeps the pelvic organs well supported in their normal physiological relationships. When it sags, so do the pelvic contents, altering the angle of the urethra as it exits from the bladder and favoring prolapse of the bladder and uterus.

During pregnancy the pressure of the enlarging fetus puts an extra burden on the pelvic floor muscles. Unless proper prenatal exercises are performed regularly, the pelvic floor begins to collapse under the increased weight. During labor the pelvic floor must stretch to allow delivery of the baby. If these muscles are already lax the pelvic floor can become permanently weakened. If postnatal pelvic floor exercises are also ignored, or done for too short a time, stress incontinence may result.

After the menopause, as hormone levels fall, a weakness in this area may become even more evident, resulting in prolapse of the bladder or uterus through the vagina. Women who have had several children, prolonged labors, large babies, large tears, or a forceps delivery are the most severely affected.

Lack of abdominal tone, overweight, and visceroptosis (drooping abdominal contents) place a further burden and more pressure on the pelvic contents, aggravating a latent incontinence condition. Often, incontinence will only first become apparent as abdominal tone slowly weakens in later years.

Treatment

Much surgery is performed to help correct incontinence. Much of this surgery could have been prevented by the simple adherence to properly prescribed prenatal and postnatal exercises. This is particularly important when the far-reaching psychological effects of incontinence are considered. Many women seclude themselves from normal activities for fear of losing urine control, with its consequent embarrassment.

Exercises

Pelvic exercises must begin during early pregnancy or before, and continued just after the birth, regularly, for at least 3 months or longer postpartum. All the following exercises are forms of what is commonly called the "Kegal" exercise, named after Dr. Arnold Kegal, professor of obstetrics and gynecology at the University of California at Los Angeles. He was the first to popularize the necessity of pelvic floor exercises in preventing and treating incontinence. The pelvic floor group of muscles not only helps support the pelvic contents, but when contracted they restrain urine flow and prevent bowel movements. Since the anal sphincter is already very strong, we are concentrating on the vaginal and urethral sphincter to help exercise the pelvic floor muscles.

EXERCISE 1

Practice slowing urine flow and eventually stopping it to gain a sense of which muscles are involved. Later, practice stopping urine flow, hold for 1 to 2 seconds, and repeat six to eight times as you urinate. Eventually you should be able to stop urine flow quickly, without any leakage. And slowly relax the pelvic floor muscles in stages from full contraction to full relaxation.

EXERCISE 2

Use the same muscles that you mastered the control of in the first exercise to contract the pelvic floor throughout the day. Do this whenever and wherever possible. This may be repeated six to eight times during each session and 50 to 100 times a day. Hold the contraction 2 to 5 seconds and then relax.

EXERCISE 3

Contract the pelvic floor muscles while making love. Ask your partner to tell you when he can feel the difference. Repeat many times whenever the opportunity arises.

In these exercises do not hold your breath, bear down (thus pushing down on the pelvic floor), or contract the buttocks, inner thighs, or abdominal muscles. It is best to learn to localize the contraction to the pelvic floor muscles entirely. Do not exhaust the pelvic floor muscles in the early stages. Do only as many contractions at a time as you can do at your maximum contraction, and then two to three more. As contractions weaken, discontinue at that time and build the muscle strength slowly, as is done with any other muscular exercise.

Diet

General whole food diet.

Physiotherapy

- Alternate hot and cold sitz baths (postnatal)
- Ice-cold sitz baths (postnatal)
- Abdominal exercises (prenatal and postnatal)
- Swimming—breast stroke/frog kick
- Bicycling

(Note: For a complete book on prenatal and postnatal exercise I suggest *Essential Exercises for the Child Bearing Year*, by Elizabeth Nobel, Houghton Mifflin Co., Boston, 1976.)

INDIGESTION (see Digestive Disorders)

INFERTILITY

Definition and Symptoms

Inability or reduced ability to produce offspring. The condition may affect the male or female partner.

Etiologic Considerations

Female

- Immature or abnormal reproductive system
- Failure to ovulate
- Fallopian tube incompetency
- Nutritional
    Low protein diets
    Nutritional deficiency
- Marathoner's amenorrhea
- Toxicity
- Emotional causes

Male

- Immature or abnormal reproductive system
- Impaired sperm production
    Toxic causes, including heavy metal poisoning, radiation exposure, and prolonged drug use
    Traumatic or infection-related atrophy of testicle
    Prolonged fevers
    Undescended testes
    Varicocele
    Endocrine disorders
    Nutritionally related causes
- Obstruction of the seminal tract
    Congenital
    Prostatitis, orchitis, epididymitis, or other local inflammatory processes
- Defective delivery of sperm
- Impotence
- Low sperm count
- Reduced sperm motility or viability

Discussion

Due to the large number of physical causes of infertility, all patients and their partners should undergo a complete diagnostic evaluation if conception fails to occur within 2 to 3 years. Once the problem area has been diagnosed, treatment can be directed more specifically. Certainly not all causes of infertility can be influenced by natural therapies; however, the cases that can be are very rewarding. When nothing can be found to prevent conception in either partner, the individualized naturopathic approach is the only course available, and certainly can do no harm.

Treatment

A very common cause of female infertility is blocked or partially blocked fallopian tubes. This is usually due to previous pelvic infections. Some of these cases may be treated successfully with a combination of strict dietary regimens, nutritional supplementation, and vigorous hydrotherapy. Often the tube is inflamed. These measures may reestablish the delivery route for the ovum. All negative health factors are identified and removed, including coffee, alcohol, drugs, and cigarettes. Adequate pelvic exercise is encouraged through daily swimming. Local circulation and nutrition is enhanced by twice-daily alternate hot and cold sitz baths. This hydrotherapy is the most important part of the regimen, and is very effective in removing internal inflammation and congestion. Diet should be as wholesome and fresh as possible. Periodic fasting on vegetable juices for 3 to 5 days is useful, with periods of 2 to 4 weeks on an adequate protein but mostly vegetarian diet. Fish and dairy foods are the only animal proteins allowed. The diet should include plenty of raw and conservatively cooked vegetables, seaweed, seeds, nuts, beans, and whole grains.

The following supplements are useful for the female partner.

Protein Supplements

Vitamin A: 50,000 IU one to two times per day.

Vitamin B complex: 50 mg one to two times per day.

Vitamin B_{12}: 1 mg intramuscularly per week.

Folic acid: 1 to 10 mg per day.

Vitamin E: 400 to 800 IU per day.

Males may respond to a similar dietary and physiotherapy regimen, but differ in their supplement needs to include the following:

Selenium: 200 mcg per day (essential for sperm production).

Brewer's yeast: 1 to 3 tsp per day.

Zinc: 25 to 50 mg one to three times per day (normalizes testosterone production, increases sperm count in some cases).

L-Carnitine: 300 to 800 mg per day.

L-Lysine: 500 to 1000 mg per day.

Vitamin C: 2 to 4 g per day (increases sperm motility).

Vitamin E: 400 to 800 IU per day.

Obviously, individual case histories will indicate other, more specific nutrients. Spinal manipulation is a useful adjunctive therapy to help establish better circulation and local nutrition.

INSECT BITES

Some people are violently allergic to insect bites and require epinephrine treatment for even minor bites, to prevent severe reactions, and even death.

The following recommendations are not for these hypersensitive individuals, but rather for the person who develops average or slightly above average sensitivity to insect bites. Inflammation and pain from insect bites may be lessened and shortened in duration through some of the following measures:

Remove stinger if present; then immediately apply ice to area.

Apis tincture: 25 drops in a small amount of water four to six times per day. Homeopathic dilutions (6 ×) also used.

Tobacco: Chew and apply to sting.

Ice water plus baking soda soaks

Clay packs

Vinegar plus lemon juice applications

Onion (topical)

Green papaya skin juice (topical)

Honey poultice

Plantain poultice

Vitamin C (topical) and internal: 4 to 5 g just after bite, and 1 g per hour until resolved.

INSOMNIA

Definition and Symptoms

Difficulty falling asleep, or awakening from sleep prematurely with subsequent inability to return to sleep. Irritability, depression, emotional disturbances, poor memory.

Etiologic Considerations

- Physical tension
- Emotional or mental stress or preoccupation; overstimulation to nervous system
- Overeating
- Caffeine drinks
- Excess salt: Increases blood volume, heart output, and blood pressure
- Food additives, preservatives, and colorings
- Allergy: Increased heart rate follows exposure
- Refined carbohydrates, sugar, soda, ice cream, or other sweets
- Vitamin B complex deficiency
- Calcium deficiency: Poor absorption of calcium or true deficiency
- Iodine excess
- Irregular sleeping hours
- Out of biorhythm
- Menopause
- Hypo- or hyperthyroidism
- Pain
- Smoking
- Alcoholism
- Poor mattress
- TV
- Heavy metal poisoning
- Unfounded fears
  Fear of not falling asleep
  Fear of not waking

- False insomnia: Light sleeper syndrome, never sure if sleep occurred
- Psychological
- Acute trauma

Discussion

Approximately 8.5 million Americans are presently taking prescription sleeping pills regularly. An additional 30 million dollars are spent yearly on nonprescription over-the-counter sleep aids. These figures not only emphasize how extensive the problem of insomnia is, but should also be taken as an expression of how drug-oriented our society has become. Apparently, millions of people care so little about their health, or are too lazy to become well-enough informed about the insidiously detrimental effects of these medications.

To begin with, over-the-counter sleep aids have been carefully studied in controlled experiments, and it has been found that these medications are no more effective in inducing sleep than a placebo.* The medicine tested was Sominex, but many other over-the-counter sleep aids (Nytol, Sleep-Eze, Compoz, Nite Rest, Sure-Sleep, etc.) contain the same "inactive" ingredients. Worse than this multimillion dollar farce, however, is the fact that while these medications do no real good, they certainly may do harm. A recent recall (1979) of sleep aids containing methapyrilene, an antihistamine, due to its carcinogenic "side effect" makes this fairly clear. Manufacturers promptly added a similar antihistamine, pyrilamine, to fill the gap, which is not known to cause cancer since it has not as yet been tested. (I wonder how all you guinea pigs out there feel when you read this little tidbit!) This really is only the tip of the pill-poppers' nightmare. Sleep studies show clearly that many nonprescription and almost all prescription sleep medications drastically alter sleeping cycles, suppressing REM (rapid eye movement) sleep. This certainly is true for any barbiturates and benzodiazepines, which are the major sleep medication ingredients. To fully understand why suppression of REM sleep is harmful, we must first delve into the normal sleeping cycle.

In the early presleep phase, body temperature falls and alpha rhythm brain waves are prominent. Stage 1 of sleep is usually heralded by "myoclonic jerks," or muscle spasms, followed by a slowing of the pulse and muscle relaxation. Stage 2 is entered after about 5 to 10 minutes. The brain waves become larger and the eyes roll side to side. After another 20 minutes Stage 3 is entered. Brain waves now become slow and fairly large. Muscles are relaxed and breathing is slow and even. Stage 4 then follows. This stage is called delta sleep and lasts about 20 minutes or so. After this time the sleeper enters the lighter REM sleep

---

*Kales, Anthony and Joyce, "Are over the counter sleep medications effective?" *Current Therapeutic Research*, 13:143–151, 1971.

characterized by rapid eye movements. The heartbeat is irregular and the brain waves are similar to the waking state. Of the time in REM sleep, 80 percent or more is spent dreaming. REM sleep lasts 10 or more minutes and then the sleeper enters Stage 2, 3, and finally again delta sleep in a cycle lasting about 90 minutes. Delta sleep lasts longer in the early part of the night, with more REM sleep taking place toward morning. This order of sleep cycles seems to be essential for health. Subjects deprived of REM and delta sleep become irritable, depressed, aggressive, angry, restless and/or apathetic. Once allowed to re-enter REM sleep, subjects spend more time than usual there, apparently making up for lost cycles. If this REM sleep has been suppressed by sleeping pills, health begins to suffer. Once the pills are discontinued the sleeper experiences light, restless, unpleasant sleep with plenty of nightmares. This REM withdrawal sleep, a built-in result of taking medication to *aid* sleep, is usually severe enough to disturb sleep and convince the poor uninformed "insomniac" that he or she still needs sleep medication, thus starting the cycle all over again.

Insomnia can be properly treated only if its true cause is recognized and removed. Frequently the cause is easy to identify, such as excess caffeine, an obvious stimulant found in coffee, tea, chocolate, and some sodas. More difficult to correct quickly, but usually easily diagnosed, is simple muscular tension due to emotional or mental stress and overstimulation.

Dietary factors other than caffeine may also be involved. The excess use of salt has been frequently associated with insomnia. Many sufferers are completely cured by this diet change alone. Overeating before bed is another common fault that is easily corrected. Deficiency of many of the B complex vitamins is associated with general stress syndromes and insomnia. This may be due to the overconsumption of refined carbohydrates which require B complex for their metabolism while being stripped of their own intrinsic B complex components found in the fiber and germ coatings. Stress itself depletes B complex, among other vitamins, as the body's glandular system, particularly the adrenal glands, are overstimulated. Calcium deficiency due to poor absorption or true nutritional deficiency is a common factor in insomnia. Calcium supplementation at bedtime frequently cures sleep disorders. Any food allergy may cause poor sleeping and insomnia. Foods causing allergic reactions are known to increase the heart rate among other actions, causing or aggravating insomnia. Food additives, colorings, preservatives, and pesticides may cause a similar allergic response. Heavy metal poisoning is a well-documented cause of nervousness, mental confusion, irritability, emotional disturbances, and sleep disorders. Many smokers find that their sleeping difficulties are removed once they stop smoking. This is not surprising since nicotine stimulates the sympathetic ganglia and also the adrenal glands, which then secrete Adrenalin. This leads to increased heart rate and elevated blood pressure, and hyperreactivity at the neuromuscular junction, the opposite effect desired for sleep.

The use of alcohol as an evening nightcap may not always be either successful or beneficial. Many people respond to alcohol as a stimulant, which it is at low blood levels. Alcohol also has a similar effect on sleep cycles as other sleep aids, reducing the REM cycle.

Another major cause of insomnia is improper or irregular sleeping habits. There is a great deal of evidence detailing the existence of internal biological clocks or rhythms. If we chronically live out of phase with our intrinsic cycles, health begins to suffer. We have all known people who call themselves "day" or "night" people, who claim they think and work best either in the morning or late at night. This may not be simple preference, but our intuitive awareness of the dictates of our biological rhythms. With the advent of electric lighting modern society has placed new and unusual demands on our inner clocks. Many workers now must force their bodies to perform, even in the middle of their biological sleep time.

Evidence shows that these inner clocks can be made to shift as the need arises, but this takes anywhere from a few days to a few weeks. For workers on rotating shifts, biological rhythms are in constant chaos. This is especially true for pilots and crew members on commercial airlines with their truly cacophonic schedules. Stress, fatigue, and insomnia are the common results of such lifestyles.

Treatment

In dealing with a "sleep disorder" it is important to recognize that not all people have the same sleeping requirements. As a person gets to be 50 or 55, he or she usually will require less sleep. Some people can get by quite nicely with 4 to 6 hours' sleep at night and a catnap during the day. The real criterion as to whether a person is getting enough sleep is his or her general health and energy level. If a person complains that he cannot get to sleep until 1 or 2 in the morning, but feels normal, he does not have an insomnia problem, but rather a biorhythm misunderstanding. The worst thing for such a person to do is to lie in bed fretting and worrying about why he can't sleep. He must be active until sleep is desired, as it probably would be if he continued at his normal pace until the time sleep normally came.

Daily tension and stress are major obstacles to falling asleep. Unfortunately, most insomniacs spend most of their time complaining to others about their problem, and little or no time reversing its true causes. The cause of such tension is a complete lack of self-knowledge and self-control. Tension is present only if you allow it to be present.

The only real cure is first to become aware of the problem, find its cause, and then slowly and steadily remove or counteract it. We are dealing here with the basic cause of almost all disease—our improper attitude toward life and lack of knowledge and awareness of ourselves. I often see obviously tense individuals who do not recognize even the gross chronic muscular spasms of their bodies. When asked to be totally relaxed and allow their bodies to go limp like a rag doll, I often find patients completely unable to let go. If I raise their arms, they stay in the air; if I touch their legs they jerk uncontrolledly. These people are truly surprised to discover that day in and day out their bodies are in constant muscular contraction, even at so-called rest! Think how much less aware these individuals must be of the mental or emotional causes of this physical tension, and you will begin to understand why sleep does not come easily.

To correct such a situation several avenues are available, depending on the psychological inclination of the patient. Relaxation exercises can help the patient gain an awareness of physical tension and help relax chronic muscular tensions. Several methods are commonly used.

PROGRESSIVE CONTRACTION/RELAXATION EXERCISES

In this method the subject lies comfortably on a bed and relaxes as much as he or she normally can. Three or four deep, slow breaths aid in reaching this state of maximum normal relaxation. An attempt is made to ignore, or pay no attention to, any thoughts or feelings, with the entire attention gently concentrated on the relaxation procedure at hand. The subject begins by contracting the face and neck into a horrible grimace, holding the contraction for 1 to 2 seconds, and then suddenly letting go and relaxing. Next the upper arms and chest are contracted, then relaxed, followed by lower arms and hands, abdomen, buttocks, thighs, lower legs, and finally the feet. End with a final convulsive contraction of every muscle in the body all at once. This whole cycle is repeated two or three times. This preliminary exercise should be ended with three slow, deep breaths. Deeper relaxation techniques may then follow.

This technique allows the person who has little knowledge of his or her physical tensions to physically reverse the process by reeducating the various muscles as to what is the state of contraction and relaxation. It is useful for the person who has not yet developed a very subtle awareness of muscular tension, or is unable to release tension by a mental command.

"DRAINING" EXERCISE

This technique is an excellent aid to relaxation for the person a little more aware of his or her tension level. Begin by sitting in a comfortable chair and getting as relaxed as normally possible. Imagine that your body is like a bathtub filled with liquid tension, with your fingers and toes being the drain. Start at the very top of your head and imagine that the liquid tension is draining down toward your head and face. Feel the tension as it passes down into your jaws and cheeks, upper neck, and then shoulders. Sense the freedom from tension and your relaxation as it passes out of your head and neck into your shoulders and upper arms. Keep your mind relaxed and dismiss any other thoughts or feelings. Attend only to the "draining," with a gentle concentration on the passage of the liquid tension down into the abdomen and lower arms. Feel the tension level lowering and draining into the lower back and buttocks, and beginning to tingle as it enters your hands and fingers. You will feel the tension tingle and flow out of your fingertips, leaving your upper body totally relaxed. Continue observing this draining process into your pelvic region and sex organs, then thighs, knees, calves, and ankles. Finally, feel the tingling as the last bit of the liquid tension drains out of your toes. Finish the exercise with three cleansing breaths, consciously feeling new vitality enter your body with each breath, relieving the old, worn-out, and toxic liquid tension you have just eliminated.

You may find that after you have finished with this exercise, or even partway through it, tension has once again begun to accumulate in your body. Disregard this and finish the exercise to its end, and then begin all over, if necessary. If this exercise is done twice daily for 15 to 30 minutes, you will find it becomes easier and more complete. If done regularly, over a period of 3 to 6 months you will notice deeper and deeper states of relaxation. Soon you will notice a steady flow of powerful currents passing through your body at the end of each session. Slowly you will discover that you have learned to recognize your physical tensions throughout the day and you will find it easy to drain them away quickly, even as you sit or stand in your ordinary daily activities.

This draining exercise is an excellent preliminary step before meditation. In meditation you will come more and more in contact with the center of yourself, revealing many things about why physical, mental, and emotional tension exists within you.

Biofeedback

This is a fairly new technique used in relaxation therapy and other applications. As applied to insomnia and tension, the subject is taught to recognize tension in the forehead through audible and/or visual feedback from an EMG (electromyograph). Once the person has learned to control the forehead muscles, he or she then is taught by a similar process with an EEG (electroencephalogram) to produce alpha brain waves that precede sleep.

Hypnosis

This method of curing insomnia works well for many. The usual method is to teach the subject self-hypnosis slowly, allowing him to relax and then sleep.

Diet

The diet must exclude all caffeine beverages (coffee, tea, colas) or foods (chocolate). Stimulant drugs, cigarettes, or alcohol should also be avoided. All refined carbohydrates, especially sugar, are excluded. Food additives, preservatives, colorings, and pesticides may also need to be eliminated, as well as all canned foods or other sources of toxicity or heavy metals. Specific allergies may need to be traced down and eliminated. The evening meal should be moderate in size. Overeating at supper may cause sleeping difficulties and nightmares. The foods eaten should be soothing in nature, with simple, compatible food combinations and sufficient sources of B complex and calcium. A large glass of warm milk may be helpful just before bed, due to its tryptophan content, an amino acid found useful in inducing a safe, natural sleep without suppressing the REM and delta cycles.

Sleeping Habits

Try to find out what time sleep comes most naturally and follow the dictates of your body. If sleep is easiest at 2 A.M. don't attempt to sleep sooner. Six hours of sleep taken in the proper cycle are much more refreshing than tossing and turning for hours, waiting for sleep to come. Keep to a regular sleep schedule, always going to bed at the same time to establish a good sleep habit. Make sure your mattress is firm and supportive.

Daily Activities

Try to maintain a relaxed and positive attitude toward life and your daily tasks. Most stress and tension states have their roots in poor attitudes. Most of us tend to blame outside events (our job, our boss, working conditions, the weather, etc.) for our tension. We must slowly come to realize that we have the ability to control our inner state and need not let external factors influence us in a detrimental way. If the conditions in which you live and work are definitely too difficult for you to handle, first try to change yourself. If this is beyond your present abilities, you must make changes in your environment. If necessary, find a new job. Your health is much more important.

Physiotherapy

- Hot foot baths: These draw the blood away from the head, making sleep easier.
- Warm baths: These are generally relaxing. Make sure the bath is not too hot or it will become a stimulant in nature.
- Foot massage
- General massage
- Alternate hot and cold showers or head baths (tonic)
- Cold baths (a daily tonic)
- General exercise, plus fresh air

- Meditation
- Candle gazing
- Relaxation techniques
- Spinal manipulation
  Cervical
  Upper thoracic
- Hops-filled pillow
- Breath holding: Take three deep breaths and hold as long as possible. Repeat three times, then concentrate on breathing shallowly.

Therapeutic Agents

VITAMINS AND MINERALS

Vitamin B complex: 50 mg two times per day.*
Vitamin B₆: 100 mg two times per day.*
Vitamin C: 500 to 1000 mg three times per day.*
Pantothenic acid: 250 mg per day.
Inositol: 1000 to 1500 mg taken 2 hours before bed.*
Calcium: 800 to 1000 mg per day.*
Magnesium: 400 to 500 mg per day.*
Zinc: 15 to 25 mg two times per day.
Manganese: 1 to 5 mg per day.

OTHERS

Tryptophan: 500 mg—1 g three times per day with one dose 45 to 90 minutes before bed.*

Lecithin: 4 capsules three times per day and a lecithin protein drink before bed. Blend 50% apple juice, 50% water, 12 almonds, and 1 to 2 tbs lecithin granules; or drink milk plus lecithin.

Brewer's yeast*

Tranquil Forte (Seroyal)*

BOTANICALS

Chamomile tea (*Anthemis nobilis*): Mild sedative.

Hops (*Humulus lupulus*): Mild sedative.

Passion flower (*Passiflora incarnata*): Sedative. Dose: 30 to 60 drops tincture 45 minutes before bedtime.*

*Asterisks indicate the most frequently used therapeutic agents.

Skullcap (*Scutellaria lateriflora*).

Valerian (*Valerian officinalis*): Strong sedative.

IRRITABLE COLON (see Colitis)

KIDNEY DISEASE: Nephritis, Pyelitis, Pyelonephritis, Glomerulonephritis

Definition

Acute or chronic diffuse, often bilateral inflammation and infection of the kidneys. Each specific term refers to the main area affected—i.e., nephrons, pelvis, kidney, or glomeruli.

Symptoms

Chills, fever, low back pain, bladder irritation, pain on urination (dysuria), frequency, and possibly edema. Each acute episode causes some permanent kidney damage.

Etiologic Considerations

- Ascending infection common (cystitis, urethritis)
- Same considerations as Cystitis
- Obstruction (stone, tumor, prostate)
- Diabetes
- Pregnancy
- Diet: Excess animal proteins, cow's milk
- Allergy
- Drug damage

Discussion

The same considerations that apply to other genitourinary diseases apply to kidney disease (see Cystitis). Always remember that the true cause of disease comes from within. Even Pasteur realized the basic importance of the healing power and vitality of the body when he wrote that "the germ is nothing, the soil is everything." By this he meant that the most important element in the cause or prevention of disease is the state of the tissues of the body, not the presence of pathogenic bacteria.

It is very important to get prompt treatment for all kidney infections since even mild infections can cause some tissue damage. Pyelonephritis is a medical emergency best treated with antibiotics. Antibiotics will usually rid the body of the immediate bacterial infection. Frequently, however, the infection will recur within 2 to 8 weeks unless the original causes of the lowered tissue vitality are removed. The worst cases I see in my practice, and the most difficult to treat, are those which have received multiple courses of antibiotics over a fairly prolonged period of time due to chronic and recurrently acute kidney infections, without an attempt being made to deal with the deeper causes of the disorder.

Treatment

Diet:

In acute cases the best dietery therapy is to fast on the following liquds:

Cranberry juice	Parsley tea
Mullein tea	Barley water
Watermelon seed tea	Watermelon juice
Potassium broth	

This is followed by a transitional low-protein vegetarian diet. A low-protein (35 to 40 g per day), low-salt diet must be followed up to 2 to 3 *years* for complete cure of chronic cases. Adequate protein homeostasis must be monitored during this period.

In chronic cases of kidney disease a different approach is usually necessary. While periodic fasting as above may be useful, a slightly higher protein diet is often more beneficial. Raw goat's milk is an ideal mono diet; or combined with noncitrus fruits and vegetables. Certain foods have proven very beneficial in the healing of kidney disease and should be incorporated into the dietary regimen:

Garlic	Horseradish
Asparagus	Raw honey
Parsley	Raw goat's milk
Watercress	Apples, pears
Watermelon	Potassium broth
Celery	Cucumber
Papaya	Mango
Potato skins	Parsnips

> Dandelion greens
> Turnip greens
> Carrot, celery, and parsley juice
>
> Kale
> Kidney beans plus pods

Spinal Manipulation

Thoracic/lumbar junction T6 to L5, to stimulate nerve, blood, and lymph flow.

Hydrotherapy

Turpentine stupes: Take 2 oz spirits of turpentine (not the turpentine in hardware stores. This is available through the Edgar Cayce cooperating pharmacies listed in Appendix II). Add to 1 quart hot water. Soak three to four thicknesses of heavy toweling in this solution and apply over the kidney area in the back. Keep the towels warm for 15 to 20 minutes by repeating the application frequently or using a hot water bottle or hydro-colator pack. Do not burn the skin. Repeat two to three times and apply two to four times daily.

Trunk packs

Hot and cold compresses

Massage

Massage the following mixture across the kidney area and abdomen with either:

1 oz dissolved mutton tallow with added:
20 drops spirits of gum turpentine
40 drops camphor
20 drops benzoin
3 drops sassafras

Or:

Camphoderm (Cayce product), mutton tallow, turpentine, and camphor.

Therapeutic Agents

VITAMINS AND MINERALS

Vitamin A: 50,000 to 75,000 IU—helps heal mucous membrane. Larger doses may be needed for a short period. *Use any dose of vitamin A over 50,000 IU per day with medical supervision only.*[*]

Vitamin B complex: 25 to 50 mg two to three times per day.[*]

---

*Asterisks indicate the most frequently used therapeutic agents.

Vitamin C plus bioflavinoids: 500 to 1000 mg two to six times per day or to bowel tolerance. Any infection needs excess vitamin C; it acidifies urine. *

Vitamin B$_6$: 100 to 250 mg one to three times per day; especially where duct blockage by stone is the predisposing cause for the kidney disease; diuretic. *

Vitamin D: Reduces aminoaciduria due to defective amino acid reabsorption, due in part to vitamin D deficiency in chronic kidney disease. *

Vitamin E: 400 IU one to three times daily. *

Choline: 250 mg four times per day. May be made from methionine, but in rapid growth (young children) this amino acid is needed in large amounts, and so is not available for conversion to choline. A diet deficient in choline and low in protein in the very young will favor nephritis. Choline causes the body to smell very fishy. Concentrated phosphatidyl choline (lecithin), however, contains much choline and leaves no fishy odor. Use 2 to 4 capsules three to six times daily. *

Magnesium: 400 to 600 mg per day.

Niacin

(Note: With diuretic therapy these supplement doses may need to be increased.)

OTHERS

Garlic

Lecithin: 3 to 6 tbs daily helps protect kidneys from atherosclerosis. Contains choline. *

Raw thymus: Immune support. 2 tablets up to every 1 to 2 hours. *

BOTANICALS

Bearberry (Arctostaphylos uva-ursi): Diuretic, gastrointestinal antiseptic. Dose: Tincture, 20 to 40 drops three to four times per day.

Buchu (Barosma betulina): Diuretic, antispasmodic. Dose: Tincture 10 to 15 drops three to four times per day. *

Chamomile (Anthemis nobilis)

Couch grass (Agrobyram): Mild diuretic: demulcent.

Coneflower (Echinacea angustifolium)

High-bush cranberry, or cramp bark (Viburnum opulus): Juice. *

*Asterisks indicate the most frequently used therapeutic agents.

Horsetail (*Equisetum arvense*): Astringent to urinary tract. Dose: Tincture 10 to 40 drops two to four times per day.

Juniper (*Juniperus communis*)

Parsley (*Petroselinum sativum*): Diuretic.*

Pipsissewa (*Chimaphilia umbellata*): Renal antiseptic.

Mullein (*Verbascum thapsus*)

Stinging nettle (*Urtica urens*): Diuretic. Dose: Tincture 10 to 40 drops three to four times per day.

Watermelon seed tea (*Citrullus vulgaris*): Diuretic, purifies kidneys. 3 to 4 cups per day.*

KIDNEY STONES (Nephrocalcinosis)

Definition

Gravel or stone formation in the kidneys. Composition of stones is usually calcium oxalate but urates, phosphates, and cystine may be present.

Symptoms

May be symptomless or with intermittent, dull, dragging pain in the low back, testicle, groin, or leg, usually aggravated by motion. Hemorrhage and renal colic occur when stone enters ureter, causing sudden sharp pain, which may last hours or even days. Pallor, frequency of urination, nausea, vomiting, and severe agony occur.

Etiologic Considerations

Diet

- Vitamin B_6 deficiency or dependency
- Calcium deficiency or phosphorus excess
- Magnesium deficiency
- Nutritionally induced secondary hyperparathyroidism
- Excess acid (oxalate plus urate stones)
- Excess alkaline (phosphate stones)
- Excess purines as in gout (uric acid)

*Asterisks indicate the most frequently used therapeutic agents.

- Milk-alkali syndrome (ulcer diet plus treatments—i.e., milk and sodium bicarbonate)
- Excess dairy products
- Excess meat-based protein
- Excess soft drinks
- Excess oxalates
    Chocolate
    Cocoa
    Tea
    Spinach
    Rhubarb
    Chard
    Beet tops
- Excess sugar and refined carbohydrates
- Vitamin A deficiency
- Some macrobiotic diets
- Excess coffee
- Excess meat
- Deficiency of fluids
- Excess fluid loss
    Occupations leading to sweating
    Living in tropics
    Runners are at risk
- Chronic urinary infections
    Stagnation of urine
    Increased salt concentration
    Lesion site instigates formation
- Hypercalciuria
    Idiopathic (of unknown cause)
    Prolonged bed rest
    Excess salt intake
    Excess protein intake
    Hyperparathyroidism
    Cushing's syndrome
    Vitamin D excess
    Sarcoidoisis (a chronic disease characterized by nodule formation in lymph
        nodes, lungs, or bones.
    Multiple myeloma (malignant tumor of plasma cells)

- Hereditary
    Congenital hyperoxaluria or cystinuria
- Excess aspirin use increases stone formation

Discussion

Normal urine contains many constituents that are present in a supersaturated solution. To maintain this excess solubility, urine also contains certain substances which form complexes to keep these otherwise insoluble salts in solution. Other factors or substances either decrease the output of some of the major constituents of kidney stones or speed their removal from the kidneys. Among these substances are polypeptides, mycoproteins, citric acid, magnesium, and vitamin B_6. The amount of urine produced is also a factor and generally the larger the urine output the less chance kidney stones have to form. If a person has a deficiency of the substances that help keep insoluble salts in a solution, or if fluid intake is restricted relative to fluid loss, stone formation is favored.

Recent evidence has appeared to link vitamin B_6 and magnesium deficiency with some kidney stones. Vitamin B_6 helps control the body's production of oxalic acid and increases oxalate excretion. Magnesium helps increase the solubility of oxalates in the urine. Both factors are important in preventing calcium oxalate stones, which are by far the most common. Although oxalates are found in some foods such as chocolate, cocoa, tea, rhubarb, spinach, chard, and beet tops, this usually amounts to only 2 percent of the total body oxalates. The rest are endogenous, being produced internally by the body. A 24-hour urine sample will reveal if oxalates are in excess. If so, vitamin B_6 and magnesium therapy has proven very effective in preventing future stone formation, especially when combined with proper diet and other naturopathic preventive therapies.

Some diets predispose to stone formation. A strict macrobiotic diet composed primarily of grains and little fruit or vegetables causes the urine to become very concentrated and may cause stones. However, not all or even most people on strict macrobiotic diets get kidney stones.

Much more common than the strict macrobiotic diet in causing stone formation is the typical American diet having an imbalance in the calcium-to-phosphorus ratio. The ideal calcium-to-phosphorus ratio in the diet is near 0.7 parts calcium to 1 part phosphorus. Meat, for example, has anywhere from 20 to 50 parts phosphorus to one part calcium. Carbonated beverages and refined foods are also very high in phosphorus. This mineral imbalance stimulates a nutritionally caused secondary hyperparathyroidism that causes increased calcium resorption from bones. This causes weak bone structure and excess calcium being handled by the kidneys, leading to stone formation. Serum calcium levels do not reflect this type of calcium deficiency–phosphorus excess syndrome, since the blood levels are kept in the normal range by the calcium taken out of the skeleton.

Excess dietary intake of protein foods high in the sulfur amino acids also can be a problem. These break down in the body to sulfate and organic acid that leads to an excess acidic environment in the kidney, which causes a reduction in calcium resorption and increased calcium excretion. This further reduces the body's calcium levels, disrupting proper calcium-phosphorus levels.

Salt is another common offender, causing an increase in calcium excretion and inhibiting renal calcium resorption, leading to a net calcium loss. Table salt as a condiment is an obvious source; more insidious, however, is hidden salt as found in most refined or convenience foods.

High vitamin C intake for therapeutic reasons has been suggested as a cause of kidney stones. This is disputed by many studies. Anyone on a high vitamin C intake (10 g or more per day) should also increase the supply of magnesium and vitamin B_6.

Diets high in sugar and refined carbohydrates increase calcium in urine and decrease magnesium reabsorption, creating an imbalance between calcium and magnesium, leading to stones. High fiber diets composed of unrefined carbohydrates lower calcium in urine and reduce the chance of stones.

Gout is associated with uric acid stones that may be aggravated or caused by improper diet (see Gout).

Kidney stones are also common among those who sweat excessively. Occupations that cause extreme water loss or sports such as running can cause the urine to become too concentrated and lead to stone formation.

Treatment

With kidney stones, the best results are obtained when the practitioner knows exactly what type of stone is present. A 24-hour urine test will show levels of oxalate, phosphate, urate, cystine, calcium, and magnesium, which will help identify the problem. If the problem lies with uric acid, then a gout-type regimen is beneficial. If, however, oxalate levels are high and magnesium low, in all probability the vitamin B_6 plus magnesium plus diet therapy will be very successful. Excess phosphorus and calcium deficiency is best determined by computer dietary analysis.

Diet

The following diet has been very successful in either acute or chronic kidney stones, as well as many other kidney complaints. Stage 1 is to be used in the acute phase until all pain has ceased for at least 24 to 48 hours.

Stage 1: Follow the diet set out below for 3 to 14 days:

On Rising	Choose one of the following: Mullein tea, watermelon seed tea, cranberry juice (unsweetened), potassium broth
Breakfast	Choose one of the following: Watermelon 2 oz fresh parsley juice in 4 oz carrot, celery, and cucumber juice Fresh watercress, parsley, carrot, and celery juice
Midmorning	Any of the above drinks. Alternate these two groups of liquids at 2-hour intervals. Try to have *at least* 2 cups of watermelon seed tea daily in *all* stages of this diet. Drink as many fluids as possible during this regimen.

Stage 2: Proceed to a diet made up of only raw foods and drink at least 2 to 3 pints of fresh fruit juice and/or vegetable juices throughout the day.

On Rising	Choose from the following: Fresh noncitrus fruit juice (especially cranberry juice) Any drink under Stage 1
Breakfast	Fresh noncitrus fruit, especially watermelon, papaya, banana
Midmorning	Any liquid under Stage 1
Lunch	A raw grated salad composed primarily of leafy green vegetables such as lettuce, celery, watercress, parsley, cucumber, cabbage, etc. You may also include carrots, onions, and cooked asparagus. Alfalfa sprouts or other sprouts may also be added. A simple olive oil, or sunflower oil dressing with plenty of lemon juice, garlic, and herbs may be used. Raw goat's milk yoghurt (in later stages of diet)*
Midafternoon	Same as midmorning
Supper	Same as lunch, or in later stages of diet: steamed vegetables, tofu, legumes, brown rice or millet, miso, seaweed, fish, baked potato
Evening	Same as midmorning

RECIPES IN DIET

POTASSIUM BROTH:

Take outside ¼ in of potato with skin, carrots, onions, garlic, cabbage, celery, and any other greens and vegetables on hand. Prepare the broth by

*Asterisks indicate the most frequently used therapeutic agents.

washing and chopping the vegetables and then simmer in large covered pot of water for not more than 30 to 40 minutes. Strain and drink essence only, flavored if desired with pure vegetable concentrate. Excess may be stored in glass containers in refrigerator for up to 2 days.

WATERMELON SEED TEA:

Grind a handful of watermelon seeds. Steep in hot water for 10 to 15 minutes, strain. Add a little honey and drink.

The basis of the long-term diet is eating foods having a better calcium-to-phosphorus ratio. Include plenty of fresh vegetables, fruit, legumes, whole grains, and fermented dairy products. Salt is strictly controlled and total protein kept at between 45 to 60 g per day. Increased fluid intake is encouraged.

Physiotherapy

- Mullein Poultice. Obtain a large amount of mullein herb. Moisten 1/4 in. of herb with very hot water, lay on a large piece of gauze and cover with gauze or cloth. This poultice should be large enough to cover the area from the umbilicus to the pubic region in front, or over the kidney area in back. Apply the poultice and cover with hot wet towels. Keep these as warm as possible, either by replacing the towels with a second set of heated wet towels, or use a hot water bottle or other source of heat. Keep this poultice on for 30 minutes.

- Spirits of Gum Turpentine Pack. Alternate the mullein poultice with this pack. Mix 2 oz spirits of turpentine with 1 1/2 qt hot water. Saturate a folded towel and apply to the prescribed area (bladder to pubic area in front or kidney area in back). Apply hot wet towels as above. Apply this pack for 30 minutes at the interval prescribed. (Every 1 hour, 2 hours, or 4 hours.)

- Hops and Lobelia Poultice, for severe pain: Mix 1 to 2 oz of the herbs and apply as per directions for mullein poultice.

- Hot Epsom salts compress.

- Hot sitz bath for pain, to help urine flow.

- Alternate hot and cold sitz bath; tonic in chronic cases.

Therapeutic Agents

VITAMINS AND MINERALS

Vitamin A: 10,000 to 25,000 IU three times per day in acute cases; one to two times per day for chronic cases. *Use any dose of vitamin A over 50,000 IU per day with medical supervision only.* *

*Asterisks indicate the most frequently used therapeutic agents.

Vitamin B complex: 25 to 50 mg two to three times per day.

Vitamin B_6: 50 to 200 mg two times per day. Some patients have a biochemical block in oxalic acid metabolism, due to a B_6 dependency. These patients need 1000 mg of B_6 or more per day to correct this problem. Please note the high doses of B_6, if taken for a prolonged time by subjects who do not need these very high doses, can be toxic.*

Vitamin C: Less than 10 g per day.*

Vitamin E: 200 to 400 IU two to three times daily.*

Essential fatty acids

Magnesium: 100 mg two to four times per day. Helps keep calcium in solution, mobilizes calcium from stone.*

OTHERS

Apple cider vinegar (to dissolve)

Hot water and lemon juice (to dissolve)

Olive oil (to help pass stone)

BOTANICALS

Aphanes (*Aphanes arvensis*)

Bearberry (*Arctostaphylos uva-ursi*): To ease stone passage.

Birch tea (*Betula* spp.): Dissolves stones, removes uric acid.

Chamomile (*Anthemis nobilis*): Reputed to help dissolve stones.

Cleavers (*Galium aparine*): To help prevent recurrence. Dose: 10 to 15 drops two to three times per day.

Couch grass (*Agropyrum repens*): Used for phosphate stones. Dose: Tincture, 5 to 30 drops three to four times per day.

Gravel root (*Eupatorium purpureum*): Use decoction. 1 cup two to six times per day to clear kidneys and dissolve stones.

Horsetail (*Equisetum arvense*)

Parsley (*Petroselinum sativum*)

Yarrow (*Achillea millefolium*): To dissolve.

Therapeutic Suggestions

The patient must increase liquid intake to 6 to 8 glasses per day to prevent a recurrence. More is needed if the person sweats heavily during work or sports,

*Asterisks indicate the most frequently used therapeutic agents.

causing excessive water loss. The magnesium supplement with vitamin B_6 is the most proven active ingredient of the regimen.

LEG CRAMPS

Discussion and Treatment

Leg cramps are an extremely common and disturbing problem. They may affect the young or old, and may occur while walking, or even while in bed. In their simplest form, the cause is a single mineral imbalance. Athletes often get leg cramps due to excessive exercise and sweating, which leads to a mineral depletion. A common mistake is to replace water lost in sweating by drinking water and taking salt tablets. Although salt is lost in perspiration, it certainly is not the only complex of minerals lost. The proper replacement for such mineral loss is fresh fruit and vegetable juice. I know of one marathoner who swears by watermelon juice. Bananas are a good source of potassium. The best prevention of leg cramps due to athletic exertion and exercise perspiration is a diet high in fresh fruits, fresh vegetables, and whole grains. Potassium broth (see Appendix I) is also a useful electrolyte source.

Other forms of leg cramps are more complicated. Older age groups may suffer leg cramps associated with arteriosclerotic changes in the circulatory system and should be evaluated by a doctor well trained in cardiovascular disease. A diet similar to that found under Heart Disease is useful for long-term care. Specifically, vitamin E, 600 to 800 IU per day, has been found very effective in this type of condition.

Another common cause of leg cramps involves mineral imbalances in the body. Excess phosphorus in the diet from too much meat or soda drinks can be a factor, causing a relative calcium deficiency. To normalize calcium, magnesium, and phosphorus levels, reduce milk and meat proteins and increase vegetables. Hydrochloric acid deficiency may be one reason for poor calcium absorption. Calcium deficiency is often associated with leg cramps. Those with dentures who find eating vegetables difficult are especially prone to magnesium and calcium deficiency and leg cramps. The only recourse in these cases is vegetable soups, potassium broth, and raw vegetable juices daily. The following supplements may be of use:

Vitamin B_6: 100 to 250 mg per day.
Vitamin C: Up to bowel tolerance.
Bioflavonoids: 300 to 1000 mg per day.
Vitamin E: 600 to 800 IU per day.
Calcium: 1000 to 1500 mg per day.

Magnesium: 500 to 1000 mg per day.
EPA (Eicosapentaenoic acid): 1 to 2 capsules two to three times per day.
Hydrochloric acid: 5 to 60 grains with meals.

LOW BACK PAIN:
Sciatica, Lumbar Disc Herniation or Prolapse

Definition

Sciatica: Neuralgia and neuritis of the sciatic nerve.
Lumbar disc herniation: A bulging of the nucleus pulposus against a weakened segment of the annulus fibrosus.
Lumbar disc prolapse: An actual breach of the annulus fibrosus by nuclear material.

Symptoms

Pain or ache in the low back; pain, ache, or altered sensation in the buttocks, thigh, calf, and foot. Muscle wasting may occur late in course, along with reduced reflexes and muscle weakness.

Etiologic Considerations

- Poor body mechanics and posture
    Improper lifting, sitting, standing, carrying
    Lumbar lordosis
    Weak abdominal muscles
    Visceroptosis
    High heels

- Obesity

- Improper heavy lifting, intermittent heavy lifting

- Insufficient stretching out before working or lifting

- Sedentary life, lack of exercise, and weak muscles

- Poor nutrition
    Protein deficiency
    Calcium deficiency
    Green vegetable deficiency
    Poor bone, cartilage, ligament, and muscle development

- Bone alterations
  - Osteoporosis
  - Ankylosing spondylitis
  - Spondylolisthesis
  - Congenital abnormalities
  - Osteoarthritis
  - Gouty arthritis
  - Rheumatoid arthritis
  - Paget's disease
- Trauma
  - Fracture
  - Ligament or muscle strain
  - Overuse
  - Microtrauma
- Short leg syndrome (real or apparent)
- Iliopsoas syndrome
- Spinal lesion
  - (Lumbar, lumbar-sacral, sacroiliac)
  - Facet lock syndrome
  - True disc lesion
- Spinal imbalance
  - Flat feet
  - Ankle, knee, hip disorders
  - Sacroiliac
  - Lumbar
  - Thoracic
  - Cervical
  - Iliopsoas, gluteals, paravertebral muscles, plus others
  - Hypomobility or hypermobility
- Referred pain
  - Menstrual, gynecological
  - Kidneys
  - Bladder
  - Prostate
  - Colon
  - Ulcer
  - Appendix
- Metabolic (calcium/mineral loss)
  - Adrenals
  - Pituitary

      Parathyroids (hyperparathyroidism)
      Rickets
      Menopause
- Infection (local or systemic)
- Emotional
- Tumor
- Pregnancy

Discussion

Backache with or without sciatica is one of the most common complaints a doctor deals with in his or her practice. As a spinal specialist I see more in my practice than most. As you can see from the above list of possible causative factors, back pain is far from a simple disorder. A complete individual case history is essential to allow for proper diagnosis and treatment.

To simplify this discussion I would like to concentrate on back pain related primarily to the osteopathic spinal lesion (see Spinal Manipulation section under Tools of Naturopathy), and also that caused by a true disc herniation or prolapse. We will omit back pain due to congenital abnormalities, degenerative arthritis, infection, metabolic disorders, cancer, referred syndromes, and so on. These, however, must always be considered when dealing with acute or chronic back pain.

Although two main syndromes of back pain exist (i.e., spinal lesion and disc), their causes are often similar. To understand more about why a good back turns bad, first we have to learn a little about how the back is designed to function. The spinal column is basically a stack of specifically designed bones separated by resilient disc cushions. Each disc is made up of a firm, fibrous outer covering, the *annulus fibrosus*, and a softer gelatinous inner core, the *nucleus pulposus*. Each vertebra is uniquely shaped according to its relative position in the spine and its function. There are two areas called *apophyseal facets* where the vertebra approximates the vertebra above and two facets for the approximation below. These facets allow the vertebrae to glide across each other and by their shape and location limit them to certain ranges of motion. Thus, in the neck, these facets allow good overall mobility with relative freedom in rotation, flexion, extension, and side bending, while in the lumbar region the angles of the facets allow free flexion and side bending but severely restrict movement of rotation.

Further controls are placed on spinal movements by strong ligaments that connect adjacent vertebrae together and also bind together groups of vertebrae and ultimately the entire spine. Strong muscles also interconnect the spine to provide both support and the possibility of motion. A series of thirty-one spinal nerves pass out of spaces between each vertebra.

The problem in the typical bad back involves one of two processes. Either the vertebral functional unit (two adjacent vertebrae and their connective-tissue components) is in distress and no longer relating to each other as designed with the disc remaining normal; or the functional unit distress may include disc damage. The difference in severity of these two syndromes is extreme. Any back disorder that includes disc damage is much more difficult to cure and has a higher likelihood of recurring and causing prolonged disability.

Many people with bad backs report only trivial motions as the initial cause of their complaint. These include bending over to pick up a dime, touching their toes, opening a window, or even washing their faces. These minor incidences are, however, not the real cause, only the "last straw" in a long list of spinal stress. Except in the case of severe, acute trauma, the real cause of most spinal complaints has less to do with what you did today or yesterday and more with what you have been doing or *not* doing over the last 5 to 10 years.

The most influential factors in developing a weak back are poor spinal mechanics accompanied by poor muscle tone. The body was designed to function according to clearly defined principles established by the shape of our vertebrae and the manner in which they fit together into three distinct spinal curves. These curves, the cervical (neck), thoracic (midback), and lumbar (low back), allow us to function in the upright position and give us a degree of stability. They are essential to maintain a good center of gravity and to help balance and compensate for carrying our heads erect. Without properly balanced spinal curves, the human frame would be incredibly unstable, capable of toppling over with a strong wind.

In the normal posture, the spinal curves leave the vertebrae and their muscular supports in what can be called a neutral condition. The vertebrae are floating free under no pressure and all supporting muscles are in their gently tonic state. If, through habitual slouching in sitting or standing, walking with high heels, obesity, or by a weakening of the muscles of spinal support, the spinal curves become exaggerated (or reduced), a series of extremely important changes takes places. Muscles which previously were at ease must shorten or lengthen to accommodate for this new position and some must actively contract to counterbalance changes in weight distribution. Ultimately, prolonged contraction of any muscle leads to a shortening and hardening of the muscle fibers, creating ropy fibrous bands instead of healthy flexible muscle.

Over a period of time even the individual vertebra will change in shape in an attempt to minimize stresses. These changes cause localized or referred pains in the manner of the osteopathic lesion (see Spinal Manipulation section under Tools of Naturopathy). The disc also is placed under unusual stresses, which seem to be a factor in its premature degeneration, leading to less elasticity and loss of fluid content. This accelerated wear and tear, along with weakened ligaments and muscles, allows the gelatinous inner nucleus to push against and cause a bulge in the outer fibrous covering (herniation). Eventually, the inner nucleus breaches this barrier, forming a true disc prolapse when an extra burden is placed on the spine, as in improper lifting or bending. The result is usually an acutely painful and debilitating nerve pinch, most commonly of the sciatic nerve, causing both local and referred pain, or altered sensations in the gluteal region and down the leg.

Treatment

Even a normal spine can suffer acute injury due to a fall, auto accident, sudden, unusual or extreme movement, or other traumatic cause. The cause of pain may simply be a result of muscle or ligament strain, in which case rest and proper physiotherapy are all that is needed. Many cases, however, are complicated by what is often called "facet lock syndrome." What occurs here is that the vertebrae become fixed in the extremes of their normal physiological motion and are splinted in place by muscle spasm. The pain is usually severe and sudden but often becomes less severe after a week or two if left untreated. Unfortunately, this lessening of pain is often misinterpreted by the patient to mean that full cure is soon to follow. In reality, what is occurring is that the acute "hot" lesion is now "cooling" to become a chronic one. If proper spinal manipulation is not received, this area can be a cause of future distress locally and in referred areas related to the nervous supply of that segment. Secondary changes in other spinal levels will also occur as the body attempts to reestablish a semblance of spinal balance. For example, if a vertebra in your neck becomes fixed in its rotation to the right, your body might accommodate by fixing one of your other neck, midback, or lumbar vertebrae to the left to keep your head pointing forward. A good rule to go by is that if a minor sore back does not significantly recover with rest after 24 to 48 hours, then it needs professional treatment. All severe back complaints need to be seen as soon as possible. In general, the longer you wait for treatment, the longer that treatment will take to restore health.

Acute low back pain may also be caused by disc herniation or prolapse. This may have a well-recognized cause, such as attempts at lifting a heavy object, such as a refrigerator or piano, or it may result from trivial motions such as those mentioned earlier. Irrespective of the amount of effort responsible for the actual disc rupture or prolapse, the symptoms are the same. The onset of pain may be gradual over several hours or sudden. The most commonly affected discs are between L3 to L4, L4 to L5, and L5 to sacrum. Common symptoms include pain and numbness in low back, buttocks, thighs, calf, and foot; muscle weakness in thigh, calf, or foot; reduced reflexes; muscle wasting in thigh or calf; and if severe, disorders in function of either bowels or bladder. Most cases of acute disc lesions are preceded by a history of chronic backache. If this structural distress had been listened to and preventive measures begun, no disc rupture would probably have occurred. The only way to prevent back disorders is to keep the body in good muscle tone, and in proper spinal mechanics and use.

The muscles that support the back span from head to toe. If any one group of muscles becomes lax or overtight, other bone and muscle relationships elsewhere in the body will be altered. Even flat feet may be the primary cause in the history of a low back complaint. This is why I recommend full-scale body stretching and toning to prevent back problems. In practice, however, specific muscle groups are more important than others. Certainly, the muscles of the back and gluteal region are important, but most people are surprised to find out that one of the main supports for the back is found in the *front*—the abdominal muscles. The most common muscular weakness found in the average back patient is weak abdominal tone.

The following exercises have been used quite successfully in treating and preventing back complaints. It is difficult to emphasize adequately just how essential they are. Along with rest, proper physiotherapy, and appropriate spinal therapy performed by a qualified spinal specialist (osteopath, chiropractor, or naturopath), these exercises are responsible for saving millions from extremely expensive, often ineffective spinal surgery.

BACK EXERCISES

Be careful not to overdo these exercises in the beginning, especially if you are presently suffering from an acute low back complaint. Do not be alarmed if the exercises cause some mild discomfort which lasts for a few minutes. If the pain is more than mild and persists for 10 to 20 minutes, stop their use and consult your doctor. Do the exercises on a firm surface covered with a thin foam cushion or folded towel. As the old proverb says, "Perseverance brings good fortune."

• Standard position: Lie on back with a small pillow under your head and both knees bent.

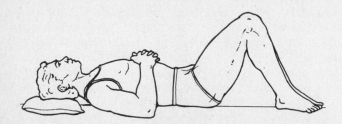

• Knee to chest: Draw your knee slowly to your chest as far as possible without excessive pain. Hold for 5 seconds and then return to starting position. Repeat four times with each leg individually, and then with both legs simultaneously. Use your legs, not your arms, to raise legs to chest. The arms are for balance and slight stretching. This exercise stretches the entire low back.

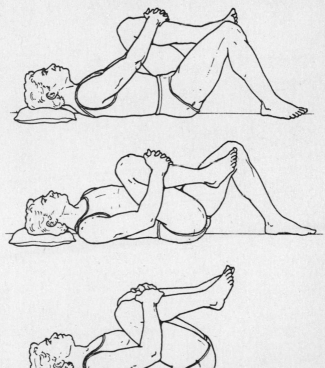

• Pelvic tilt: While lying in the standard position simply tighten your buttock muscles and tilt your pelvis up. This will flatten the low back against the floor. Do not try to flatten the spine by contracting your abdominal muscles or legs, but confine the exercise as much as possible to the gluteal (buttock) muscles, squeezing them together tightly. Each contraction is held 5 seconds and then relaxed, gradually working up to ten or more repetitions. This exercise strengthens the buttock muscles and helps reduce swayback (lordosis).

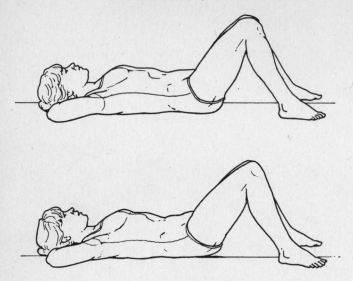

• Trunk stretch:

Start in the standard position. Cross right leg over left just above the knee and use this weight as a lever to help rotate leg toward the floor as far as comfortably possible. Hold for 5 seconds. Repeat with other leg. Repeat exercise five times for each leg. Always keep the upper back flat against the floor. This exercise stretches the muscles on both sides of the spine.

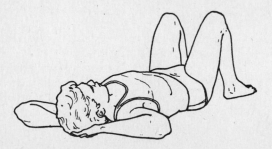

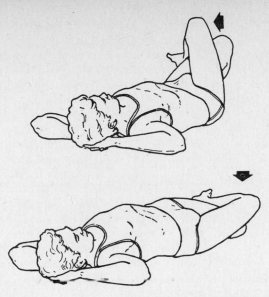

• Raised pelvic tilt: Lie in standard position and perform the pelvic tilt, but continue the contraction to include the buttocks and abdominal muscles so that the hips raise off the floor. Hold for 6 to 8 seconds and slowly relax. Repeat five to ten times.

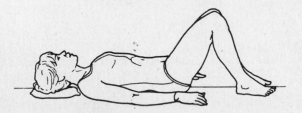

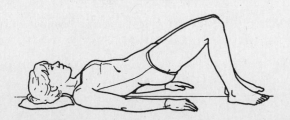

• Sit-ups:

Begin in the standard position and slowly raise head, neck, and upper torso, reaching for your knees. Do not raise mid- or lower back. Maintain this position with hands positioned gently on the knees for 5 to 6 seconds and slowly relax. Do not grasp knees. Repeat five to ten times. As these sit-ups become easier to perform, place your lower legs up to the knee on the seat of a chair, making a right angle with your thighs. Keeping your arms across your chest, do half sit-ups that cause your low back to barely rise off the floor, but no further. You do not have to hold this sit-up. Try to do 150 to 300 of this type of sit-up daily—half in the morning and half in the evening. Of all the back exercises I know, this is the most effective, if done as prescribed. I have seen very bad back complaints improve dramatically. Time and perseverance are essential.

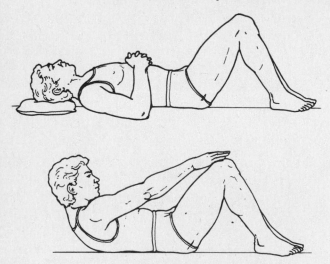

• Hamstring stretch:

Starting from the standard position stretch out the right leg flat against the floor. Slowly raise the leg as far as you can until a sensation of pain or tightness occurs in the back of your thigh. Hold for 5 seconds and slowly lower leg. Repeat five to ten times with each leg. Make sure to keep the back flat against the floor and do not use hands or arms as leverage.

This exercise helps stretch the hamstring muscles, which get very tight with all back problems.

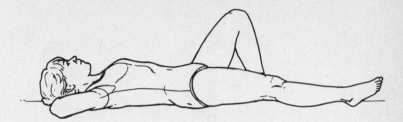

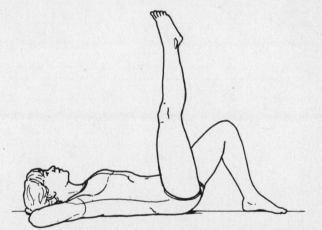

• Knee to nose: From the starting position bring one knee slowly to the chest, clasp it with both hands and extend the opposite leg until it lies flat on the floor. While keeping the low back flat to the floor, slowly raise head, neck, and upper shoulders forward until the nose touches the knee, or as far as comfortably possible. Hold 5 to 6 seconds and slowly relax. Repeat with both legs five to ten times. This exercise helps stretch the flexors of the hip on the opposite side of the leg used and also will help strengthen the abdominal muscles.

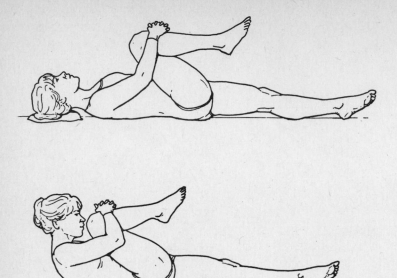

• Hamstring and Achilles stretch: Begin in the sitting position with one knee bent and the other leg flat against the floor with sole of foot firmly placed against the wall. Slowly bend forward until a stretch is felt behind your leg. Hold 5 to 6 seconds and relax. Repeat five to ten times with each leg.

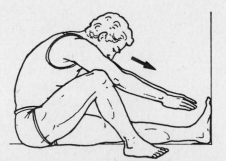

• Standing calf and
  Achilles stretch:

Place front half of foot across a thick book placed 1 to 2 ft from the wall. Place arms against the wall, and with legs kept straight, lean forward toward the wall until the calves and Achilles tendon begin to stretch. Hold 5 to 6 seconds. Repeat ten to fifteen times.

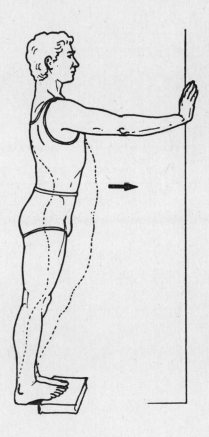

ADVANCED EXERCISES

- Standing hamstring stretch:

From a standing position place the heel on a low chair. Keeping both legs straight, slowly lean forward until you feel the hamstring muscles stretch. Repeat with both legs five to ten times.

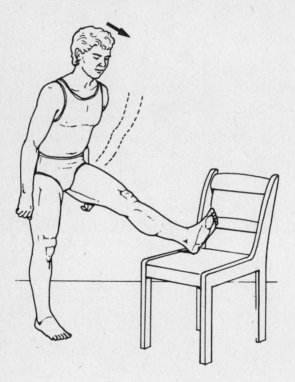

- Iliopsoas stretch:

From a standing position place one foot forward as far as you can with knee bent. Make sure front and rear feet point forward. Rock forward, stretching out the anterior thigh muscles, hip, groin, and iliopsoas muscle.

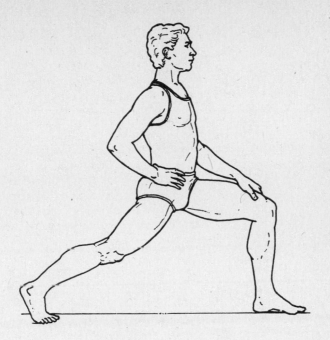

• Hyperextension of hip: Lie on stomach and raise one leg, with knee un-
flexed. Hold 4 to 6 seconds and slowly lower. Repeat
five to ten times with each leg. This exercise helps
strengthen low back and buttock muscles.

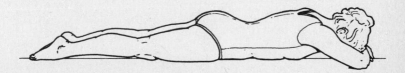

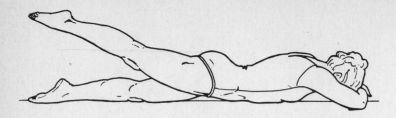

• Low back extension: Lie on stomach with hands along the side. Slowly raise the head and chest from the floor. Hold 4 to 6 seconds and then slowly lower. Rest and repeat ten times. An advanced form of this exercise is to place a pillow under the hips and perform the same exercise.

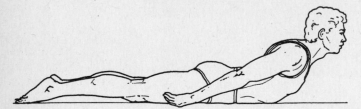

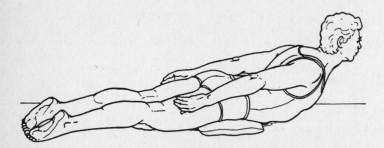

• Hip roll: Lie on the back with arms out at your sides. Bend
                                    knees with feet close to buttocks. Slowly roll both
                                    knees to one side toward the floor while keeping
                                    knees close to chest. Slowly return to starting po-
                                    sition and repeat on opposite side. Repeat entire
                                    exercise four to eight times.

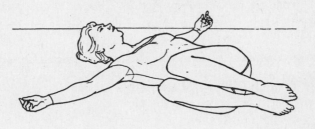

Physiotherapy

• Complete rest: Many acute low back complaints, and especially those with
disc lesions, require complete bed rest for the first 24 to 48 hours after the
injury. Do absolutely *nothing* except go to the bathroom. Make sure bowels
stay loose and prevent constipation by following a light diet with laxative-type
foods. Straining will aggravate the condition. Make sure the bed is extremely
supportive, or lay the mattress directly on the floor.

• Ice packs: Usually the application of ice in the first 24 hours will be the most
beneficial. Make sure not to apply this for too long a period and thus injure
the tissues. Ice should be applied for 10 to 30 minutes with 10 to 30 minutes
between applications.

• Heat: Local moist heat will help in later stages to loosen tight spinal muscles
and give pain relief. Ready-made hydrocolator packs are the most convenient
applications but they are not always available. For home use apply hot moist
towels, folded several times. These may be placed steaming hot over two to
four dry layers of towels and then covered with several more layers to retain
heat. The thicker the folded wet towel, the longer it will retain its heat. Lie
on your back with a large pillow under your knees and a thin one to support
your lower back; or on the side with legs drawn up in the semi-fetal position.
Care must be taken when applying heat to prevent the tissues from becoming
congested with blood. Follow heat applications with the gentle spinal stretching

exercises previously described. In later stages alternate hot and ice-cold applications will be useful to stimulate circulation and healing.

- Hops and lobelia hot compress: For pain relief.
- Ultrasound: This physiotherapy modality has been found very useful in the acute stages of low back pain.
- Diathermy
- Warm Epsom salts baths (see Appendix I): These are very relaxing and antispasmodic.
- Olbas rub
- Inversion: One of the best forms of controlled spinal traction is now available for home use for inversion at varying degrees. Several units are available to enable you to hang upside down from the feet or hips. This gives gentle traction to the spine and dramatically helps with some disc lesions and other back complaints. This can be done several times a day for 3 to 10 minutes in the acute phase and once or twice daily as preventive care. Although the foot hanging units are specifically designed so that you hang with your back to the apparatus, I find that by hanging on the stomach with several pillows placed under the hips and stomach places the back in a better position for traction with an acute disc disorder.
- Spinal manipulation and/or McMannis style traction.

Therapeutic Agents

VITAMINS AND MINERALS

Vitamin B complex: 25 to 50 mg two times per day.

Vitamin B_1: 100 mg, plus B_{12}, 1 mg intramuscular injection two times per week for 2 weeks, then once a week.

Vitamin C: 3000 to 10,000 mg per day, or to bowel tolerance. Essential for health of connective tissue (disc).*

Vitamin E: 400 IU two times per day.*

Calcium/magnesium in ratio of 2:1 (i.e., 800 mg calcium to 400 mg magnesium).*

OTHERS

Bromelain: 2 to 3 tablets three times per day.

DL-Phenylalanine: Analgesic, better than aspirin for pain. Increases release of endogenous endorphin-like substances.*

*Asterisks indicate the most frequently used therapeutic agents.

GENERAL

Lose weight.

MASTITIS (Acute)
(Not included in this section is Fibrocystic breast disease, sometimes called cystic mastitis)

Definition

Inflammation of the breast and milk duct system, usually due to infection by staphylococci invading a fissured or cracked nipple.

Symptoms

Pain, redness, hard swelling, fever, abscess, and possibly swollen cervical and/or axillary lymph nodes.

Etiologic Considerations

• Engorged breast, early postpartum or on weaning
• Incomplete emptying in feeding
• Shallow grip on nipple by infant
• Blocked duct
• Nipple fissure with secondary infection
• Poor nipple care and hygiene
• Irritating clothing
• Lack of proper nipple preparation prior to lactation

Discussion

Acute mastitis is most common during lactation and usually is due to invasion of a cracked nipple by bacteria. It occurs frequently in the first week postpartum, due to the combination of poor nipple preparation in the final 2 to 3 months of pregnancy, breast engorgement due to incomplete emptying, and excessive sucking by the newborn. A further major cause is a blocked milk duct, which may occur at any time during lactation and cause localized engorgement, inflammation, and infection.

Prevention and early treatment of mastitis is essential to avoid the need for antibiotics. Prevention of mastitis begins even before the baby is delivered. For a period of 2 to 3 months the prospective mother must get her nipples ready for lactation. She should massage her nipples daily with chickweed ointment. Vitamin E also may be used. She should also perform the "nipple pull" several times daily during a shower and dry off with a semirough towel.

As soon as the baby is born, the mother must be careful not to feed for overly long periods, to avoid maceration of her tender nipples. Be sure to break suction of infant's mouth on breast by inserting a finger into the corner of infant's mouth, not just pulling nipple out of infant's mouth. After her feeds, she should empty her breast manually or with a breast pump until supply and demand reach an equilibrium. Nipple cleanliness is important and nipples should be gently washed after each feed, if possible. Obviously this is not always possible. Clothing worn next to the breast should always be soft and nonirritating.

Treatment

Prompt and energetic treatment is essential to prevent abscess formation and the use of antibiotics. The essentials of treatment involve mostly botanical medications, both internal and external. Apply *Phytolacca* (pokeroot) (highly toxic; see p. 62) ointment frequently (every 2 hours) externally to all but the nipple itself. *Phytolacca* tincture should also be taken internally. The usual dose is 25 drops diluted in water, four to six times per day. Hot compresses of calendula lotion or calendula lotion plus *Phytolacca* should be applied every 2 to 4 hours. You may also wish to apply a calendula compress continually for extended periods of 4 to 6 hours or all night. This may be done by diluting calendula lotion in warm water (50/50 or a higher concentration), saturating a gauze or cotton diaper with the solution, and applying it to the breast.

Other herbal treatments include:

Clay packs
Jaborandi (*Pilocarpus*) for blocked duct, internal and external
Castor oil: Massage of blocked duct. May also use warm packs.
Dandelion (*Taraxacum*) plus onion bulb poultice
Plantain poultice
Barberry (*Berberis vulgaris*)
Dandelion (*Taraxacum*) and coneflower (*Echinacea*): Internal
Green onion poultice
Coneflower (*Echinacea angustifolium*): 25 drops of the tincture three or four
    times daily. Best taken with *Phytolacca* (highly toxic; see p. 62).

Therapeutic Agents

VITAMINS AND MINERALS

Vitamin A: 10,000 to 25,000 IU two to six times per day. *Use any dose of vitamin A over 50,000 IU per day with medical supervision only.* *

Vitamin C: High doses, 500 to 1000 mg four to eight times per day. *

Vitamin E: Internal, plus external massage. *

Thymus tablets

(*Note:* Opinion is divided as to the advisability of breastfeeding during the infection. Each case must be evaluated individually; however, I usually feel that continuation of breastfeeding will cause no harm to the infant and is the most efficient method of emptying the breast. Should the breast remain full after feeding, or the infant go off the breast voluntarily, it must be emptied by a breast pump.)

MEASLES (see Childhood Diseases)

MÉNIÈRE'S DISEASE

Definition and Symptoms

A recurrent and usually progressive disorder characterized by severe vertigo, progressive deafness, ringing in the ears (tinnitus), and a sensation of fullness in the ears.

Etiologic Considerations

The cause is considered unknown. Edema of the membranous labyrinth has been found in autopsy. Other postulated factors include allergy; viruses; infections, toxic or accumulative; or hormonal intolerances. Symptoms exactly like Ménière's disease can be caused by a cholesteotoma (a tumor-like growth that can erode into the central nervous system from the middle ear if not diagnosed soon enough). Anyone with the symptoms of Ménière's disease should be examined by a specialist to rule out other causes.

*Asterisks indicate the most frequently used therapeutic agents.

Discussion

The only clear pathological condition found in these cases has been swelling of the membranous labyrinth, with upsets of the balance center. Naturopathic treatments often can help reverse such congestion through diet and lifestyle changes, local physiotherapy, spinal or cranial adjustments, and homeopathy.

One interesting note on Ménière's syndrome is that occasionally this condition may be a misdiagnosed case of salicylism from excessive self-medication of aspirin. This causes deafness, ringing in the ears, dizziness, headache, vomiting, confusion, and hyperventilation in later stages. It is easy to see how these symptoms could cause confusion. I personally have seen several elderly patients with arthritis who had been diagnosed as also having Ménière's disease, only to find that on aspirin withdrawal all the Ménière's symptoms were relieved.

Treatment

Diet

A general cleansing regimen is usually greeted with rapid results. Fasting for 3 to 7 days on vegetable juices every 6 weeks is alternated with a diet high in nutrient-rich foods, composed of plenty of raw and cooked vegetables, seaweed, sprouts, seeds, nuts, beans, low-fat yoghurt, and fish. Although this diet is what can be called nonspecific, it is also very effective. I suspect irritants in the diet such as coffee, salt, fried foods, alcohol, and any drugs, and routinely remove these from the diet. The general tonic influence of this diet regimen, along with a better calcium-to-phosphorus ratio, can only benefit health. Often all that is needed to reverse a health disorder is the removal of obstacles to the body's own self-regulating healing powers.

Physiotherapy

- Exercise must be gradually increased, to increase circulation to the head. Any exercise will do as long as it aims at increased respiration and improved blood flow.

- Alternate hot and cold head baths taken once or twice daily will help local circulation and drainage. Use two bowls of water, one very warm and the other ice-cold. Immerse the entire upper head up to and including the ears and jaw area in the warm water for 30 seconds to 1 minute. Follow with the ice-cold immersion. For severe cases, for the elderly, or for anyone with a heart condition, begin with less extreme water temperatures and gradually build up to the ice-cold water.

- Spinal and/or cranial manipulation should be done once or twice weekly, to help improve local circulation, enervation, and nutrition.

Therapeutic Agents

VITAMINS AND MINERALS

Vitamin A: 25,000 to 50,000 IU one to two times per day. *Use any dose of vitamin A over 50,000 IU per day with medical supervision only.*

Vitamin B complex: 50 mg one to two times per day.

Vitamin B₃: 400 to 800 mg per day, time release (will cause flushing sensation).*

Vitamin B₆: 100 to 400 mg per day.*

Bioflavonoids: 300 to 1000 mg per day.

Vitamin C deficiency problems are coincidental: 4 to 6 g per day.

Vitamin E: 400 to 800 IU per day.

OTHERS

Lithium: 2 to 3 mg per day.

MENOPAUSE (Change of Life, Climacteric)

Definition

The transitional change in a woman's life when menstrual function ceases. Menopause occurs generally between the ages of 45 to 50, as a result of failure of estrogen and progesterone production by the ovaries.

Symptoms

These may include amenorrhea, irregularity, increased flow, vasomotor instability, hot flushes and cold sweating, palpitation, vertigo, tingling, chills, nervousness, excitability, depression, fatigue, irritability, insomnia, headaches, muscle and bone aches, and gastrointestinal or urinary disturbances. Later there may be osteoporosis, urinary frequency, stress incontinence, unwanted hair, and drying of vaginal secretions resulting in painful coitus and vaginitis; also, obesity, pruritus, dry skin, reduced breast size, and loss of vaginal elasticity.

Etiologic Considerations

- Adrenal exhaustion
  Hypoglycemia: Refined carbohydrates, sugar, coffee, stress

*Asterisks indicate the most frequently used therapeutic agents.

- Diet deficiency
  Calcium, vitamin D, magnesium, and phosphorus
  Vitamin B complex
  Vitamin E
  Others

- Thyroid malfunction
  Thyroid/parathyroid imbalance

- Lack of exercise

- Psychological factors

- Poor absorption and digestion
  Hydrochloric acid deficiency

- Surgical menopause
  Causes most severe menopausal symptoms

Discussion

The menopause, or "change of life," was also called the *climacteric* by the ancient Greeks. By this they meant "a step in the ladder." Their understanding of the cycles of life in periods of 7 years coincides with many Asiatic beliefs. Accordingly, the climacteric was simply another normally occurring 7-year cycle where gradually and gracefully a woman was relieved of the burden of bearing children.

Much has been written about the female menopause and unfortunately most of this has been about its most negative aspects. This negative education has done much harm in establishing fears about menopause that soon become self-fulfilling prophecies by the power of suggestion.

The fact is that menopause was intended by nature to be a gradual process of reduced estrogen output by the ovaries with few, if any, side effects. In the normal, healthy, well-nourished and active woman, the pituitary then sends signals to the other glands such as the adrenals, to increase their estrogen output. This backup system helps to keep some estrogen in the circulation, and helps further maintain a portion of the secondary sexual characteristics. It is only when the adrenal glands are exhausted from poor diet, diet deficiency, hypoglycemia, and stress that this backup system may fail, leading to the sudden and severe physiological changes now accepted as "normal" for a menopausal woman.

The psychological symptoms of menopause distress are caused by previous emotional instabilities which were present prior to menopause. These may be aggravated by insecurities resulting from much negative education about "the change," and fears of a loss of natural feminine attractiveness.

Estrogen has been used in various forms as medication to help halt the menopausal syndrome. Not only does estrogen therapy merely postpone symptoms and mask real problems, it also has been linked to a drastic increase in cancer of the uterus and breast (five to twelve times more), cardiovascular disease, stroke, and alterations in the balance of a number of natural vitamins and minerals in the body. It increases the body's need of vitamin B complex, pyridoxine, and vitamin E, and reduces zinc levels. Recent studies have even questioned its effectiveness, let alone its safety. In double-blind studies where estrogen was used in one group and a placebo in another, there was no significant statistical difference in the groups, as far as effectiveness in relieving most menopausal complaints. It appears that receiving *any* tablet from the doctor will help relieve many menopausal complaints as long as you believe it will work.

Certain physiological changes do, however, occur in varying degrees as estrogen levels are reduced. The most predictable of these are a slight reduction in vaginal elasticity, and a lessening of its natural lubrication. For some women this can cause some pain with sexual intercourse. This is easily corrected by using an artificial lubricant, and should not limit sexual activity in the least. Far from reducing sexual drive, menopause often increases sexual desire by making the clitoris more sensitive, even though it often does reduce in size. Hot flashes and cold sweats due to vasomotor instability may be corrected by proper diet, exercise, and vitamin E supplements.

One common problem of postmenopausal women is osteoporosis, or weakened bones. When estrogen production is reduced, calcium tends to be lost from the bones. This effect may be influenced by a preexisting thyroid and parathyroid imbalance. Certainly, women who have a previous history of thyroid disorders have a higher risk of having severe menopausal complaints, including osteoporosis. Other factors that affect the body's calcium metabolism and bone density are lack of dietary calcium, or excess phosphorus, magnesium deficiency, poor absorption with hydrochloric acid deficiency, and lack of exercise. Similar causes are responsible for menopausal arthritis, a fairly common condition.

Treatment

Diet

Treat for hypoglycemia (refer to diet in that section). See also section on Premenstrual Tension Syndrome.

Diet should also include:
Seeds and nuts (especially sunflower seeds)
Wheat germ
Vitamin B complex, iodine, iron, calcium foods
Brewer's yeast
Protein supplements

Lecithin granules
Seaweed

Physiotherapy

• Cold water walks
• Daily exercises—muscle work*
• Daily walks
• Hot and cold alternating showers
• Sauna
• Wet grass walks

Therapeutic Agents

VITAMINS AND MINERALS

Vitamin A: 25,000 IU one to two times daily. *Use any dose of vitamin A over 50,000 IU per day with medical supervision only.* *

Vitamin B complex: 25 to 50 mg two to three times per day. Intramuscular injections once a week with severe symptoms. *

Vitamin C: 250 to 1000 mg three to six times per day or more to bowel tolerance.

Vitamin E: 400 IU one to three times per day. *

Calcium: 800 mg one to two times per day.

Magnesium: 400 mg one to two times per day.

Pantothenic acid

PABA (para-amino benzoic acid)

Zinc

OTHERS

Atomodine (with doctor's prescription) or 636 (Cayce Products)*

Bee pollen

Brewer's yeast: 1 tsp two to three times per day.

Essential fatty acids (GLA, EPA, and oil of evening primrose)*

Kelp: 2 to 4 tablets two to three times per day. *

Raw glandulars (thyroid, pituitary, adrenal, ovarian): With doctor's prescription. *

*Asterisks indicate the most frequently used therapeutic agents.

Royal jelly
Wheat germ oil: Use concentrated forms.*

BOTANICALS

Angelica (*Angelica archangelica*)
Dong quai (*Angelica sylvestris*)*
False unicorn root (*Helonias dioica*): Contains estrogen*
Ginseng and Fotitieng (*Panax ginseng and Polygonum multiflorum*)*
Lady's slipper (*Cypripedium pubescens*): For anxiety, insomnia, hysteria
Licorice (*Glycyrrhiza glabra*): Estrogen derivative
Mother's wort (*Leonurus cardiaca*): Dry vagina
Oat (*Avena sativa*) and St. John's wort (*Hypericum perforatum*): Neurosis
Passion flower (*Passiflora incarnata*)
Blazing star (*Aletris farinosa*)
Squaw vine (*Mitchella repens*)

MENSTRUAL DISORDERS (Amenorrhea, Dysmenorrhea, Metrorrhagia, Oligomenorrhea, Premenstrual Tension)

Definition and Symptoms

Amenorrhea: Absence or suppression of menstruation. Normal prior to puberty, during pregnancy, during lactation, and after menopause.
Dysmenorrhea: Painful or difficult menstruation. Cramplike pains or steady, dull ache 24 to 48 hours prior to menstruation, persisting for variable periods of time.
Metrorrhagia: Bleeding between periods.
Oligomenorrhea: Infrequent or scanty menstruation.
Premenstrual tension: Symptoms occurring just prior to and in some cases during menstruation, including depression, irritability, edema, sore breast, abdominal distension, and nausea.

Etiologic Considerations

- Poor body mechanics
- Visceroptosis [dropped abdomen and pelvic contents due to lumbar lordosis (sway back)] or weak abdominal tone.

*Asterisks indicate the most frequently used therapeutic agents.

- Spinal lesions have a specific action on pelvic organs or act secondarily through altered spinal mechanics and visceroptosis.

- Weak abdominal tone leads to dropped abdominal and pelvic contents, congestion, poor circulation.

- Lack of exercise leads to weak abdominal and pelvic muscles and ligaments, poor circulation.

- Improper diet leads to nutritional deficiencies of B_6, folic acid, B_2, B complex, calcium, iron, vitamin K, and protein. Consumption of junk foods [refined foods, coffee, tea, soda, excess salt and excess meat (high phosphorus levels causing calcium deficiency)] results in nutritional deficiencies.

- Extreme diets:
    Fruitarianism
    Protein deficiency, excess dieting, anorexia

- Hypoglycemia

- Methylxanthines (coffee, tea, chocolate, cola): These are associated with dysmenorrhea and premenstrual syndrome.

- Stress/ Psychological
    Anxiety
    Depression
    Fear, of pregnancy, of maturity
    Sudden shock
    Sexual problems
    Estrogen therapy; "the pill"

- Pathology
    Cancer
    Endometriosis
    Fibroids
    Misplaced womb
    Salpingitis
    Cervical lesion

- Other diseases
    Endocrine disorders
        Pituitary
        Thyroid
        Ovary
        Liver
    Hypertension

    Diabetes
    Blood disorders
    Anemia
    Kidney disease
    Syphilis
    Scurvy

- Abortion or miscarriage

- IUD

- X-ray therapy—suppression

- Sudden change of climate

- Marathoner's amenorrhea

- Puberty, pregnancy, lactation, menopause

- Aspirin: Destroys vitamin K; K antagonist

- Oral antibiotics

- Allergy

Discussion

Menstrual disorders have many causes, as can be seen in the list of Etiologic Considerations. The first consideration should always be to exclude any pathology or disease process that may be the causative factor. Any bleeding between periods should be investigated for possible cancer, fibroids, cervical lesions, or other pathology prior to attempting the general therapeutic recommendations found under Treatment. Most menstrual problems can be caused by hormonal imbalances and a 24-hour urine sample may be used as a simple method of evaluating estrogen levels. Evidence of ovulation may also be found by keeping a morning temperature chart. This will aid evaluation and help direct therapy.

Probably the most effective way to upset the entire hormonal balance is to take the birth control pill. This convinces the body that it is pregnant. After stopping the pill many women fail to regain normal periods for varying periods of months to several years. Amenorrhea following use of the birth control pill is very common.

Other hormonal disorders involving the pituitary, adrenals, or thyroid may also produce amenorrhea or abnormal bleeding cycles. This may be physiological, as with hypothyroidism due to iodine deficiency; or psychological, affecting first the hypothalamus then pituitary, thyroid, and ovaries. Stress or the birth control pill may also profoundly affect the adrenal glands, which produce 20 percent of the total estrogen output. These glands are very sensitive to changes in blood sugar levels, so that hypoglycemia may depress adrenal function over time (see Hypoglycemia).

Extreme diets, such as strict fruitarianism, very low protein diets, or repeated strict weight loss regimens, often cause amenorrhea. This has been recognized for years. On these restricted diets, the levels of circulating hormones fall until a normal menstrual cycle is no longer possible and pregnancy unlikely. Many women on these diets have been told and sincerely believe that to no longer menstruate is a sign of purity and is the normal state for women. All I can say is that if this is normal, then so is sterility. If everyone lived on these diets, the human race would probably die out within one or two generations. These people are, unfortunately, led solely by emotion—not intellect or common sense.

Not listed above is anorexia nervosa. This disorder is a psychological problem leading to extreme weight loss and amenorrhea. My strong remarks above are not meant for sufferers of this disorder, who need psychological counseling to cope with their problem, which often results from an inability to adjust to sexual maturity.

Another major cause of menstrual abnormality is poor body mechanics. In the woman with normal posture, with strong abdominal muscles and pelvic supports, the female organs are suspended unencumbered within the pelvis. If, however, the abdominal muscles are weakened, or there is an excess lordotic curve in the low back, the abdominal contents prolapse and put pressure on the pelvic organs. This may result from simple lack of demanding exercises, spinal lesions causing an increase in the lumbar curve, or something as common as habitual wearing of high-heeled shoes, which increases the lumbar curve. Constipation and loaded bowel syndrome may also cause intestinal prolapse.

Failure to do sufficient prenatal and especially postnatal exercises may lead to weakening of the supporting ligaments of the female organs. This is a common finding in menstrual disorders. The resultant prolapse interferes with normal blood and lymph flow, resulting in congestion and reduction in local tissue vitality.

Certainly, diet may play a major role in menstrual problems. As previously mentioned, a protein-deficient diet will produce amenorrhea and infertility. Hypoglycemia, nutritional anemia, iodine deficiency, and hypothyroidism are some of the more widely accepted nutritional causes of menstrual disorders. Vitamin B complex deficiency and calcium deficiency are also now being recognized. Certainly, calcium deficiency related to cramps is fairly well proven. Vitamin B_6 deficiency is also associated with the premenstrual tension syndrome of irritability, cramps, fluid retention, and acne flare.

Stress and psychological problems may profoundly affect menstrual flow. It is not uncommon for amenorrhea to follow a severe psychological and physical trauma, such as rape. Fear of pregnancy may also be a common factor in menstrual disorders of all kinds. Less obvious psychological problems may also be the cause and should be sought through careful questioning.

An interesting type of amenorrhea has recently been coined "marathoner's amenorrhea," found exclusively among those females who regularly run long distances.

Treatment

Many doctors routinely recommend dilatation and curettage (D&C) for abnormal menstrual bleeding. It is not entirely certain how curettage works, but many hypothesize that removal of a probably hypertrophied endometrium lining the uterus allows a newly formed, normal endometrium to be produced. There is no question that the D&C is effective for some permanently, while others receive only temporary relief, or no relief at all, even after multiple curettages.

Estrogen combined with progesterone will usually stop excessive bleeding. This, however, is not curative and must be repeated at intervals. Estrogen is also routinely used in cases of amenorrhea. This is not reserved for patients with reduced ovarian function, but also commonly used in patients with normal estrogen levels. This has no proven therapeutic results and only induces a menstrual period by what is called "estrogen withdrawal" when the course of medication is stopped. This form of therapy has been much abused by physicians who have accepted the credit for restoring temporary menstrual function without making it clear to the patient that estrogen withdrawal bleeding is not the same as restoration of normal menses.

The naturopathic approach to menstrual disorders attempts to restore normal function by removing the cause and increasing both local and general vitality.

Diet

Although fasting is employed in some cases, especially where toxicity has been a factor, I find a full dietary regimen as for anemia or hypoglycemia the best initial approach. This may be intermixed with short fruit and vegetable juice fasts of 3 to 7 days. Obviously, amenorrhea due to protein deficiency should not be treated through fasting. The diet should contain foods high in calcium, vitamins A, B complex, C, E, K, and iodine, zinc, iron, and protein. Extra vitamin and mineral supplements are required in the early stages of treatment. The diets outlined under Hypoglycemia or Anemia, stressing vegetarian or fish protein sources with less meat, are best for these conditions.

Physiotherapy

• Alternate hot and cold sitz baths: This is the most effective method of removing pelvic congestion and restoring ovarian and uterine health. These baths should be taken two times daily, if possible. There is no substitute for sitz baths.

- Ice pack to uterus and pubic region or sacral region for excessive bleeding or pain. Hot compresses may also be applied at the same time to the legs and feet to enhance the action of removing blood from the pelvic region.

- Spinal manipulation: Lower thoracic, lumbar, and lumbar/sacral, once weekly for 6 to 8 weeks. Rest a few weeks and repeat.

- Slant-board exercises

- Abdominal exercises

- Prenatal-type exercises

- Outdoor exercises; swimming

- Depletion pack

Therapeutic Agents

VITAMINS AND MINERALS

Vitamin A: 10,000 to 25,000 IU one to two times per day. *Use any dose of vitamin A over 50,000 IU per day with medical supervision only.* *

Vitamin B complex: 50 mg one to three times per day. Intramuscular injection may be useful. *

Vitamin B_6: For premenstrual tension and acne; 100 mg three to four times per day, initially, then two times per day.

Folic acid: 25 to 50 mg per day—especially with abnormal PAP smears. *

Vitamin C plus bioflavonoids: For excess bleeding. 1000 to 2000 mg two or more times per day, up to bowel tolerance.

Vitamin D: 400 to 1000 IU per day. Increases calcium absorption along with acidic environment (hydrochloric acid, vitamin C, cider vinegar, lemon juice, etc.). Take care in prescribing extra vitamin D; it is often taken in excess in the diet, and can have toxic effects. A prescription for plenty of sunshine is safer.

Vitamin E: 400 IU one to two times daily.

Vitamin K: For excess bleeding; antihemorrhagic (alfalfa, seaweed, spinach, cabbage, and other vitamin K foods).

Calcium: Levels are lowest just before menstruation begins. Low calcium may be related to premenstrual tension syndrome, along with vitamin B_6. Calcium is especially useful with cramps and heavy blood loss. 1 to 2 tablets per hour are taken in acute cases. 1000 to 2500 mg per day as regular dose. Higher doses in individual cases.

*Asterisks indicate the most frequently used therapeutic agents.

Iron: Even one heavy period may use up the entire month's supply of iron. Heavy blood loss always requires iron. 25 to 50 mg per day.

Magnesium: 200 mg two to three times daily, or 1 mg for every 2 mg of calcium.

Zinc: 25 mg one to two times daily.

OTHERS

Brewer's yeast*

Lecithin

Choline/inositol

Garlic

Kelp*

Alfalfa

Essential fatty acids (GLA, oil of evening primrose)

EPA (eicosapentaenoic acid): 3 to 10 g per day

Chlorophyll: 2 to 3 tbs four to six times per day

Protein supplements*

Tryptophan

With doctor's prescription, prescribed according to individual case

Atomodine or 636 (Cayce products)*

Raw thyroid tablets*

Raw pituitary tablets*

Raw adrenal tablets*

Desiccated thyroid

BOTANICALS

Amenorrhea

Angelica (*Angelica archangelica*)

Black cohosh (*Cimicifuga racemosa*): Ovarian pain; cramps.

Blazing star (*Aletris farinosa*): For low ovarian function, hypoestrogenism. Dose: Tincture, 10 to 30 drops three times per day.*

Blue cohosh (*Caulophyllum thalictroides*)

Elecampane (*Inula helenium*)

*Asterisks indicate the most frequently used therapeutic agents.

False unicorn root (*Helonias dioica*)

Licorice root tea (*Glycyrrhiza glabra*)

Life root (*Senecio aureus*): Uterine tonic; increases local circulation. Dose: Tincture, 10 to 30 drops two to four times daily.*

Mother's wort (*Leonurus cardiaca*)

Pennyroyal (*Hedeoma pulegioides*): Strong infusion, three or four times per day.*

Pulsatilla (*Anemona pulsatilla*): 10 drops three times per day; especially if due to stress, apprehension, or other emotional suppression.*

Tansy (*Tanacetum vulgare*)

Dysmenorrhea

Angelica (*Angelica archangelica*)

Black cohosh (*Cimicifuga racemosa*)

Black haw (*Viburnum prunifolium*): Antispasmodic; useful with menstrual cramps. Dose: Tincture, 15 to 30 drops three to four times per day.*

Blue cohosh (*Caulophylum thalictroides*)

Cramp bark, or high-bush cranberry (*Viburnum opulus*): uterine sedative.*

Chamomile tea (*Anthemis nobilis*): Mild calmative.

False unicorn root (*Helonias dioica*): A uterine tonic used in ovarian dysmenorrhea.

Ginger root (*Zingiber officinale*)

Lady's slipper (*Cypripedium pubescens*): For hysteria.

Life root (*Senecio aureus*): Uterine tonic, useful in atonic conditions. Dose: Tincture, 15 to 30 drops three times per day.*

Mother's wort (*Leonurus cardiaca*)

Pulsatilla (*Anemona pulsatilla*)

Red raspberry (*Rubus strigosus*)

Squaw vine (*Mitchella repens*): Used in dysmenorrhea, especially of menarche.*

Valerian (*Valeriana officinalis*): Sedative.

Wild yam root (*Dioscorea villosa*): Cramps; ovarian neuralgia.

Oligomenorrhea

Blazing star (*Aletris farinosa*)

Catnip (*Nepeta cataria*)

Chamomile (*Anthemis nobilis*)

Lady's slipper (*Cypripedium pubescens*)*

Pipsissewa (*Chimaphila umbellata*)

Pulsatilla (*Anemona pulsatilla*)*

Red raspberry (*Rubus strigosus*)

*Asterisks indicate the most frequently used therapeutic agents.

Skullcap (*Scutellaria lateriflora*)
Squaw vine (*Mitchella repens*)*

Menorrhagia/Metrorrhagia

Amaranth (*Amaranthus hypochondriacus*): Astringent. Dose: tincture, 15 to 25 drops three to four times per day.*

Angelica (*Angelica archangelica*)*

Cinnamon (*Cinnamomum zeylanicum*): Use infusion, 1 cup two to three times per day.

Cramp bark or high-bush cranberry (*Viburnum opulus*)

Geranium (*Pelargonium* spp.): 15 to 20 drops tincture.

Life root (*Senecio aureus*): Uterine tonic, useful in atonic conditions. Dose: tincture, 15 to 30 drops three to four times per day.*

Red raspberry (*Rubus strigosus*)

Shepherd's purse (*Capsella bursapastoris*)

Solomon's seal (*Polygonatum multiflorum*)

Squaw vine (*Mitchella repens*)*

Strawberry leaf tea (*Fragaria vesca*)

White oak bark (*Quercus alba*): Astringent.

Witch hazel (*Hamamelis virginiana*): Astringent.

Yarrow (*Achillea millefolium*)

General

Dong quai (*Angelica oylvestris*): All menstrual problems.

MIGRAINE (see Headache)

MINIMAL BRAIN DAMAGE (see Hyperactivity)

MONONUCLEOSIS (see Immune Deficiency)

MULTIPLE SCLEROSIS (Disseminated Sclerosis)

Definition

A widespread, progressive degenerative disease of the central nervous system characterized by scattered areas of destruction of the myelin sheath covering nerves in the brain and spinal cord. Periods of exacerbation and remission occur.

*Asterisks indicate the most frequently used therapeutic agents.

Symptoms

Onset is usually between 20 to 30 years of age, with peak incidence in the late 20s. First signs are minor and include minor visual disturbances, transient visual loss, double vision, or ocular palsy; fatigue; weakness; slight stiffness or weakness of an arm or leg; minor incoordination; dizziness; temporary loss of bladder or bowel control; numbness; or mild emotional disturbance. These may come and go with more severe symptoms occurring later, such as tremor; lack of motor coordination; nystagmus; slow, slurred speech; seizures; paralysis; and mental disturbance. Most die due to complications of respiratory infections.

Etiologic Considerations

- Allergy
  Celiac (gluten)
  Yeast
  Wheat
  Milk
  Eggs
  Any food or chemical
- Hypoglycemia
- Excess saturated fats
- Deficiency of unsaturated fats
- Refined foods
- Glandular disturbance
  Liver
  Gallbladder
  Adrenals
  Pancreas
- Deficient assimilation
- Toxicity
- Heavy metal poisoning
- Pesticides, fungicides, additives, etc.
- Vaccinations
- Vitamin dependency

Discussion

Multiple sclerosis is found predominantly in civilized nations. It is most common where the diet is high in saturated fats and refined carbohydrates. The fats involved are not just the obvious ones such as meats, cheese, milk, cream, and butter, but also hidden fats in pastries, baked goods, cookies, cakes, fried foods, and even peanut butters or margarines made with hydrogenated oil. Fats consumed with sugar or other refined carbohydrates are particularly dangerous. Societies such as the Eskimos who consume a high amount of saturated fats show no evidence of multiple sclerosis until refined carbohydrates are introduced into their diet. The same fact applies to many other tribal cultures. Hypoglycemia, a condition due primarily to the consumption of refined carbohydrates, is commonly found in subjects with multiple sclerosis.

Not only are refined carbohydrates suspected by naturopaths in the causation of multiple sclerosis, but also in some cases any gluten-containing grain. These include most grains except brown rice and millet. Multiple sclerosis has been arrested in some cases simply by following a totally gluten-free diet (see Celiac Disease). Other food allergies may be a factor, including eggs, milk, or literally any food.

Heavy metal toxicity, especially lead, but others as well, has been associated with some cases of multiple sclerosis. Toxicity or hypersensitivity to pesticides and food additives, colorings, or preservatives may also be a factor. Glandular disturbances of the gallbladder, liver, pancreas, thyroid, and adrenal glands may be related, causing poor assimilations and interactions between the endocrine and central nervous systems. Many naturopathic physicians suspect that previous vaccination with smallpox, measles, and other inoculations may be associated with multiple sclerosis. These inoculations can cause profound changes within the body years after their introduction.

Treatment

Multiple sclerosis is a degenerative disease and as such must be treated vigorously, generally, consistently, and over a prolonged period of time before true healing may begin. The longer a person has had multiple sclerosis, the less likely is complete cure, since the demyelinated areas of the nerves become scarred and calcified, causing permanent debility. Long-lasting remissions are possible, however, with perseverance in some cases.

Diet

The initial basic diet must be a gluten-free, dairy-less, completely nonsaturated fat regimen. This implies complete vegetarianism, even excluding dairy products. Some therapists in the field allow 10 to 15 percent saturated fats and dairy products such as low-fat goat's yoghurt. I advise a period of at least 6 months if not a year totally free of saturated fats. This effectively eliminates all meats, dairy foods, eggs, and hydrogenated fats. Fried foods are also prohibited. Some followers of typical gluten-free diets include nongluten flour in baking bread. I feel these products are generally abnormal and should be avoided. Since yeast is also highly suspect, I advise absolutely no yeast products. All foods must be free from additives, pesticides, colorings, or preservatives. No coffee, alcohol, salt, or sugar is to be used. No smoking, either! I know all these "No's" sound terribly forbidding, but the diet isn't really that bad. In fact, when the reality of the situation is considered, all I am recommending is a good, wholesome vegetarian diet without eggs, yeast, wheat (gluten grains), or dairy products.

Allergy tests (RAST, cytotoxic, and pulse) should be performed to diagnose any other specific allergens. The foods suggested, all organic and unrefined, are as follows:

Raw and cooked vegetables, vegetable juices

Raw fruits, fruit juices

Sprouted seeds such as alfalfa, sunflower, red clover, etc.

Sprouted beans

Cooked beans, tofu

Nuts and seeds, especially sunflower and pumpkin seeds; nut butters, stone fruit seeds (i.e., apricot kernels, peach kernels, etc.)

Brown rice and millet

Seed yoghurts

Cold pressed unsaturated oils

Periods of raw vegetable juice fasting of 3 days to 2 weeks should be undertaken periodically throughout the regimen.

Physiotherapy

- Spinal manipulation: Weekly treatments are advised.

- Massage: Use a combination of:
  2 oz peanut oil
  2 oz olive oil
  Oil of sassafras
  ½ oz lanolin
  Oil of pine needles
  Massage all along spine nightly just after using the Cayce wet cell device (see below).

- Cayce wet cell appliance (with gold): Apply 45 minutes per day. For in-depth information see "Two electrical appliances described in the Edgar Cayce readings," available from the ARE Press, Virginia Beach, Va. (see Appendix II).

Hydrotherapy

- Alternate hot and cold showers daily
- Alternate hot and cold compresses or sprays to spine
- Hair analysis: Check all cases for toxic metals and then detoxify (see Heavy Metal Toxicity).
- Outdoor exercise
- Sunshine
- Ocean swimming
- Outdoor living

Therapeutic Agents

VITAMINS AND MINERALS

Vitamin A: 10,000 to 25,000 IU one to two times per day; more used in some cases. *Use any dose of vitamin A over 50,000 IU per day with medical supervision only.*

Vitamin B complex: 50 mg three times per day (nonyeast source if yeast allergy is suspected).*

Vitamin B_1: 10 to 15 g per day, plus 1 g intramuscular injection, one to two times per week, with 1 mg B_{12}.*

Vitamin B_3: 500 mg up to 20 g.

Vitamin B_6: 100 to 250 mg one to three times per day.*

Vitamin B_{12}: Oral dose and intramuscular injections used.

Inositol/choline (lecithin)

Folic acid

Pantothenic acid: 100 mg per day.*

Vitamin C: Up to 10 g or more.*

Vitamin D: Take care not to exceed toxic levels.

Vitamin E: 800 to 2000 IU per day.

Essential fatty acids: 2 to 4 capsules two to three times per day.*

Calcium/magnesium: In 2 to 1 ratio.

Manganese

*Asterisks indicate the most frequently used therapeutic agents.

Selenium: 200 mcg per day.

Zinc: Serum zinc levels low in MS; 25 to 50 mg two times per day.*

Trace minerals

OTHERS

Adrenal*

Atomodine

Cod-liver oil: 2 to 4 capsules three times daily.*

EPA: 2 to 10 capsules three times per day.

Kelp: 2 to 4 tablets two to three times per day.

Lecithin: Concentrated phosphatidyl choline; 3 to 4 capsules three times per day, or more.*

Oil of evening primrose—gamma linoleic acid (GLA): 2 to 4 capsules three to four times per day or more.*

Pancreatic enzymes to aid digestion.*

SOD (superoxide dismutase): 2 to 5 tablets three times per day.

Spirulina

Wheat germ oil: Large doses.* Use octacosanol.

MUMPS (see Childhood Diseases)

NAIL ABNORMALITIES

The condition of the finger- and toenails is a useful diagnostic aid. The following are some of the more common associations between nail health and nutritional status:

Absent half moons: Protein deficiency

Nail ridges: Protein deficiency, vitamin A deficiency

Pale nail beds: Anemia

Peeling nails: Vitamin A deficiency

Poor nail growth: Zinc deficiency

*Asterisks indicate the most frequently used therapeutic agents.

Splitting nails: Sulfur amino acid deficiency

Spoon-shaped nails: Iron deficiency

Thin, brittle nails: Iron deficiency, calcium deficiency, vitamin D deficiency, hydrochloric acid deficiency

Washboard ridges: Iron deficiency, calcium deficiency, zinc deficiency

White nails: Liver disease, copper excess

White spots: Zinc deficiency, thyroid deficiency, hydrochloric acid deficiency

NEURITIS AND NEURALGIA

Definition

Irritation or inflammation of a nerve.

Symptoms

Local or referred pain; altered sensation (burning, tingling, numbness); muscle weakness and later atrophy; possible visceral symptoms; sensory, motor, reflex, or vasomotor symptoms.

Etiologic Considerations

- Spinal lesion
  Cranial
  Temporomandibular joint (TMJ) syndrome
  Cervical
  Brachial outlet syndrome
  Thoracic outlet syndrome
  C7 rib
  Intercostal neuralgia
  Sciatica
  Etc.

- Disc lesion

- Trauma
  Blow
  Compression
  Stretching
  Exposure to cold

- Referred from viscera
- Herpes zoster
- Nutritional deficiency
  B_1 deficiency
  B_{12} neuropathy
  Anemia
- Alcoholism
- Diabetic neuropathy
- Circulatory
  Angina
  Migraine
- Toxic
  Lead, arsenic, mercury, chemicals, pesticides, others
- Viral
- Lupus
- Leprosy
- Cancer
- Arthritis

Discussion

The most frequent causes of neuritis and neuralgia are conditions related to the bony and other connective-tissue elements of the body where these may put direct or indirect pressure on nerves. In these cases a proper diagnosis by an osteopath, chiropractor, or naturopath is essential to determine if spinal or soft tissue therapy should be applied. This may include spinal manipulation or mobilization, cranial techniques, soft-tissue techniques (massage, neuromuscular therapy, friction, etc.), physiotherapy, exercise therapy, postural reeducation, and others. If you need to be seen by a neurologist or orthopedic specialist, they will refer you.

Neuritis and neuralgia may also result from less obvious causes. This includes referred pain from internal visceral complaints such as pain in right shoulder and shoulder blade with gallbladder disease, midback pain with ulcers, or low back pain in menstrual complaints. Post-herpes zoster neuralgia can be a painful problem for months or even years following the original viral skin lesions. Other viruses are also known to cause muscle paralysis and weakness along with nerve irritation.

Severe nutritional deficiencies, especially of the vitamin B complex group, cause well-recognized neuropathies. Vitamin B_{12} neuropathy is becoming increasingly apparent as many young people convert to vegetarian or vegan diets without adequate understanding of essential nutritional requirements. Informed vegetarianism is an extremely healthful diet. However, if proper care is not taken to provide sufficient B_{12}, a severe and permanent nerve degeneration may occur (see Anemia).

Alcoholism and diabetes are also associated with nerve disorders, as are several other systemic chronic degenerative diseases (i.e., lupus, leprosy, cancer, or heart disease). Often an otherwise untraceable neuritis or neuralgia will be found to stem from toxic causes. This may be heavy metal poisoning, chemical exposure, pesticide exposure, or an imbalanced and acidic bloodstream. Similar dietary causes as those found under Arthritis, with which neuritis and neuralgia are often associated, are frequently a factor.

Treatment

Diet

Nearly all cases of neuritis or neuralgia will benefit by an initial elimination regimen. A 3-day fast or mono diet on subacid fruit juice or fruit such as apples may be used in some cases, while a longer carrot-based vegetable juice fast may be of more benefit to others. The diet regimen found under Arthritis is an excellent outline to follow to help alkalize the bloodstream in a steady and gentle manner. Emphasis should be placed on raw green vegetables, seaweeds, seeds, and seed or bean sprouts.

Physiotherapy

- Spinal therapy, as needed
- Massage
- Muscle reeducation
- Hot Epsom salts baths (see Appendix I)
- Alternate hot and cold showers
- Alternate hot and cold compresses
- Alternate hot and cold local baths
- Poultices
  Mullein
  Mustard
  Hops plus lobelia for pain relief (antispasmodic)

Mullein plus lobelia
Chamomile

Therapeutic Agents

VITAMINS AND MINERALS

Vitamin B complex: 25 to 50 mg two to three times per day.*

Vitamin B_1: 100 mg one to two times per day, plus 100 mg intramuscularly per week.*

Vitamin B_6: 250 to 500 mg one to two times daily (carpal tunnel syndrome).*

Vitamin B_{12}: 25 mcg two times per day, plus 1 mg intramuscularly per week.*

Folic acid: 400 to 800 mcg per day.

Vitamin C: To bowel tolerance.*

Vitamin E: 400 IU two to three times per day, especially with post-herpes zoster syndrome.*

Essential fatty acids: 1 to 2 tbs cold pressed oils daily.

Inositol: 1000 mg one to two times per day (diabetic neuropathy).*

Iodine: Atomodine.

Calcium chelate or lactate: 400 mg two to three times per day.*

Magnesium: 200 mg two to three times per day.*

OTHERS

Brewer's yeast

Bromelain: Anti-inflammatory.

Desiccated liver

Kelp: 2, three times per day (not to be taken with Atomodine)

Lecithin: 4 capsules three times per day, or as granules, 1 to 3 tbs per day.*

Wheat germ oil*

BOTANICALS

Aconite (*Aconitum napellus*) Homeopathic doses.

Betony (*Betonica officinalis*)

---

*Asterisks indicate the most frequently used therapeutic agents.

Blue cohosh (*Caulophyllum thalictroides*)

Bryony (*Bryonia alba*)

Catnip (*Nepeta cataria*)

Hops (*Humulus lupulus*)

Jamaica dogwood (*Piscidia erythrina*): For facial or sciatic neuralgia.*

Myrrh (*Commiphora myrrha*)

Oregon grape root (*Berberis aquifolium*)

Passion flower (*Passiflora incarnata*)

Pulsatilla (*Anemone pulsatilla*)

St. John's wort (*Hypericum perforatum*)

Skullcap (*Scutellaria lateriflora*)

Valerian (*Valeriana officinalis*)

Wintergreen (*Gaultheria procumbens*)

OTHERS

Myrrh plus capsicum external

Menthol ointment external

Olbas oil combination external

Peppermint oil external

Wintergreen oil external

Deadly nightshade (*Atropa belladonna*): *Use with medical supervision.* Topical application in neuralgia, 6× dilution internally for pain.*

NUTRITIONAL DEFICIENCIES

Clinical states of single nutritional deficiencies are, fortunately, fairly rare. This is not to say that even in the developed nations cases of the more well-known nutritional deficiencies such as vitamin A deficiency (night blindness), vitamin B deficiency (beriberi), vitamin B₃ deficiency (pellagra), vitamin C deficiency (scurvy), or vitamin D and calcium deficiency (rickets) do not occur. They do, and in some cases their incidence is on the rise rather than the wane, due to our devitalized western diet. But the relative infrequency of these easily

*Asterisks indicate the most frequently used therapeutic agents.

recognizable deficiencies in no way represents the incredible frequency, perhaps as high as 50 percent or more of the general population, of subclinical multiple nutritional deficiencies. The average medical doctor looks at the infrequency of reported clinical nutritional deficiencies and draws the false conclusion that our diets are adequate without supplementation.

This oversight is not usually the doctor's fault. The blame lies in orthodox crisis care medical education and philosophy. Unless something can be shown by a series of tests to be definitively wrong, then everything is fine. A disease is not a disease until someone is sick, and sickness is defined clearly in medical texts that do not discuss subclinical nutritional states. Only within the past 10 years or so have some medical doctors expanded their vision of disease to include the early calling cards of disease—the subtle yet significant subjective and objective symptoms and signs of suboptimal nutrition. Health is no longer simply the absence of disease, but rather the perfect freedom of expression of the individual on all his or her three planes of function—the body, mind, and emotions. Any interference and blockage among any of these three facets contain a possible clue to nutritional deficiency. Certainly not all signs or symptoms within the body, mind, or emotions can be traced to nutritional causes; however, all these clues involve nutritional factors. If a person experiences prolonged stress, worry, fear, or anxiety, a close interaction occurs within the body that affects the nutritional state. Think a thought and you invariably move a muscle; feel an emotion and you secrete a host of hormones and initiate hundreds of biochemical reactions. The body and emotions are all connected, and until we can see this, no true healing will take place.

On a more practical level is the purely statistical evidence that a significant proportion of the western population is clearly nutritionally deficient. If we accept the fact that between 1 to 2 percent of the population has an increased need over the recommended dietary allowance (RDA) of a particular nutrient (a reasonable assumption, since the manner in which RDAs are established is based on standard statistical evaluation with usually 1 to 2 percent of the sample falling either above or below the acceptable range), and if we then multiply this 1 to 2 percent by the fifty or so known essential nutrients, vitamins, minerals, and trace elements, we arrive at the conclusion that any given individual has between a 50 to 100 percent chance of being deficient in at least one of these life-sustaining factors. This assumes that all of us are already getting the recommended RDAs in our diet, an assumption proven wrong by study after study. Nutritional deficiencies are not the rare, insignificant phenomena we have been led to believe, but rather a prevalent cause of disease in the civilized nations today.

Recent studies have made this picture even more grim. In animal studies it has been found that some single nutrient deficiencies (i.e., zinc) in the mother during pregnancy can lead to nutritional deficiencies, nutritional dependencies, and immune malfunction in not only the immediate offspring but to a lesser degree for three generations, in spite of a normal diet.* Although these animal studies do not directly apply to humans, they help suggest explanations for several clinical observations. Studies dating back to the end of World War II recorded cases of severe malnutrition in prisoners of war that resulted in vitamin dependency in later years. In this particular case, these people required doses 50 or over 100 times the recommended dose of vitamin B_3 to maintain proper physical and mental health.

Similar observations have been made with other vitamins. These findings further reinforce the idea that individualized requirements for specific nutrients can be affected not only by genetics as previously recognized, but may also be acquired within one's lifetime. I am sure that more research in this direction over the next 10 years will help explain why even the best of diets may no longer supply adequately all nutritional elements for all individuals.

I think this is a particularly important breakthrough in our knowledge of the possible cause of nutritional dependency disease. It also emphasizes the little-understood concept that the pattern for our health and the strength of our immune system may be laid down by our parents or even grandparents. This may explain why, in spite of positive changes for the better in diet and nutrition by many of the population, true health is still hard to obtain. Our health foundation is weak, and it may take generations for this weakness to be corrected.

OBESITY

Definition and Symptoms

Excess fat storage.

Etiologic Considerations

- Excess refined carbohydrates and saturated fats
- Allergy
- Lack of demanding exercise
- Hormonal imbalances
  Hypothalamus
  Pituitary
  Pineal
  Thyroid
  Adrenal
  Pancreas

---

*"Initial zinc deprivation affects three generations," *Science*, 218:469–471, 1982.

- Incoordination of assimilation or elimination
- Improper feeding as infant and child
- Hereditary predisposition (familial?)
- "The pill"

Discussion

Obesity is not merely a cosmetic problem, but a severe threat to health and longevity. The old proverb stating "The longer the belt, the shorter the life," is entirely accurate. Associated with obesity are diabetes and heart disease, two of the major killers of modern civilization.

The origins of obesity often lie in early childhood. Statistically, children who are overweight by the age of 2 turn into fat adults more frequently than their lean playmates. Early feeding patterns set the stage for adult obesity. The most common mistake is fattening the child with excess starch and cow's milk. Most infants receive starchy foods as their first solid foods, around 4 months of age. This is far too early for proper digestion, and sets the stage for later allergies, as referred to in other sections of this book.

More importantly, however, in causing obesity, these grains cause rapid weight gain. This is in part due to the fact that most grains are of the refined variety of empty calories, stripped of their fiber and bran. Rather than grains being given early and regularly as a first food, they should be introduced relatively late in the weaning process and less frequently, to avoid rapid weight gain. Cow's milk is another cause of rapid weight gain. Its composition was designed for the rapid growth of cows, not children. The fact that most cow's milk given is homogenized, making the fat particles easier to assimilate, is another aspect of milk that favors obesity. Raw unhomogenized goat's milk is a far better food for human infants over 6 months of age and does not cause rapid weight gain since the composition is closer to that of mother's breast milk. Always make sure your goat's milk comes from a reliable dairy and that the milk has been bottled under proper antiseptic conditions. Prior to 6 months of age, all liquids given to an infant should be boiled to prevent gastroenteritis.

Breastfed infants have far less chance of becoming obese than formula-fed babies. I have, however, seen enough quite obese infants who were totally breastfed not to reinforce this commonly quoted statistic too dogmatically. I have seen infants up to 32 lb by the age of 1 who were totally breastfed by mothers on "whole food" diets. In most of these cases, but not all, these mothers themselves were, if not obese, at least full-bodied and a little plumpish. Most of the infants demanded the breast nearly every 2 hours day and night, and were allowed fairly unrestricted access. From these observations I feel fairly certain that the cause of such breastfed obesity is a combination of milk of an unusually fattening nature, and too-frequent feedings.

It seems obvious that all mother's milk is not identical and I suspect the mother's own biochemistry goes a long way in affecting the type of food she produces for her infant. I do not generally like the idea of restricting feedings to set times or hours, but see the need for some restraint in these cases. There is also the possibility that the infant is feeding more for psychological reasons than hunger, and pleasant distractions might break the pattern. I do admit this is no easy task, but the dangers of obesity make it worth the effort.

In this discussion I have not mentioned the obvious fact that if the breast-feeding mother is herself on an improper diet of excess refined carbohydrates, sugar, and excess animal fats, she is not only laying the foundation for infant obesity, but also for a generally unhealthy child.

In many cases, the child fortunately passes through childhood without growing fat. Two possibilities can be the cause. The first is that the child, being lucky enough to have parents with some common sense, has been "deprived" of all kinds of sweets, pastries, white bread, soda, sweetened and refined cereals, or other junk foods and given only wholesome unrefined foods. These children then pass into adult life having the least chance of becoming obese and the best chance of a long, healthy life. The second possibility is that the child has been given a typical junk food diet in his or her growing years, but due to an abundance of childhood play and exercise, has been able thus far to avoid weight gain or other obviously noticeable complaints except possibly a tendency to get sick frequently or possibly to have behavior problems.

In fact, if nothing "obvious" is taking place outside, something insidious is taking place inside, as we shall see. As the child passes into adult life the general activity level usually decreases markedly, but the diet does not, except maybe to include alcohol, which is certainly not an improvement. The body has already become accustomed to a diet of quickly absorbed refined carbohydrates and internal biochemical changes have been made to deal with these more or less as demanded. The pancreas now knows it must act fast at the first signs of sugar in the system since from experience it knows a flood of it will soon be in the bloodstream. Refined carbohydrates are, after all, very quickly absorbed. This increased sugar sensitivity may then progress into a clinical case of hypoglycemia (low blood sugar), especially with the added burden of alcohol, which, next to refined sugar, is the ultimate refined carbohydrate. Couple these dietary influences with the addition of stress from a job or new family life, which depletes the adrenal glands, the co-manager of our blood sugar level along with the pancreas, and we see how profoundly our internal chemistry has been abused.

It is no small wonder then that the chemistry of an obese person is found to differ from the average person of normal size. Most obese people show abnormal glucose tolerance and have raised blood levels of cholesterol, triglycerides, and free fatty acids. Many overweight people report quite honestly that they do not eat any more than other people and yet still gain weight. Although this statement is occasionally born out of a lack of awareness of true eating habits, more often than not it *is* true. Fat people often *don't* eat more than thin people. Often, the reverse is true with some thin people eating far more without gaining weight. This does not necessarily mean that the thin person has a healthier biochemistry, but he or she certainly has a different one. Often, both are suffering from the insidious results of the same refined diet, but have made different biochemical adjustments, depending in part on hereditary predisposition, or the state of their organs of elimination, endocrine system, or nervous system.

The basic problem in obesity then is an abnormal biochemistry caused by a diet of excess refined carbohydrates and saturated fats, and a reduction in activity level when reaching adult life.

The common answer to this problem is usually "eat less and exercise more." This advice is both right and wrong at the same time. Certainly, weight loss can be obtained by a calorie-restricted diet and an increase in exercise. The problem, however, is in preventing weight gain after the diet is over. If an obese person stores fat better than a thin person on the same diet, something must be done to change the inner controls or else the obese person will be doomed to a lifetime of ridiculously limited diet and self-reproach for each minor incident of leniency.

No real progress will ever be made along these lines unless the actual bio-chemistry of the obese person is changed. The answer to the dietary aspect of obesity is not necessarily to eat less, but to eat properly. Certainly, refined carbohydrates will cause weight gain and these must be totally excluded from the diet and replaced by unrefined high-fiber carbohydrates such as brown rice, millet, barley, buckwheat, wheat berries, bulgur, corn, and other whole grains. These should be cooked only enough to make them chewy but not soft. In the early stages of weight loss and weight maintenance they should not even be ground up or used in flour form, as in bread. The reasons for these changes are simple. A person can eat a much larger amount of refined starches and grains than their whole grain counterparts. The refined grains are also much easier to digest and absorb. By eating whole grains cooked very conservatively one can eat only a fraction of the amount previously eaten and can thoroughly digest even less. The difference is obvious if we compare the stool contents after several meals of cornbread as opposed to corn on the cob. A similar difference exists between white rice and brown rice, or between white bread and whole wheat bread. With unrefined grain the person eats much less but the stools are much larger. To prove this, first eat an entire loaf of white bread at one meal and try to eat an entire loaf of whole wheat bread at another meal. You will soon see what I mean.

One step further than the concept of refined vs. whole food is the concept of "unaltered whole grains," which works even better with the obese. A similar comparison between bread made from white flour and bread made from whole wheat flour can be made between whole wheat bread and whole wheat berries. If the whole grain itself is eaten and has not been ground up into flour by powerful grain mills, much less can be eaten and still less digested and absorbed. For this reason the best diet approach for the obese is a balanced diet of fresh fruit, raw vegetables, protein, especially vegetarian protein, and unaltered, unrefined, high-fiber carbohydrates.

To change the biochemistry exercise is needed, but not as usually suggested. Weight loss due to caloric benefits of exercise is not all it is made out to be. Walking may use up to 120 calories per hour while actual jogging burns only 440 calories per hour. The average obese person is incapable of doing enough exercise to expend sufficient calories to affect profound weight loss. In reality, the best way to lose weight would be to exercise and play as actively as when we were young children—in other words almost constantly, but this is clearly impossible. The second best is to exercise as if one were to train for a demanding sport such as football or boxing. Clearly this is also pretty impossible for the average person with a job or a family.

As explained in the excellent book *Fit or Fat?* by Covert Bailey (and which I recommend to everyone who is overweight), the only type of exercise of real significance for the obese is aerobic exercise. Bailey points out clearly that only through a regimen of sufficiently prolonged *aerobic* exercise can the biochemistry of the body be altered. He shows the futility of most of the weight loss diets, since the real problem is not one of overweight, but "over fat." What this means is that an obese person has more fat, not only in the normal subcutaneous fat reserves, but also more fat content in the muscles. The average percentage of fat in muscles is somewhere from 12 to 22 percent, depending on body type, occupation, and sex. Athletes tend to have much lower muscle fat, even down to 5 to 6 percent, while females tend to be on the upper part of the scale. The obese person, however, has a higher than normal percentage of muscle fat. What seems to occur in the fattening process is that as we grow out of our active childhood into adult life, we use less of our muscles in our daily duties. If the diet is improper and the body has developed abnormal responses to dietary carbohydrates, alcohol, or fats, these unused muscles begin to accumulate fat. Initially, no weight gain is noticed since fat is merely being substituted for muscle, but eventually obesity begins to develop. Normal diets to lose weight only reduce fat stores or even worse, protein weight, and do not significantly affect muscle fat. For true weight loss a biochemical change is necessary, and once again the way is through aerobics.

What are "aerobic" exercises? To quote Bailey,

> The word Aerobic means air, but more specifically refers to the oxygen in the air. The muscles need oxygen to function and their need for oxygen goes up

dramatically when we work them. We can measure how hard a muscle is
working by how much oxygen it is using (or burning). As you exercise harder,
you need more oxygen and the heart rate goes up. Increases in your heart rate
due to exercise are an indirect measure of how hard your muscles are working.*

Baily recommends steady, nonstop aerobic exercise for a duration of not less
than 12 to 20 minutes, depending on the exercise, at 80 percent of the maximum heart rate, providing there are no health complications to make this in-
advisable.

The type of exercises considered "aerobic" are nonstop exercises such as those
performed in aerobic exercise classes, fast walking, jogging, running, rope jumping, calisthenics, jumping jacks, bicycling, rowing, cross-country skiing, roller
skating, etc. Swimming is an aerobic exercise but is not advised for weight loss
since the water temperature is usually colder than body temperature and signals
the body to store fat for insulation, clearly not what is desired. As a cardiovascular
exercise, or for the entire body tone, however, it is excellent.

Many people feel that they get plenty of exercise on their job or about the
house, but this is not "aerobic" exercise and therefore has little or no real effect
on true weight loss. Even if you work with your body all day long (as a carpenter,
for instance), the activity is usually intermittent and rarely calls for 100 percent
use of your muscles.

True aerobic exercise changes the body on a biochemical level, altering the
deeply ingrained way the obese handle carbohydrates and fat. These exercises
also stimulate the endocrine system, which may be a factor in weight gain in
the first place. Certainly, thyroid disorders have been implicated in obesity, as
have disorders of the hypothalamus, pituitary, pineal, pancreas, adrenals, and
sex glands.

Patients often ask me what their ideal weight should be, or how much weight
they need to lose for their height. All the height vs. weight charts that have ever
been written are totally useless in determining proper weight, since they in no
way take into consideration what proportion of the body is fat, and which is
toned muscle. Two people of the same height can weigh the same, while one
is composed of muscle and the other of fat. Even if you start with fat and through
dieting end up fitting into the weight charts, what good is it if you look skinny
with sagging skin? What you need is to replace fat with muscle. Get *in* shape
rather than just get *out* of a bad one.

In the final analysis all you need is a mirror and a large water source to
judge your weight accurately. The mirror will show general body shape. If you
look more like a blob than a figure eight, you have a way to go. You don't need
a medical degree to know what a shapely body looks like. If you float easily in

*Bailey, Covert, *Fit or Fat?* Houghton Mifflin Co., Boston, 1977, p. 42.

water, it means you still have plenty of fat. When you begin to sink easily on exhalation you are getting there.

Treatment

Diet

The basic diet includes the following:

- *Raw fruit:* Moderate amounts of raw citrus and subacid fruits are allowed. No sweet fruits such as grapes or dried fruits should be consumed. Fruit juices are also forbidden since these are in essence "refined," being devoid of their pulp and roughage. The only exception is diluted red grape juice taken ½ hour before all meals. This helps decrease the appetite, allowing the subject to eat less, and does not signal a weight gain. Bananas also are not allowed.

- *Raw vegetables:* These are allowed almost without restraint. A raw salad meal should be taken once or twice each day, alone, or with other compatible foods such as protein or unrefined starch.

- *Cooked vegetables:* The only cooked vegetables allowed are fresh and conservatively cooked (steamed, stewed, lightly sautéed, or baked, but not fried) fresh vegetables. No frozen, fried, or canned vegetables are to be used. The proportion of cooked vegetables consumed should be less than raw. Vegetables properly cooked are still slightly crispy. Potatoes are allowed two to three times per week but *only* if eaten with the skin.

- *Proteins:* Beans, sprouted beans, sprouted seeds, nuts in moderation, fish, chicken and turkey (wild, if possible), low-fat yoghurt, and poached eggs are the major proteins with the vegetarian sources stressed. Absolutely no pork or meat is allowed unless it is from wild game, which has far less fat content.

- *Carbohydrates:* All refined carbohydrates are absolutely forbidden. This means sugar, alcohol, white flour and its products (bread, pastry, macaroni, etc.), quick oats, most packaged cereals, and any other processed starch. Eat only conservatively cooked, unrefined brown rice, millet, barley, rye, buckwheat, wheat berries, bulgur, corn, and any other whole grain. These should be taken in their natural state and not ground into flour for bread or cooked cereal. Let your teeth do the grinding.

- *Fats:* Cold pressed unsaturated oils are allowed for salad dressings with lemon juice plus herbs, or when needed in cooking in very small amounts.

Obviously, one should not overeat, a tendency that may be carried over from days of eating unrefined carbohydrates. Until the stomach adjusts to its proper size, some restraint in the diet is obviously required. It is also far better to eat four to five smaller meals than two or three large ones. A useful rule to eliminate habit snacking is to eat only while eating. In other words, when eating, concentrate only on the meal or snack at hand. No talking, reading, listening to the radio, watching TV, or any other mental distraction is allowed. This eliminates the tendency to munch incessantly and requires that the person be hungry enough to discontinue all other activities to eat. A simple diet might be as follows:

¹/₂ hour before breakfast	6 oz glass of diluted grape juice, 2 to 1 with water, sipped slowly
Breakfast	Fresh raw fruit (especially citrus) or fresh raw fruit with low-fat yoghurt *or:* Fresh raw fruit and a small handful of nuts *or:* Poached eggs and fruit *or:* Poached eggs and whole grain such as brown rice or millet *or:* Forever Lite diet plan* *or:* Salad *or:* Salad and nuts *or:* Salad and low-fat yoghurt
Midmorning	Fresh vegetables such as carrot or celery sticks Apple One fruit plus eight to twelve almonds Herb tea Dandelion coffee Raw or baked tofu (teriyaki tofu or other)
¹/₂ hour before lunch	Diluted red grape juice
Lunch	Always have a raw mixed salad composed of at least three vegetables that grow above the ground for each that grows below In addition, choose from: Beans

*Available from Forever Living Products, P.O. Box 29041, Phoenix, AZ 85038.

	Fish
	Turkey or chicken (two times per week only)
	Wild game meat
	Tofu
	Whole grain
	Baked potato with skin (two to three times per week only, in any meal)
	Nuts or seeds (pumpkin, sunflower, etc.)
Midafternoon	As midmorning
$^1/_2$ hour before supper	Diluted red grape juice
Supper	Raw salad or cooked vegetables
	Protein and whole grain (1 cup cooked) individually cooked and served as a casserole dish

I suggest obtaining several good salad and whole food cookbooks. Variety and interest must be maintained. With a little experience you will learn to make nearly anything out of whole foods. Use your imagination, but use whole foods. In addition to the basic diet, take 1 tbs raw bran with one to two glasses of water 10 to 15 minutes prior to each meal. This tends to reduce appetite.

Another approach to weight loss for relatively short terms (1 to 3 months) is the modified protein-sparing fast/diet. During the normal fasting state the body first mobilizes glycogen stores in the liver and tissue stores. These are converted to glucose and supply the brain and tissues with this vital energy source for the first 12 to 24 hours of the fast. Following this period, the body begins to convert both fat and protein into glucose to maintain an adequate supply in the blood to sustain life. Without a steady supply of glucose the brain cannot function.

Unfortunately, with the conversion of fat to glucose, by-products are produced, which, if allowed to build up in the blood, cause a state of acidosis and toxicity. This is one of the reasons many people suffer varying degrees of unpleasant symptoms such as headaches, mental lethargy, and foul breath during the first two or three days of a fast. Fortunately, the body has the ability to stimulate the release of hormones not normally present in the brain that are capable of utilizing as a new source of energy the previously toxic substances (ketones), resulting from the conversion of fat to glucose. This biochemical trick only occurs during the fasting state and is the reason why most people experience a feeling of renewed vigor and even a slight euphoria on or shortly after the third day of a fast. Finally, the brain has guaranteed itself a steady supply of glucose. This new source of energy is not, however, sufficient for the total body need for energy and therefore protein initially from the muscular system, and much later from organs, is utilized to fulfill this need. This protein conversion to glucose causes muscle wasting, certainly not the desired result of a weight loss regimen, which is aimed at fat deposit mobilization. To prevent this protein loss and still mobilize fat from its stores, causing generalized weight loss without at the same time losing muscle, the modified protein-sparing diet is used. On this regimen a person fasts on a well-balanced instant protein powder, such as Ultrabalance or Forever Lite. This is consumed three times per day in 6 to 8 oz of diluted juice or low-fat milk. Two or three tbs of the protein powder are taken with each liquid meal, to equal approximately 50 g of protein per day. This satisfies the body's protein need and spares the body mobilizing its own protein sources. By not consuming large amounts of glucose directly in the form of carbohydrate, the brain continues to produce enzymes capable of utilizing ketones for energy and this fat is still mobilized. The urge to eat is very small since hunger is partly controlled by the blood glucose levels which will remain fairly constant throughout the diet.

To maintain bowel function in the absence of solid food, a hydrophilic bulking agent is taken two to three times per day, with a glass of water. This swells in the stomach as water is absorbed, providing a nondigestible "meal" that not only keeps the bowels functioning regularly, but also provides a sensation of fullness in the stomach. This is felt by the stomach, which sends impulses to the brain, basically saying "I'm full, thank you, no need to feel hungry right now."

Water should be taken regularly to total 6 to 8 large glasses per day. This helps the bulking agent swell adequately and helps dilute the many toxins provided by the breakdown of proteins and fats for energy; also toxins stored within the fat stores which are liberated as the fat stores melt away. One small salad meal per day is eaten with no dressing.

A good multivitamin, multimineral supplement should be taken on this diet. It would also be beneficial to drink three cups of warm potassium broth (see Appendix I) per day, and eat as much celery as desired.

On this regimen you should expect to lose 4 to 5 lb per week, possibly more initially. This regimen should be followed by a calorie-reduced high-fiber diet coupled with aerobic conditioning. A weight loss of 20 lb in 4 to 5 weeks is not uncommon. The diet may safely be continued to 1 to 3 months with proper supervision. It is essential to have medical supervision on such a diet if it is followed for over 3 weeks. In the past, several deaths have resulted because overzealous dieters have followed a liquid protein diet from nutritionally inadequate sources for extremely prolonged periods of time. Ultrabalance and Forever Lite are advocated by respected biochemists as safe if used according to instructions.

Physiotherapy

• Aerobic exercise: Continuous for 12 to 20 minutes minimum at 80 percent maximum heart rate (see *Fit or Fat?* by Covert Bailey), six times per week.

• Saunas to be taken whenever possible one to six times per week.

- Alternate hot and cold showers stimulate the circulation and endocrine system.
- Spinal manipulation and massage: one to two times per week.

Therapeutic Agents

VITAMINS AND MINERALS

Vitamin B complex: 50 mg one to two times per day.*

Vitamin B_6: 100 mg one to two times per day for fluid retention problems.*

Vitamin C*

Essential fatty acids (GLA, EPA, oil of evening primrose)*

Multivitamins

OTHERS

Amino acids: Taken before meals will reduce hunger and total intake.*

Atomodine (Cayce product): Hypothyroid.

Bran: 1 tsp with 1 glass water 10 to 20 minutes before meals; reduces appetite.*

DL-Phenylalanine: Appetite suppressant, 100 to 300 mg per day.*

Garlic*

Kelp

Lecithin*

Raw pancreas tablets*

Raw pituitary tablets

Raw thyroid tablets

BOTANICALS

Fucus (bladderwrack): For obesity due to hypothyroid condition.

Pokeroot (*Phytolacca decandra*) (highly toxic; see p. 62): Infusion of poke berries two times per day or poke berry tablets, two to three times per day.*

OSTEOPOROSIS

Definition

Decrease in bone mass and density with loss of mineral and protein components.

*Asterisks indicate the most frequently used therapeutic agents.

Symptoms

Back pain, pain on weight-bearing (T8 and below), kyphosis, loss of height, spontaneous fractures, muscle spasms.

Etiologic Considerations

- High-protein diet: Induces calcium deficiency if the protein excess is animal in origin.
- Poor calcium absorption: Calcium absorption decreases with age.
- Menopause
- Excess sweets and refined carbohydrates: Stimulate alkaline digestive juices, making calcium insoluble (calcium is more soluble in an acid medium).
- Hydrochloric acid deficiency, enzyme deficiency
- Lactose deficiency
- Postoperative ulcer, stomach removal, dumping syndrome
- Prolonged stress
- Alcoholism
- Pregnancy, lactation, menstruation, repeated births
- Heavy metal toxicity: Excess aluminum or cadmium is associated with bone loss.
- Hormonal imbalance
    Parathyroid
    Thyroid
- Phytic acid
- Oxalic acid
- Drugs
- Steroids
- Antibiotics
- Lack of exercise
- Vitamin D, magnesium, and calcium, and protein deficiency
- Poor dentures, leading to reduced green vegetable intake
- Distilled water, soft water
- Extreme vitamin C deficiency
- Sodium fluoride in water binds calcium

- Excess bicarbonate of soda
- Malabsorption syndromes
- Cushing's syndrome
- Hyperparathyroidism
- Acromegaly
- Excess cigarette smoking
- Bedridden: Lack of movement and disuse leads to atrophy.
- Aluminum excess: Causes pseudohyperparathyroidism.
- Stress
- Magnesium deficiency: 80 percent loss in refining of grains.
- Phosphorus excess (excess meat, soda drinks, processed foods)

Discussion

Bone is not, as many people believe, an unchanging material. In fact, each of the body's bones is constantly being remade. No single bone strut is ever permanent. Osteoblast and osteoclast cells are constantly dissolving and reforming bone. In addition, bone acts as a reservoir of calcium plus other minerals. When the blood level of calcium begins to fall, calcium is mobilized from the bones.

It has been estimated that over 30 percent of the American population suffer from calcium deficiency. The recommended adult minimum daily requirement (MDR) for calcium has been set at 800 mg per day. Many people, especially the aged, get 450 mg or less. To maintain calcium balance, the body mobilizes calcium from the bone by the action of parathyroid hormone (PTH). This mobilization is most pronounced at night.

Pregnancy, lactation, and growth also demand extra amounts of calcium. In pregnancy and lactation the MDR is raised to 1200 mg. With infants it is 540 mg.

Calcium need increases with age due to multiple factors, including poor digestion, lack of dentures which results in an altered diet (lack of green vegetables), hydrochloric acid deficiency, lack of exercise, and others. Calcium absorption is fairly inefficient, with up to 70 to 80 percent being excreted in the gut. This percentage is even reduced in cases of hydrochloric acid lack in the digestive juice.

Unfortunately, calcium lack does not show itself early. Often the first sign of osteoporosis is a broken bone, or is seen on a routine chest x-ray. Calcium deficiency will show itself on x-ray only after 30 percent of the bone is lost.

Excessive consumption of meat is another factor leading to calcium deficiency. Meat contains twenty to fifty times more phosphorus than calcium. This leads to a loss of calcium from the bones to keep a proper phosphorus/calcium ratio in the blood. Aggravating this situation even more is the excessive meat eater who also smokes cigarettes. Cigarettes increase the acidity of the blood, which inhibits conversion of vitamin D into its active form, leading to a pseudohyperparathyroidism with bone demineralization.

Many people believe they consume enough milk and cheese to prevent calcium deficiency. Unfortunately, however, calcium absorption from these sources may be very poor in cases of dairy intolerance. A far better source of calcium is to be found in raw green vegetables which are high in both calcium and magnesium. It is the general lack of raw vegetables in the diet that predisposes many people to osteoporosis. Vegetarians have less incidence of osteoporosis. The calcium-to-phosphorus ratio is much more favorable in vegetables than in dairy or meat products. This may be one factor explaining this observation.

Certain foods have also been implicated in inducing calcium deficiency and osteoporosis. Foods containing calcium oxalate bind calcium and thus make it unavailable. These foods include spinach, chard, beet greens, and chocolate. Recent research, however, questions this conclusion. The amount of calcium oxalate in these foods appears only capable of binding approximately the amount of calcium within these foods themselves, and not other foods taken in the same meal. Still, caution is suggested, to avoid excessive use of these foods in the diet.* Phytic acid found in wheat and oats also will bind calcium. Wheat, however, contains the enzyme *phytase*, which acts in the leavening process to split phytic acid, rendering it incapable of binding calcium. This occurs only in the leavening process. A diet high in unleavened bread can inhibit uptake of zinc and calcium and cause rickets or osteoporosis. This seems to be a problem only for those on severely restricted diets.

Oats, however, contain very little phytase and some studies have associated a high incidence of rickets and osteoporosis in Scotland with habitual consumption of porridge. Other studies, however, stress the ability of the gut to acquire the capability to split phytic acid if accustomed to oats over several generations.†

An interesting note on milk in relation to calcium absorption is that lactose, the sugar in milk, has been found to favor calcium absorption in people of northern European stock. These people seem to have a larger amount of lactase, the enzyme needed to digest milk. This seems to be a survival factor in countries with little exposure to sun.

*Passwater, Richard A., *Trace Elements, Hair Analysis and Nutrition*, Keats Publishing Co., New Canaan, Conn., 1983, p. 45.
†Ibid., pp. 45–47.

Several drugs have been found that definitely will cause osteoporosis. These include the steroids and many antibiotics. Of these, steroids are the most important, since these are frequently taken over a period of years. A frequent finding in cases of rheumatoid arthritis with steroid medication is osteoporosis with spontaneous fractures.

Estrogens are frequently used as therapy for osteoporosis in postmenopausal women. However, not only does estrogen therapy have many dangerous side effects, including cancer, but many studies reveal that it has no more effect in correcting osteoporosis than do simple calcium and mineral supplementations; in addition to which calcium has no side effects. It appears that the best preventative of postmenopausal osteoarthritis is adequate calcium levels prior to menopause. This means attention to proper diet long before menopause begins.

Treatment

Diet

The diet should have an excess of green leafy vegetables and adequate sources of protein, especially vegetarian in origin. A meat-free diet is best with plenty of fruits, vegetables, legumes, whole grains (such as brown rice, barley, and millet), nuts, sprouted seeds and beans, and fermented dairy foods such as kefir and yoghurt; in short, a vegetarian or lacto-vegetarian unrefined diet. Taking extra calcium foods just before bed is useful. Salads should contain lemon juice or cider vinegar dressing to increase calcium absorption. Contrary to popular belief, milk and dairy sources are *not* a very good source of *absorbable* calcium and should not be increased in the diet. In fact, some cases may require reduction of dairy intake to establish proper mineral balance.

Physiotherapy

• Sun bathing daily if possible

• Sea bathing

• Daily exercise

Therapeutic Agents

Vitamins and Minerals

Vitamin B complex: 25 to 50 mg two to three times per day.

Vitamin C: 1000 to 2000 mg two to four times per day.*

*Asterisks indicate the most frequently used therapeutic agents.

Vitamin D: 400 to 1000 mg per day.*

Calcium orotate: 1000 to 1500 mg per day, best source.*

or: Calcium lactate: with no milk intolerance.

or: Calcium glucomate

or: Chelated calcium: 800 mg two times per day.

Magnesium: 400 mg two times per day.*

Pancreatic enzymes

Hydrochloric acid: if hypoacid.

Cod-liver oil*

Silica*

Vitamin E: 400 to 800 IU per day.

Apple cider vinegar, water and honey: one to two times per day.*

Note: (Some dolomite sources have recently been found to have not only calcium and magnesium, but also unusually high levels of toxic minerals such as lead, arsenic, mercury, and aluminum. Who wants to eat rocks anyway!)

BOTANICALS

Comfrey (*Symphytum officinale*)*

Horsetail (*Equisetum arvense*)*

PARKINSON'S DISEASE

Definition and Symptoms

A chronic, slowly progressive disorder of the central nervous system characterized by hypokinesis (impairment of movement); muscle weakness; rigidity; tremor; unsteady, shuffling gait; and an expressionless look on the face (Parkinson's mask). First sign is usually a hand tremor which is present at rest, but may disappear during purposeful movement. Speech is monotonous and handwriting is cramped. Muscle cramps and pain often occur.

Etiologic Considerations

• Reduced dopamine levels in central nervous system
• Encephalitis may precede disease

*Asterisks indicate the most frequently used therapeutic agents.

- Cerebrovascular disease

- Trauma

- Syphilis

- Tumor

- Drugs

- Heavy metal poisoning

- Nutritional deficiency or toxicity

- Food allergy

- Unknown

Discussion

Parkinson's disease and Parkinson's-like symptoms may occur following encephalitis, trauma, cerebrovascular disease, or drug usage, or may accompany syphilis or tumor. These cases, however, cannot explain the large proportion of Parkinson's sufferers who show no apparent cause for their disorder.

Most cases show a clear abnormality in the brain. The areas of the brain affected are the *globus pallidus* and *substantia nigra*. This damage interferes with central nerve connections responsible for visual and proprioceptive information essential for normal postural maintenance and movement.

On the biochemical level the brain has been found to show a reduced level of dopamine, usually found in high concentration within the substantia nigra. The drug L-dopa has been used therapeutically. This precursor to dopamine penetrates the brain, is converted into dopamine, and helps relieve some of the symptoms of Parkinson's disease, such as slowness in movement, rigidity, and tremor. Other biochemical factors are probably involved, also, since L-dopa does not correct all the disease's symptoms.

Some promising results, however, come from the clinical application of strict naturopathic principles to Parkinson's disease. Like so many other difficult-to-understand degenerative diseases, a drastic lifestyle change and internal detoxification often have shown remarkable results. With so much to gain and absolutely nothing to lose, the naturopathic approach given below should be tried for at least 6 months to 1 year, or longer. The only side effect will be improved health.

The treatment of Parkinsonism is best managed by or with a neurologist, or well-trained internist, and the patient *must* be referred if the symptoms persist or worsen.

Treatment

Begin therapy with a hair analysis test and any allergy tests available. Specifically test favorite foods.

Diet

It is always best to begin any treatment of a serious degenerative disease with an initial period of rebuilding. The best rejuvenation regimen in these cases is the raw foods lacto-vegetarian diet. This includes unlimited fruits, vegetables (especially greens), vegetable juice (carrot), seaweeds, sprouted grains, raw seeds (i.e., sunflower, pumpkin), and yoghurt. The object of this diet is to supply an abundance of vitamins, minerals, trace elements, essential fatty acids, and proteins to replenish the weakened body and strengthen the general vitality.

After this rejuvenation regimen is followed for a period of 4 to 6 weeks the patient will be ready for his or her first major elimination, which takes the form of a 7-to-14-day vegetable juice fast emphasizing carrot, beet, and green vegetable juice combinations. *Spirulina* or wheat grass juice may also be added. Enemas should be taken on days 1, 2, 3, 5, 7, etc. This fast is broken by 1 to 2 days on grated apple and yoghurt and followed by a diet similar to the initial rejuvenation regimen, with the addition of seafoods. Shellfish are not allowed, only small ocean reef fish. It is essential to obtain organically grown foods whenever possible, and to avoid all canned, frozen, preserved, or otherwise poisoned or devitalized foods. Over the next 6 to 12 months alternate this rejuvenation diet with periods of fasting for 3 to 7 days every 4 to 6 weeks.

Physiotherapy

- Alternate hot and cold showers
- Alternate hot and cold head douches
- Saunas followed by massage and spinal therapy
- Outdoor exercise
- Sun and ocean baths
- Wet cell appliance (gold)—(Cayce product)

Therapeutic Agents

VITAMINS AND MINERALS

Vitamin A: 25,000 IU one to two times per day. *Use any dose of vitamin A over 50,000 IU per day with medical supervision only.*

Vitamin B complex: 50 mg two to three times per day.*

---

*Asterisks indicate the most frequently used therapeutic agents.

Vitamin B₁

Vitamin B₃: 100 to 500 mg per day.

Vitamin B₆: 150 mg to 2 g per day (Do not take B₆ if you are taking L-dopa, since it will interfere with its action).

Vitamin B₁₂: 1000 mcg intramuscularly one to two times per week.

Vitamin C: 500 to 2000 mg three to four times per day.*

Vitamin E: 400 IU two to three times per day.*

Essential fatty acids: Use GLA or oil of evening primrose.*

Zinc: 25 to 50 mg one to two times per day.

Magnesium: 400 to 500 mg per day.*

Calcium: 800 to 1000 mg per day.*

Manganese*

Selenium: 100 to 200 mcg per day.

OTHERS

Lecithin: As concentrated phosphatidylcholine, 4 capsules three to four times per day, or more.*

Note: If you are currently taking L-dopa, do not stop, and do not take vitamin B₆ in large doses since it will interfere with its action.

Raw pituitary tablets

Raw adrenal tablets*

Raw brain tablets

Tranquil forte (Seroyal)

Kelp: two to three times per day

See Heavy Metal Poisoning if aluminum toxicity is a factor.

PEPTIC ULCER (Gastric Ulcer, Duodenal Ulcer)

Definition

A circumscribed erosion of the mucous membrane of the stomach and/or duodenum.

*Asterisks indicate the most frequently used therapeutic agents.

Gastric Ulcer: Usually found on the lesser curvature of the stomach.
Duodenal Ulcer: Usually occurs on the duodenal side of the pyloric region.
Peptic Ulcer: A common name for either of the above. The word "peptic"
comes from the enzyme pepsin, which digests protein.

Symptoms

Localized gnawing, burning pain (the pointing sign), heartburn, local tenderness, pain referred to the interscapular area, nausea, vomiting, diarrhea. Pains
are related to food. Duodenal pain comes on 2 to 4 hours after meals and is
relieved by food. Patient wakes around 2 to 4 A.M. with pain. Gastric ulcer
begins just after eating, or within twenty minutes.

Etiologic Considerations

• Refined diet: Protein stripping of carbohydrates (acts as buffer to stomach).

• Improper diet: Coffee, tea, tobacco all stimulate excess acid production. Highly
  seasoned and fried foods stimulate acid production. Excess sweets cause excess
  acid; overconsumption of sweets with no protein buffer a factor.

• Acidosis: Excess acid and/or decreased mucus protection.

• Stress upsets normal digestive process.

• Constipation
    Gastric stresses
    Chronic purging

• Chronic gastritis plus indigestion
    Reflux of bile
    Alcoholism
    Low blood sugar
    Anemia (iron deficiency)
    Aspirin
    Steroids
    Parasites
    Spinal, T4 to T9

• Food allergy

Discussion

The long-held view that the primary causes of ulcers are excess acid and
stress is losing favor. While these factors often are present in many patients and
may be contributing factors, it is becoming increasingly obvious that improper
dietary habits are the primary cause in nearly all ulcer patients. Although na-

turopaths for years have stressed the importance of an unrefined diet in preventing disease, it took the efforts of a medical doctor, Dr. T. L. Cleave, to present these ideas in a form acceptable at least to a significant minority of the scientific medical community. Although I feel Dr. Cleave's insights into the causation of peptic ulcer and what he coins "the saccharine diseases," that is, diabetes, coronary heart disease, diverticulitis, obesity, and dental caries, are incomplete, they explain the role of diet and the refining of carbohydrates in the causation of peptic ulcers quite clearly.

Studies of the African Zulus of Natal, Ethiopian peasants, and natives on the Gold Coast in Africa (Ghana), where the incidence of peptic ulcers was exceedingly low or nonexistent, led Dr. Cleave to conclude that the main dietary difference between these people and ourselves is that we generally tend to eat highly processed, refined foods rather than whole grain foods. Refined foods such as white rice and white flour are all made by removing the outside germ and bran of the whole grain. This leaves mostly carbohydrate, or starch. The germ and bran, however, contain a large amount of fiber and protein. These are very important in normal digestion, as we will soon see, and also contain valuable minerals and vitamins necessary for good health.

During digestion the stomach produces hydrochloric acid which provides the proper conditions for the enzyme pepsin to break down protein in foods. The stomach itself is protected by a mucous layer, also made up of much protein. Normally, the stomach acid does not affect the stomach wall and digests only foods. The protein in our diet helps protect us from the acid in our stomach, where it acts as a buffer. This is the main reason many doctors advise a high-protein milk diet for people with ulcers. The protein in milk helps, temporarily, to neutralize or buffer the stomach acid, and gives relief from ulcer pains. Refined grains, which have lost their outer coverings, no longer contain such a large amount of protein, so that when white rice or white bread is consumed, the stomach is exposed to much acid and very little protecting protein. If this is done repeatedly for a period of months or years, the stomach slowly gets eaten away and an ulcer is the result. Coffee, tea, cigarettes, and alcohol may also aggravate this condition since each of these stimulates hydrochloric acid production.

The protein stripping of carbohydrates is even more of a problem when we consider the enormous consumption of sugary sweets in the civilized nations today. Unlike wheat, which may have lost 30 percent of its protein contents in refining, these products are completely devoid of all buffering protein. The result of their use is the stimulation of acid production for digestion, with literally nothing to be digested, except of course the stomach or duodenal walls!

Other factors in our civilized nations also affect digestion. Stress certainly is a factor, in conjunction with a refined diet, causing digestion to halt and allowing food and digestive juices to lie for long periods in the stomach. The parasympathetic nervous system, which is responsible for the function of the digestive organs, ceases to act when the sympathetic nervous system, which is very responsive to danger and stress, is stimulated. This is the main reason all naturopaths emphasize eating only when relaxed and stress-free. Overeating or eating when not really hungry will cause indigestion and predispose a person to gastritis and ulcers. The peristaltic movements are decreased and gastric emptying time is increased.

Certainly all the other Etiologic Considerations have their influence, but diet, as you can see, plays the major role.

Treatment

Diet

There are no hard and fast rules in the dietary treatment of ulcers. Initial therapy depends on individual considerations, such as the severity of the ulcer, its duration, chronic or acute, vitality of the patient, weight, previous ulcer diets, dependency on antacid medication, etc. In general, if the patient has not already lost much weight a period of liquid dieting is very useful. This allows the ulcer to heal, especially if the liquids used are all specifically prescribed with this aim in mind. The fast may continue anywhere from 3 to 21 days, depending on the case. The following liquids have been found especially beneficial:

Stage 1:

- Cabbage juice contains metioninic acid and other undiscovered ingredients. This juice helps to normalize the mucous membrane in both stomach and duodenum. Drink four to five 6-to-8-oz glasses of half fresh cabbage juice and half celery or carrot juice daily.*
- Comfrey tea (*Symphytum officinale*) contains allantoin, a cell proliferant. The tea is very mucilaginous.*
- Slippery elm tea (*Ulmus fulva*) soothes and heals mucous membranes. Also very mucilaginous.*
- Carrageen moss tea
- Licorice root decoction (*Glycyrrhiza glabra*)*
- Carrot, celery, and cabbage juice*
- Marshmallow decoction
- Raw potato juice
- Alfalfa tea

*Asterisks indicate the most frequently used therapeutic agents.

- American saffron tea
- Potassium broth
- Fenugreek tea or decoction heals and soothes inflamed mucous membranes. *

Stage 2:

This liquid diet should then be followed by the introduction of nourishing, easily digested foods, such as the Concord grape and raw goat's milk diet, taken at frequent intervals. The previous liquids in stage 1 are also continued in this diet. The following foods are useful at this stage if introduced slowly:

Ripe banana	Okra
Raw goat's milk	Parsnips
Beef juice	Baked apples
Cooked carrots	Soy milk
Papaya	Raw goat's yoghurt
Avocado	Raw egg
Yams	Gelatin

After this interim diet, finely grated raw vegetables are added to the regimen, as well as thoroughly cooked grains. The emphasis at this stage, as with previous diets, is to completely masticate each mouthful until it is liquefied; even liquids should be "chewed."

Physiotherapy

- Trunk or abdominal packs
- Ice compress (for hemorrhage)
- Hot moist compress (for pain, apply front and back)
- Spinal
    T4 to T9
- Avoid
    Sugar
    Refined foods
    Refined grains
    Alcohol

*Asterisks indicate the most frequently used therapeutic agents.

Gum
Chocolate
Nicotine
Tea
Coffee
Salt
Hot spices
Red meats

Therapeutic Agents

VITAMINS AND MINERALS

Use with discretion, depending on case. Be careful with their introduction. As with all ulcer prescriptions, *go slow.*

Vitamin A (micellized): 10,000 to 25,000 IU four to six times per day. *Use any dose of vitamin A over 50,000 IU per day with medical supervision only.**

Vitamin B complex (liquid): 50 mg two to three times per day. Intramuscular B complex and B_{12} in early stages

Vitamin C (buffered): Dose depends on condition and response to use.*

Bioflavonoids

Pantothenic acid

Vitamin E: 200 to 400 IU two to three times daily.*

Zinc: 25 to 50 mg two to three times per day.

Iron

OTHERS

Duodenal substance: 1 to 2 tablets with meals.*

Essential amino acids

Glutamine: 1.5 to 2 g per day.

Kelp

Pancreatic enzymes

Roberts Formula (Seroyal)

Spirulina: 1 tsp three times daily.*

*Asterisks indicate the most frequently used therapeutic agents.

BOTANICALS

Aloe (*Aloe vera*): Use fresh juice. 1 to 1.5 oz two to three times per day.

American saffron (*Carthamus tinctorius*)

Comfrey (*Symphytum officinale*)

Geranium (*Pelargonium* spp.): Bleeding ulcer.

Goldenseal (*Hydrastis canadensis*)

Licorice (*Glycyrrhiza glabra*): De-glycerinated.*

Marshmallow (*Althaea officinalis*)

Myrrh (*Commiphora myrrha*)

Plantain (*Plantago lanceolata*)

Pokeroot (*Phytolacca decandra*) (highly toxic; see p. 62)

Slippery elm (*Ulmus fulva*): Demulcent; ½ tsp in warm water four to six times per day.*

White oak bark (*Quercus alba*)

Therapeutic Suggestions

I usually do not advise any nutritional supplements in the early stages and rely on diet changes and mild demulcent herbs such as slippery elm. Later, as the condition improves, I advise supplements according to need. Intramuscular vitamins are useful in early stages and in severe cases. Vitamin C intravenously also may be useful to accelerate healing. Severe cases with blood in the stool; severe anemia; black, tarry stools; or severe epigastric or back pain should be referred to a sympathetic M.D.

PHLEBITIS AND THROMBOPHLEBITIS

Definition

Phlebitis: Irritation and inflammation of a vein.
Thrombophlebitis: The presence of a thrombus (clot) in a vein with irritation of the vein wall.

*Asterisks indicate the most frequently used therapeutic agents.

Symptoms

May be symptomless or show redness, edema, tenderness, heaviness, aching, slight fever, embolism. Sudden death is possible.

Etiologic Considerations

- Blood stasis
  Prolonged sitting
  Prolonged bed rest
  Inactivity
- Heart disease
- Allergy
- Obesity
- Varicosities
- Fracture
- Postsurgical
- Debility
- Injury to endothelium of blood vessels
  Trauma
  Intravenous lines
  Bacteria
  Chemicals
- Excess animal-based protein and saturated fat diet
- Increased coagulation of blood
  Oral contraceptives
  Malignancy
- Toxemia
- Pregnancy
  Enlarging fetus may cause pressure on blood vessels, reducing flow.
- Smoking may lead to vasoconstriction.
- Stress may lead to vasoconstriction.

Discussion

Phlebitis and thrombophlebitis are extremely serious conditions. A clot in a vein tends to form at areas of irregularity, trauma, or inflammation due to injury, intravenous lines, bacteria, or irritating chemicals. It begins as dense layers of platelets and fibrin, and later may become a large, friable, jellylike mass, which may break off to form an embolism, or free-floating body in the bloodstream. Embolisms may travel to the lungs, heart, or brain and occlude small blood vessels, which may have disastrous and even fatal results. Thrombophlebitis most commonly develops in the deep veins of the lower leg, but it may occur elsewhere.

Conditions causing blood stasis, which allows a thrombus to propagate, are the major causes of thrombophlebitis. Faster-moving blood helps to clear the blood vessels effectively and helps prevent thrombus formation. Postsurgical or postpartum thrombophlebitis is particularly common. Any other condition that restricts blood flow, such as prolonged bed rest, sitting, inactivity, obesity, varicosities, or heart disease may be a contributing factor.

The use of oral contraceptives has now been recognized as carrying an increased risk of thrombophlebitis and embolism. For some as yet unknown reason many malignancies show an increased coagulation of blood, causing an increased chance of thrombus formation.

A little-recognized factor, but extremely important, is the influence of toxicity in the bloodstream. This factor, along with nutritional deficiency, is probably the primary cause of the phlebitis in the first place. The worst combination of factors is a nutritionally deficient, toxic bloodstream in a sedentary individual who smokes cigarettes and is under stress.

Treatment

All cases of phlebitis and thrombophlebitis must be under the care of a physician. They are serious and possibly life-threatening problems, not to be taken lightly.

Diet

The main dietary aims are elimination and blood cleansing. Begin with a 3-to-7-day fast on citrus juice (grapefruit) and vegetable juice (carrot and others). Nightly enemas should be taken. For those unable to fast the all fruit diet (see Appendix I) will be adequate. The initial fast is followed by a raw foods diet still stressing citrus and carrot juice, but also including a large amount of green salads and sprouts. The basic diet should be as follows:

On Rising	Hot water and lemon
Breakfast	Grapefruit
Midmorning	Carrot juice

Lunch	Mixed raw green salad with plenty of sprouted seeds and beans, and a large portion of steamed onions.
Midafternoon	Carrot juice
Supper	As lunch

Five to 10 days on this gentle blood-cleansing regimen should help alleviate the problem. This diet is followed by an unsaturated fat vegetarian diet, stressing citrus, green vegetables, sunflower seeds, soy protein (lecithin), and whole grains, until the condition is completely removed. Absolutely no sugar, refined carbohydrates, fried foods, coffee, tea, alcohol, or cigarettes should be taken during this regimen.

Physiotherapy

- Alternate hot and cold compresses and showers
- Hot Epsom salts baths (see Appendix I)
- Mild exercise
- Papaya poultice
- Mullein tea poultice
- Plantain and witch hazel poultice
- Elevate foot of bed 4 in. (if thrombosis is in leg)
- Avoid
  Crossing legs
  Prolonged sitting
  Inactivity
  Constipation
  Garters, girdles, or restrictive clothing

Therapeutic Agents

VITAMINS AND MINERALS

Vitamin A: 25,000 IU two times per day. *Use any dose of vitamin A over 50,000 IU per day with medical supervision only.* *

Vitamin B complex: 50 mg two to three times per day. *

Niacin: 200 to 600 mg per day (helps dissolve fibrin). *

Pantothenic acid: 100 mg per day. *

Rutin: 100 to 200 mg per day. *

*Asterisks indicate the most frequently used therapeutic agents.

Vitamin C: 6 to 10 g per day; helps keep capillaries strong. *

Bioflavonoids*

Vitamin E: 400 IU two to three times per day. With adequate calcium it is an antithrombic agent. Helps strengthen blood vessels. *

Essential fatty acids (linoleic acid): Use GLA or oil of evening primrose; helps decrease adhesiveness of platelets.

OTHERS

Bromelain

Chlorophyll

Garlic: 2 capsules three times per day. *

Lecithin: 3 to 4 capsules four times per day (helps inhibit clotting). *

Orthophosphoric acid: Blood thinner. *

Raw spleen: Anticoagulant. *

Wheat germ oil

BOTANICALS

Comfrey (*Symphytum officinale*): Poultice.

Mullein tea (*Verbascum thapsus*): Internal.

Plantain (*Plantago lanceolata*): Poultice.

Note: The above therapies are mostly for use with superficial venous thrombophlebitis. Phlebothrombosis of a deep vein is a life-threatening situation and requires treatment in an inpatient facility.

PILES (see Hemorrhoids)

POISON IVY

Definition and Symptoms

A contact dermatitis resulting from irritation of the skin by the resin of the poison ivy plant. Within hours, or sometimes several days, the skin begins to itch or burn, followed by the eruption of small blisters which may coalesce to

*Asterisks indicate the most frequently used therapeutic agents.

cover large portions of the body. As the vesicles rupture, crusting forms, overlying a raw, oozing surface.

Treatment

Wash skin with antiseptic soap as soon after exposure as possible. Apply antipruritic skin lotions such as calamine lotion. Cooling compresses with cold water and vinegar are very useful every 1 to 2 hours. A bath in potassium permanganate may help relieve itching, as will oatmeal baths. A plaster of baking soda moistened with water is also useful. Other treatments include plantain poultices and *Hydrastis* infusion wash. *Rhus toxicodendron* and *Urtica urens* tinctures taken internally at frequent intervals will shorten the course of the rash. Salt-water swimming is very effective therapy.

Therapeutic Agents

VITAMINS AND MINERALS

Vitamin A: 25,000 to 50,000 IU one to two times per day.

Vitamin B complex: 50 mg two times per day.

Vitamin C: 1 g per hour.

Zinc: 25 to 50 mg two to three times per day.

OTHERS

Chlorophyll: Bowel detoxicant.

Raw adrenal: 2 tablets three times per day.

PREMENSTRUAL TENSION SYNDROME

Definition and Symptoms

A cyclic condition related to the menstrual cycle, characterized by tension, irritability, sudden mood swings, depression, hostility, emotional disturbances, anxiety, crying, lack of energy, sleeping difficulties, headaches, sinusitis, vertigo, faintness, fluid retention, swelling and soreness of breasts, abdominal bloating, abdominal cramps, acne flare, or craving for sweets or alcohol. Onset is usually 4 to 10 days prior to menstruation and ends abruptly after onset of flow.

Etiologic Considerations

- Hypoglycemia
  Excess sweets
  Excess coffee, tea, soda, chocolates, alcohol

- Essential fatty acid deficiency
- B complex deficiency
- Vitamin B$_6$ deficiency
- Magnesium deficiency
- Stress
  Adrenal exhaustion
  Stress-induced hypoglycemia
  Vitamin B deficiency
- Birth control pills (fibrocystic breast disorder)
- Vitamin C deficiency
- Glandular imbalance
  Estrogen excess
  Progesterone deficiency
- Water retention
- Lead or copper toxicity

Discussion

The premenstrual tension syndrome has been recognized for centuries. The fact that *some* women go through varying degrees of emotional volatility prior to their menstrual flow has been used as an excuse by some employers to exclude women as unfit for critical, high-responsibility, "level-headed" executive jobs.

Most sufferers of severe premenstrual tension are well aware that they have a serious problem. The cyclic outbreaks of uncontrolled emotions cause great distress to other family members and are often a source of deep remorse once the "witch cycle" is passed. Many women readers may be bristling with animosity toward me at this point. I think it fair to mention very early in this discussion that certainly not all women suffer from the premenstrual syndrome, and of those that do, many experience only the physiological symptoms and not the more advertised psychological ones. Much evidence, however, does support the fact that these psychological symptoms do exist for some women. The highest number of violent crimes committed by women occur in the premenstrual period, 4 to 7 days prior to menstruation. This period is the peak for women being admitted to both prison and psychiatric institutions. There also is an increased percent of female accidents and suicide attempts during this part of the menstrual cycle. Brain waves in the premenstrual period are increased in frequency and amplitude compared to those of midcycle, another indication of a true psychological alteration.

For years premenstrual tension was considered to be entirely psychosomatic in origin. Later authorities gave women a little more consideration and blamed the condition on the normally fluctuating female hormones, estrogen and progesterone. Although the exact role of these hormones in causing common premenstrual symptoms is as yet not clearly defined, certain overall patterns have emerged in PMS patients. The female hormone estrogen has been found elevated in the late luteal phase, reaching its maximal point 1 to 5 days before menstruation. By contrast, progesterone in PMS patients shows a reduction in the mid-luteal phase, compared to non-PMS control subjects, reaching its lowest relative deficiency 5 to 10 days before menstruation. Other studies have implicated increased levels of follicle-stimulating hormone (FSH), aldosterone, and prolactin. Of these hormone abnormalities, those most significantly associated with the symptoms of PMS seem to be the late luteal estrogen excess, and mid-luteal progesterone deficiency.

Although repeated studies show a correlation between elevated estrogen and elevated estrogen/progesterone ratios with premenstrual anxiety, irritability, and depression, the actual mechanism by which these hormonal changes influence moods and how they may interrelate with known micronutrient deficiencies is still unclear. We know that elevated estrogens interact with brain enzymes to cause an elevation of adrenalin, which is known to trigger anxiety; with noradrenalin, known to promote hostility and irritability; and with serotonin, which helps cause nervous tension, fluid retention, and inability to concentrate. Dopamine, which is believed to balance the effects of these three amines by enhancing relaxation and mental alertness, is found to be at reduced levels.*

Irrespective of exactly which hormone or combination of hormones, vitamins, and minerals initiates the physiological or even psychological symptoms of premenstrual tension, the usual implication being made is that "women are just made that way." In other words, women are designed by nature as intellectually and emotionally unstable creatures due to their "normal" hormone fluctuations and that is all there is to it.

Obviously, this explanation is incorrect. It completely fails to explain why some women have severe premenstrual symptoms while others have mild or even no symptoms whatsoever. I do not doubt that this syndrome is mediated by one or more of the female hormones described above. Whatever the glandular "cause," which as yet is still not specifically known, the general condition of premenstrual tension is due to a hormone imbalance and this imbalance, like most other imbalances within the body, is due, I feel, to an improper mode of living. Hypoglycemia, stress, and nutritional deficiency due to improper diet seem to be the main factors causing this hormonal imbalance.

Hypoglycemia, caused by an improper diet of refined carbohydrates, sweets, pastries, coffee, and alcohol, is well known to cause bouts of emotional instability and clouded thought. PMS patients have been shown to consume more refined

*Piesse, John, "Nutrition Factors in the Premenstrual Syndrome," *International Clinical Nutrition Review*, 4(2):54–81, 1984.

carbohydrates and two-and-one-half times the amount of refined sugar than normal non-PMS controls.† It is not the hypoglycemic state itself that causes premenstrual tension. Low blood sugar affects the individual in relation to food, and not the menstrual cycle. Its symptoms disappear after food is eaten and are never prolonged for days on end. What hypoglycemia does, however, is to overburden the adrenal glands as they struggle to keep up with the roller-coaster ride of the drastically fluctuating blood sugar level. This is significant for several reasons. The adrenal glands require large amounts of vitamin B complex and vitamin C, among other nutrients, to maintain their functioning. They literally burn off a great deal of the body's supply of these vitamins when overstressed, depriving the rest of the body of these essential substances at the same time. The typical diet that produces hypoglycemia in the first place is composed of highly refined carbohydrates which are stripped of their B complex in the refining process. Vitamin B complex in turn is essential for carbohydrate metabolism. Thus we have a vicious cycle of B complex-deficient foods consumed in excess that require B complex for metabolism (therefore B complex must be obtained from elsewhere in the body for this purpose), producing hypoglycemia, creating adrenal exhaustion. The adrenals in turn require excessive amounts of B complex for their own function. If we now couple this catastrophic scenario with habitual consumption of coffee and alcohol, both of which further stimulate the adrenal glands violently and deplete B complex even further, we begin to see why B complex and B_6 in particular have been found useful to some degree in preventing and treating premenstrual tension.

Stress-induced adrenal exhaustion is another common finding in these cases. If severe, this may even lead to stress-induced hypoglycemia. Stress also is important since emotions play such a strong role in the female endocrine system, affecting first the hypothalamus, then pituitary, ovaries, and adrenal glands. Prolonged stress is also known to cause a relative dopamine deficiency. The combination of improper diet and stress is the most detrimental of all.

All of this abuse to the adrenal glands has particular importance in relation to hormonal balance. The adrenal glands also function as a backup for the ovaries, producing about 20 percent of the total estrogens.

Several other nutritional factors have been associated with this symptom. PMS patients consume four-and-one-half times more dairy products than normal controls. This correlation is interesting since it is known that saturated (animal) fats inhibit the formation of PGE_1, an anti-inflammatory prostaglandin found deficient in PMS women. PGE_1 synthesis is also inhibited by *trans* fatty acids as found in processed or heat-treated vegetable oils and margarine, alcohol, and stress-induced catecholamines. Animal fats also contain large amounts of arachidonic acid, which acts as a precursor to PGE_2, PGF_2, and thromboxane, which function antagonistically to PGE_1. This may be the reason that sources

†Ibid., pp. 66–67.

rich in cis-linoleic acid and gamma-linolenic acid (GLA), such as oil of evening primrose, which enhance PGE_1 production, have been found useful therapeutically with PMS.

Magnesium deficiency is also associated with PMS and is known to cause a depletion of brain dopamine levels. Erythrocyte magnesium levels taken from PMS patients in the mid-luteal phase have been shown to be significantly lower than in control groups. Magnesium and zinc are required for the synthesis of PGE_1, from the cis-linoleic acid pathway. Magnesium deficiency may result from lack of whole grains and vegetables in the diet, or may be the result of stress-induced adenocorticoid secretion, or prolonged diuretic use.

Interestingly, the supplementation of vitamin B_6 (pyridoxine) has been reported to normalize low erythrocyte magnesium levels. B_6 deficiency may also be a factor in low dopamine levels, since this vitamin acts as a cofactor in dopamine biosynthesis.

Other neuroactive substances that are vitamin B_6-dependent are alpha-aminobutyric acid, a brain neurotransmitter producing sedation, as well as serotonin and tryptophan. The earliest reports that vitamin B_6 therapy was useful in PMS were found in relation to women on the birth control pill, which is known to be associated with vitamin B_6 deficiency. Later studies showed its effectiveness with many PMS patients not previously on oral contraceptives. Still other reports found that vitamin B_6 was not as effective for some of the class of PMS patients whose symptoms were primarily depression. In cases where an acne flare occurring premenstrually was a symptom, vitamin B_6 was found to be up to 72 percent effective. Once again, the precise therapeutic mode of action of vitamin B_6 is not yet clear. Preliminary findings demonstrate that it increases mid-luteal serum progesterone and reduces elevated estrogen levels. It is suspected that B complex deficiencies, and in particular vitamin B_6 deficiency, may cause a lowered hepatic clearance of estrogen, causing an elevated serum level to occur.

Another very interesting nutritional factor related to PMS is the use of essential fatty acids. In double-blind placebo trials, oil of evening primrose has been proven effective in significantly relieving PMS symptoms. The postulated mode of action is the enhanced synthesis of PGE_1 from the increased supply of cis-linoleic and gamma-linolenic acid.

Vitamin E has also been found useful in the treatment of PMS with most improvement in cases where benign breast disease was a major problem. Vitamin E plays a role as antioxidant, and may help prevent adverse inflammatory reactions to dietary fats by preventing rancidity. Vitamin E may also play a role by inhibiting the formation of PGE-antagonist derived from the arachidonic acid found in animal fats. Other antioxidants, such as vitamin C or selenium, may play a role, as well as vitamin A and zinc.*

Piesse, John, op. cit., pp. 54–81.

Treatment

Diet

The most effective dietary regimen will be an integration of the diet regimens found under Hypoglycemia and Heart Disease. These emphasize elimination or drastic reduction of refined carbohydrates and simple sugars, a reduction of animal-based proteins, and an increase in unrefined whole grains and essential fatty acids. This diet combination is aimed at normalizing the blood sugar level, healing the overburdened adrenal glands, and providing a proper supply of vitamins, minerals, trace elements, and essential fatty acids. It is important to exclude coffee, tea, cola, chocolate, salt, alcohol, cigarettes, and heated or processed oils from the diet.

Stress Reduction

Even a good diet will not totally protect the body from the devastating effects of prolonged stress. Stress is often the result of an improper attitude or approach to life and its problems (challenges). Many times I hear patients say that they simply have no time to devote to relaxation exercises or meditation, even when they recognize stress as a real health problem. This attitude comes from a completely inappropriate value system and lack of self-knowledge.

One of the most valuable assets a person can have in life is the ability to be relaxed, poised, and centered. This "centering" or concentration can bring even the most difficult of tasks within your capabilities. To obtain and maintain this desirable state of being, a certain amount of effort and time is required; however, the effort, time, and energy *saved* throughout your day by more efficient and productive action more than compensates for this expenditure. In reality, most people waste a phenomenal amount of time and energy each day. Fifteen or 20 minutes once or twice a day devoted to relaxation exercises or meditation can be set aside by even the busiest person. The truth of the matter usually is that people have the time, but have so little control of their thoughts, feelings, and actions that they are *unable* to sit quietly, until completely exhausted by their day. This is all the more reason to begin disciplining the mind.

You will find a list of relaxation exercises under Insomnia. These are very useful in stress reduction, as are many forms of meditation.

Physiotherapy

• Spinal manipulation: Once weekly for 4 to 6 weeks and then once or twice per month until two normal premenstrual tensionless months pass.

• General exercise: Exercise helps stimulate and regulate the hormonal system. It also helps reduce stress.

- Outdoor fresh air walks and sun baths
- Ocean swimming

Therapeutic Agents

VITAMINS AND MINERALS

Vitamin A: 10,000 to 20,000 IU per day; 40,000 to 100,000 IU 10 days premenstrually in difficult cases. *Use any dose of vitamin A over 50,000 IU per day with medical supervision only.**

Vitamin B complex: 50 mg two to three times per day.*

Vitamin B$_6$: 250 mg two times per day, especially when an acne flare occurs with the premenstrual tension syndrome. Also used for its diuretic characteristics when fluid retention problems are severe.*

Vitamin C: 1000 to 2000 mg three times daily or more to bowel tolerance.*

Vitamin E: 400 IU two to three times per day.*

Calcium lactate or chelate: two or three times daily (total 800 mg).*

Magnesium: 400 mg one to three times per day.*

Zinc: 25 to 50 mg per day.*

Others, as found under Hypoglycemia.

OTHERS

Brewer's yeast*

Desiccated liver*

Oil of evening primrose: 1 g three times per day.* GLA may also be used.

EPA (eicosapentaenoic acid): 5 to 10 g per day.*

Parsley tablets: Diuretic.

Raw adrenal tablets*

Raw ovary tablets*

Raw pituitary tablets*

Tryptophan: with depression
Reduce liquids premenstrually

No coffee, tea, cola, chocolate, sugar, or refined carbohydrates.

No alcohol until cured, then only in moderation.

*Asterisks indicate the most frequently used therapeutic agents.

Salt: Fluid retention is the major cause of physiological symptoms. Avoid salt-containing foods such as dried fish, dried meats, soy sauce, hot dogs, pickles, salted popcorn, monosodium glutamate (MSG), cheese, bacon, ham, canned foods, butter, salted nuts, etc.

BOTANICALS

Licorice (*Glycyrrhiza glabra*)

Parsley (*Petroselinum sativum*): Diuretic

Watermelon seed (*Citrullus vulgaris*): Diuretic, use infusion of seeds

Therapeutic Suggestion

When fibrocystic breast disease is present with PMS, it is essential to stop *all* coffee and use high levels of GLA (gamma-linolenic acid) as found in evening primrose oil, vitamin E, and vitamin B_6.

PROSTATE: Benign Prostatic Hypertrophy and Prostatitis

Definition

Benign prostatic hypertrophy: Enlarged prostate gland.
Prostatitis: Inflamed, swollen prostate usually due to infection. May be acute or chronic.

Symptoms

Dysuria (painful urination), painful defecation, frequency of urination, inability to empty bladder fully, desire to urinate, incontinence of urine, possible fever, impotence, back pain, painful orgasm.

Etiologic Considerations

• Cancer must always be considered first, to exclude this as a possibility.

• Diet: Too little alkaline foods, constipation, too little fiber, excess alcohol, tea, coffee, spices, essential fatty acid deficiency, zinc deficiency.

• Congestion: Sluggish bowels, poor lymph and blood flow, toxicity of blood, poor abdominal tone.

• Sedentary occupation

• Lack of exercise

- Spinal lesions
- Excess exposure to cold surfaces
- Infection
  Gonorrhea
  Foci spread from elsewhere

Discussion

The prostate gland, present only in males, secretes a lubricating fluid which forms the bulk of spermatic fluid and aids in the transport of sperm. Not only is surgical treatment of an enlarged prostate very uncomfortable, the removal of the prostate can disrupt sex life for some people and should be resorted to as a last alternative. Fortunately, in the majority of cases many alternatives to surgery exist, which help to relieve the symptoms and slowly remove the basic causes.

In this discussion we must differentiate between benign prostatic hypertrophy and prostatitis. Prostatitis may be the result of infection. This infection can be caused by gonorrhea or may be caused by spread of infection from a foci elsewhere in the body, such as the teeth. Benign hypertrophy has multiple causes, and it is for this condition that natural therapies are the most effective.

Internal congestion is a major cause of an enlarged prostate, caused by poor abdominal tone and constipation, sluggish lymph and blood flow due to lack of exercise or a sedentary occupation, and a toxic condition of the blood. Dietary factors influence this congestive toxic state, and further add dietary deficiency to the list.

Much evidence has been reported linking essential fatty acids, vitamin B complex, and zinc deficiency with prostate disorders. As the circulation of lymph and blood is reduced in the area of the prostate due to a combination of any of the etiologic factors, the prostate becomes diseased and enlarged. This enlargement slowly puts pressure on various internal structures (especially the urethra, as it passes through the prostate gland itself) and causes the common symptoms of prostate disease. The bladder becomes increasingly more difficult to empty completely, and urinary retention may soon cause cystitis to further complicate the problem.

Treatment

Prostatitis due to gonorrhea should first be attended to with antibiotics. Once antibiotic therapy has been instituted, the general health of the prostate may be improved through many of the same therapies used for a condition of benign hypertrophy. The main contraindication is that prostatic massage should *not* be used in cases of acute prostatitis due to gonorrhea or other infection.

Benign prostatic hypertrophy should always be treated generally, as well as locally. The various causes must be removed and reversed to allow as full a recovery as possible.

Diet

The diet should be a high-fiber, noncitrus, alkaline-reacting diet, containing large amounts of raw green vegetables, essential fatty acids, and zinc. The fiber content will help correct habitual constipation and adding 1 tbs raw bran to each meal further aids in this process.

Essential fatty acids as found in cold pressed unrefined vegetable oils such as sunflower, safflower, and sesame should be included in the diet regularly. Nuts and seeds are also important sources.

Zinc foods such as oysters, herrings, clams, wheat and rice bran, wheat germ, molasses, eggs, nuts, pumpkin seeds, peas, carrots, corn, beans, brown rice, garlic, onions, and brewer's yeast should be included in the diet whenever possible. Due to the unreliability of present food sources of zinc, however, additional zinc supplements will also be needed.

It is wise to begin the dietary regimen with an internal cleansing regimen, the length and severity depending on the patient. The apple mono diet is an ideal cleansing regimen in this condition and involves eating four meals of organic apples and drinking diluted (50/50) apple juice and water periodically throughout the day when thirsty. This may be followed for 3 to 7 days or longer. 1 tbs cold pressed olive oil should be taken on the evening of the final day of this diet.

Internal massage to the prostate done by a physician will help reduce the swelling of the prostate, reduce acute retention problems, and help break down any fibrous buildup on and around the gland. This must be done repeatedly for proper results. (Note: This is contraindicated in acute prostatitis due to infection.)

Hydrotherapy

- Hot sitz baths are useful to help relieve pressure on the urethra and allow the bladder to empty fully. Chamomile tea may be added to the water to increase this effect. Used primarily in acute conditions.

- Hot compresses have an effect similar to the hot sitz bath, and are also used in acute conditions.

- Alternate hot and cold sitz baths are used to reduce congestion and increase circulation in a chronic condition, or just after the acute stage has reduced in severity.

- Alternate hot and cold perianal sponges are used with an effect similar to the hot and cold sitz baths, but are employed more in chronic conditions and as maintenance therapy, once cure has been established.

- Cold perianal sprays
- Ice-cold retention enemas
- Ice applied to perineum for pain in acute prostatitis

Physiotherapy

- Abdominal exercises to correct visceroptosis (a sagging condition of the internal organs due to weak musculature).

- Prostatic massage exercise: Lie on back with legs extended. Bend knees and hips to draw knees to chest. Spread knees apart and press soles of feet together firmly. Keep soles of feet pressed together firmly as you extend your legs to floor. Repeat 75 to 100 times per day.

- Spinal
  Lumbar
  Lumbosacral
  Sacral

- Sex life
  Avoid coitus interruptus
  Avoid prolonged intercourse
  Avoid abstinence
  Avoid excitation without natural climax

Therapeutic Agents

VITAMINS AND MINERALS

Vitamin A: 25,000 IU one to two times per day. Larger doses may be needed. *Use any dose of vitamin A over 50,000 IU per day with medical supervision only.* *

Vitamin B complex: 50 mg three times per day. *

Vitamin B$_6$: 50 to 100 mg two times per day.

Vitamin C: 1000 to 5000 mg per day or more. *

Vitamin E: 400 IU two to three times per day. *

Essential fatty acids: 2 to 4 capsules three to six times per day. *

Calcium: 800 to 1000 mg per day.

*Asterisks indicate the most frequently used therapeutic agents.

Magnesium: 400 to 500 mg per day.

Trace minerals

Zinc: 50 to 100 mg per day. At high doses this may interfere with proper zinc-to-copper ratio, and therefore 3 to 5 mg copper per day may be needed also.*

Selenium: 100 to 300 mcg per day.*

OTHERS

Bee pollen

Brewer's yeast

Chlorophyll

EPA (eicosapentaenoic acid): 2 to 4 capsules two to three times per day.

Evening primrose oil: 1 to 2 capsules three times per day.*

Flaxseed oil: 6 to 10 g per day: high in linolenic acid.*

Garlic

Glutamic acid, glycine, and alanine (Prostol Rx): Three times per day.*

Kelp: 2 tablets three times per day.

Lecithin: 1 to 2 tbs one to two times per day, or in capsule form.

Pumpkin seeds: ¼ lb per day, every day.*

Raw prostate tablets: Two to three times per day.*

Raw thymus tablets

BOTANICALS

Bearberry (*Arctostaphylos uva-ursi*): Diuretic.*

Buchu (*Barosma betulina*): Diuretic.*

Couch grass (*Agropyrum repens*): Diuretic.*

Coneflower (*Echinacea angustifolium*): Anti-infective.

Fenugreek (*Trigonella foenumgraecum*): Tea soothes and cleanses mucous membrane of urinary tract.*

False unicorn root (*Helonias dioica*): Enlarged prostate.*

Geranium (*Pelargonium* spp.): Astringent.

Gravel root (*Eupatorium purpureum*): Diuretic.*

*Asterisks indicate the most frequently used therapeutic agents.

Juniper berries (*Juniperus communis*): Diuretic.*

Marshmallow (*Althaea officinalis*): Diuretic.

Parsley root (*Petroselinum* spp.): Diuretic.*

Saw palmetto (*Serenoa serrulata*)

Therapeutic Suggestions

This condition responds best to a high zinc, high essential fatty acid regimen [i.e., cod-liver oil, evening primrose oil, EPA (eicosapentaenoic acid), essential fatty acid capsules]. Prostol is recommended in all cases. High doses of vitamins A, B, C, and E, calcium and magnesium in a balance of 2:1 are used in all cases.

Botanicals are used primarily to relieve the uncomfortable symptoms in early stages, and as prostatic tonics later on. The alternate hot and cold sitz baths are an essential part of therapy.

PSORIASIS

Definition

A chronic relapsing skin disease.

Symptoms

Skin lesions with silvery scales found most frequently on knees, elbows, and scalp. However, any skin area may be involved, including the nails. The symptoms tend to flare up acutely with remissions. Arthritis in the smaller joints is commonly associated with psoriasis.

Etiologic Considerations

- Thinning of walls of small intestine, especially the jejunum or lower duodenum
- Poor eliminations
- Emotions may play a part
- Malfunction of liver, kidneys
- Excess meat-eating: Associated with the amino acid taurine
- Immunization aftereffects
- Possible copper excess and zinc deficiency
- Constipation

*Asterisks indicate the most frequently used therapeutic agents.

- Faulty diet
- Food allergy
- Acid/alkaline imbalance
- Faulty essential fatty acid utilization

Discussion

Psoriasis has been considered practically incurable by orthodox methods. Various external applications such as coal tar, zinc paste, tar plus ultraviolet light, and steroids have been advised for years, with little success. The latest treatment in severe cases is a combination of the drug methotrexate with special ultraviolet sessions. This therapy carries the severe danger of toxic effects to the liver and bone marrow, and although somewhat successful in the short term, must be repeated frequently due to remission.

The reason these methods all fail miserably to cure this tenacious disorder is that no attempt is made to remove its cause. This is primarily due to the fact that the cause is considered unknown. Psoriasis can never be cured by external applications without removing the cause. The real cause or causes of psoriasis are internal, not external, according to the Edgar Cayce readings. The most common factor seems to be a thinning of the small intestinal walls. This allows toxins to enter the circulation system and lymph, which set up irritations on the skin. This thinning may be due to constipation, faulty utilization of fats, food allergy, spinal lesions, malfunction of liver and kidneys, previous immunizations, candida overgrowth, or other factors.

Treatment of psoriasis takes much time and perseverance for the best results. Allergy tests such as RAST, cytotoxic, or pulse tests may reveal common foods that cause allergic reactions. Rotation diets, where suspected foods, especially grains, proteins, and any other suspected foods are not consumed more frequently than every 4 to 7 days, are also very useful to desensitize the individual. Milk and wheat may also act in ways other than true allergy by means of intestinal incompatibility or enzyme deficiency. It is wise to exclude these foods for 6 months, even if allergy tests are negative. Improper weaning to cow's milk and wheat is often a major cause.

Many naturopathic physicians have observed that previous immunizations seem to be another cause of allergic skin conditions, including eczema and psoriasis. Other drugs such as antibiotics can cause long-term allergic skin reactions.

Treatment

The aim of therapy is to remove conditions that result in a loss of intestinal villi with thinning of the bowel, to remove allergens and irritants from the diet, and to provide a diet and herbs that help soothe these delicate membranes. In most cases balancing the body fluids' pH (acid/alkaline ratio) is a major aim.

Diet

Food consumed should be primarily alkaline in reaction, with at least one meal per day consisting of raw vegetables. Yellow foods are especially useful in the long term. Soybeans, tofu, and lecithin are also very useful due to their cholesterol-lowering capabilities. In general, citrus fruits should be avoided, as well as tomatoes, red meats, saturated fats, hydrogenated fats, sweets, alcohol, pastry, or carbonated beverages. If food allergy is suspected, several tests are available to help confirm this. Some commonly offending foods are meat, wheat, eggs, citrus, and dairy products. These often are excluded in initial phases of the diet.

A good procedure with which to begin therapy is the 7-to-21-day vegetable juice fast, emphasizing carrot juice. With this, if possible, add ultragreen substances such as *Spirulina*. Therapeutic herb teas should be taken frequently in addition to the vegetable juices. These include slippery elm tea, mullein tea, and American saffron tea. During this fast enemas or colonics are to be taken and a series of colonics are to follow the fast, one to two times per week for 2 to 6 weeks, in some cases.

Following the initial fast, the high-fiber, high-raw-vegetable, no-acid, no-meat diet begins. Psoriasis sufferers seem to have extreme difficulty handling saturated fats and these should be reduced to a minimum or excluded entirely from the diet. These patients often have been found to have high serum cholesterol levels. Repeated fasts may be necessary to aid further recovery and correct the lesions of the small intestine. At all times eliminations must be kept regular. This may require herbal purification, colonics, and spinal manipulation to achieve permanent results. See section on Yeast Infection if this is a suspected cause.

Foods especially useful are:

Soy
Yellow foods
Green vegetables
Seaweeds
10-day brown rice diet

Physiotherapy

- Alternate hot and cold showers to stimulate the circulation.
- Castor oil packs: Apply to lower abdomen nightly for 45 minutes to 1½ hours. Use three to four thicknesses of undyed wool. Saturate this with castor oil and wring out lightly. This is then heated in a special pot used for this purpose

only. You may reuse the same cloth twenty to forty times. Just store in the pot and add more castor oil as needed with each use. This cloth is applied as hot as the body can bear to the area from the lower right rib border over the entire right side of the abdomen, down to just above the pubic bone. The pack is then covered with an oiled cloth or plastic and kept warm with a heating pad. If necessary, the bed may also be protected by plastic. After the application, wash the area with a weak solution of bicarbonate (1 tsp to 1 quart of warm water).

Hydrotherapy

• Ocean swims and sun: As often as possible.

• Ultraviolet light given in slightly burning doses in conjunction with diet and herbs is very successful in removing obstinate lesions. Expose areas daily until pink for 2 to 3 weeks. An ultraviolet lamp may also be used with care for isolated lesions. Be careful, however, not to overuse the ultraviolet lamp as skin cancer has been associated with chronic overexposure. A 2-to-5-week session, however, should have no harmful effects.

• Colonics

• Enemas

Spinal Manipulation

To correct constipation. Adjust midthoracic through sacral region, one to two times per week.

Therapeutic Agents

VITAMINS AND MINERALS

Vitamin A: 25,000 IU two times per day or more with supervision. *Use any dose of vitamin A over 50,000 IU per day with medical supervision only.* *

Vitamin B complex (yeast-free, if allergic to yeast): 25 to 50 mg two to three times per day. *

Vitamin B_{12}: 1 mg I.M. injection once weekly.

Folic acid: 25 to 75 mg per day. *

Vitamin C: Ascorbates may be tolerated best.

Essential fatty acids: 2 to 4 capsules GLA (gamma-linolenic acid) three times per day.

EPA (eicosapentaenoic acid): 2 to 4 capsules two to three times per day. *

*Asterisks indicate the most frequently used therapeutic agents.

Zinc: 25 to 50 mg three times per day (if bowel upset occurs, reduce dose).*

Oil of evening primrose: 1 to 2 capsules three times per day.*

Hydrochloric acid: 5 to 20 grains per meal if hypoacid.

OTHERS

Cod-liver oil: 2 to 4 capsules three times per day.

Elixir of lactated pepsin: To regularize eliminations.

Lecithin (phosphatidylcholine): This is the most important additive to the diet.* Soy and soy products are also essential.

Pancreatic enzymes*

Sulfur (organic colloidal sulfur): 6 to 8 drops three to four times per day for 4 weeks; 4 drops three to four times per day until symptoms improve.

Spirulina: 1 tsp two to three times per day.*

BOTANICALS

Bergamot oil (*Citrus bergamia*): Apply oil to lesion, then expose to sun or ultraviolet lamp. Sensitizes skin to ultraviolet light.

Bloodroot extract (*Sanguinaria canadensis*)

Burdock root (*Arctium lappa*): As decoction, or 20 to 40 drops of tincture two to four times per day.*

Chamomile (*Anthemis nobilis*)

Common figwort (*Scrophularia*): 1 to 3 mL of tincture one to two times per day.*

Mullein (*Verbascum thapsus*)*

Oregon grape root (*Berberis aquifolium*)

Sarsaparilla (*Smilax ornata*)

Slippery elm tea (*Ulmus fulva*)*

Wild clover (*Trifolium pratense*)

Yellow dock (*Rumex crispus*)

Yellow American saffron tea (*Crocus sativus*)*

Therapeutic Suggestions

Psoriasis is an extremely difficult condition to cure, and great perseverance is required. This disorder in particular must always be dealt with on all levels

---

*Asterisks indicate the most frequently used therapeutic agents.

of the person, especially emotional. Look deeply into what irritates you on a psychological level, to see what may be irritating you on a physical level. Each patient responds to the regimen uniquely, and individual modifications are required. Many cases respond well to vitamin A topically, followed by sunlight, or ultraviolet exposure. Sunlight is best, whenever possible. This must be done in conjunction with the suggested nutritional changes. Essential fatty acids also are useful, including EPA (eicosapentaenoic acid) and GLA (gamma-linolenic acid) and primrose oil.

The question of essential fatty acid malabsorption or faulty metabolism is of particular interest in relation to psoriasis. Essential acid deficiency in humans causes skin rashes resembling eczema and psoriasis. Some patients receive favorable results by reducing saturated fats and increasing unsaturated fats in the diet, while avoiding commercially transformed or overheated unsaturated fats (such as margarine or fried foods), which contain harmful *trans* fatty acids known to interfere with normal essential fatty acid metabolism. Other patients appear to have a block in normal essential fatty acid metabolism, and can bypass this fault by using oil of evening primrose, high not only in linoleic acid as are the vegetable oils of sunflower, safflower, corn, soy, and flaxseed, but also containing significant amounts of gamma-linolenic acid. The only other dietary source of this is human milk, which may explain why breastfeeding seems to be protective against many cases of infantile eczema.

The use of various oils in the form of EPA (eicosapentaenoic acid) is also another way to help bypass this biochemical fault along a closely related pathway. It is my feeling that significant advances will soon be made in better and hopefully less expensive forms of essential fatty acids and their metabolic products, to help correct these very tenacious skin disorders. *

PYORRHEA (see Teeth and Gum Disease)

RHEUMATOID ARTHRITIS (see Arthritis)

SALPINGITIS AND SALPINGO-OOPHORITIS

Definition

Salpingitis: Inflammation of the fallopian tubes.
Oophoritis: Inflammation of the ovaries.

*Horrobin, David, *Clinical Use of Essential Fatty Acids*, Eden Press, London, 1982, pp. 73–89.

Symptoms

May be acute or chronic. Tenderness of fallopian tube; severe (in acute cases) abdominal pain, usually bilateral, but may affect only one ovary or tube; fever; coated tongue; vaginal discharge common; swelling; abscess possible, with later peritonitis; pain with sex; infertility common.

Etiologic Considerations

- Ascending infection more common during or due to
  Menstruation
  Postpartum
  Postabortion
  IUD

- Appendicitis
  Direct spread

- Diverticulitis of sigmoid colon, causing left salpingo-oophoritis

- IUD (intrauterine device)

- Tuberculosis of fallopian tubes

- Congestion
  Spinal
  Diet
  Lack of exercise
  Psychological
  Constipation
  Appendicitis, etc.

- Mumps
  Oophoritis

Discussion

The fallopian tubes and ovaries are anatomically open to the outside world with all its foreign infective agents by access through the vagina and uterus. Physiologically, however, these delicate inner passageways and glands are protected by built-in self-defense mechanisms and barriers. The vagina, with its acidic nature (see Vaginitis), helps protect pathogens from flourishing. The thick mucous plug of the cervix further acts as a mechanical barrier to invasion. Hairlike cilia in the uterus and fallopian tubes themselves constantly waft any debris or bacteria downward toward the cervix and vagina.

These protective measures are normally effective in preventing infection from outside. However, during menstruation, several of the mechanisms fail to operate. The mucous plug is not effective and the vagina becomes relatively alkaline. Normally, infection is still prevented, especially with a healthy flow. In the postpartum period, again, similar self-defenses are reduced. In addition there is the possibility of infection introduced from outside during delivery, from retained products of conception only slowly being eliminated or entirely retained, or tissue trauma and congestion. Coupled with the prolonged vaginal discharge that normally follows childbirth (2 to 6 weeks), these factors make the possibility of an ascending infection extremely likely. In fact, most cases of salpingitis due to ascending infection either follow birth or abortion.

An IUD is also a major cause of ascending infections, due either to septic inoculation at the time of insertion, or to mechanical irritation and congestion, creating a more favorable environment for bacterial growth.

Congestion is a little-understood cause of salpingitis. Any organ or tissue that suffers poor circulation of blood, lymph, or nerve supply will lose the ability to resist infection. It is this loss of resistance that is a central factor in so many internal infections. In the case of salpingitis, congestion may be strictly local due to a spinal lesion; confined to the pelvic/abdominal region due to constipation, diverticulitis, appendicitis, or poor abdominal tone; or more systemic because of improper or deficient diet, lack of exercise, psychological causes, or other general health factors.

Salpingitis usually is accompanied by involvement of the ovaries due to direct spread of infection, and also via the lymphatics. It may be either acute or chronic, and is classified into two types, *catarrhal* or *suppurative* (pyogenic or infective). In the catarrhal form an excess of mucus is associated with congestion of the fallopian tube walls. In the suppurative form actual infection is found. Either form may, and usually does, permanently damage the delicate inner linings, leading to adhesion formation and possible occlusion of the tubes. In many cases the fimbriated end will swell with the infection and adhesions may permanently close this opening. Any of these damaging results may lead to infertility by hindering the passage of the egg from the ovary through the fallopian tubes, where it is fertilized, and on into the uterus where implantation occurs.

Surgical repair of the tubes when possible is unfortunately only about 30 percent successful. Even if the tubal blockage is removed and the tubes are reunited, adhesions may later form due to the surgery itself, creating a new barrier. The only possibility of pregnancy left for a woman with blocked fallopian tubes is the recent development of test tube impregnation. For the large number of women with blocked tubes, I pray this technique becomes widespread, and proves itself both safe and successful for those who cannot conceive naturally.

Treatment

Antibiotics are the usual course of treatment prescribed in salpingitis. I have mixed feelings about their use in this instance. The danger with salpingitis, as previously explained, is damage to the fallopian tubes. This damage may be best prevented by quick and appropriate treatment that removes the inflammation or infection as fast as possible. In a case of suppurative or pyogenic salpingitis, if an antibiotic can quickly remove the infection to prevent damage, I am in full support. Unfortunately, this is not always the case. Too often I see women who have received antibiotic therapy for *acute* salpingitis, only to suffer from incredibly stubborn cases of *chronic* salpingitis because the true causes were never removed and antibiotics could only have a short-term effect. These cases are extremely difficult to treat, either with further courses of antibiotics or natural therapies. Whatever the cause of such a situation, the result is the same—a woman with damaged fallopian tubes and probable infertility.

The decision whether or not to use antibiotics must include a careful consideration of the patient, past history, and present complaint. In all cases where antibiotics *are* used, naturopathic treatments should also be used to help remove the primary causes. These methods are outlined below and are very effective, though they may appear extremely simple in design. In acute cases, where the patient is in general good health and has no previous history of similar pelvic disorders, the decision to use antibiotics is no easy task. These patients make the best response to both antibiotics *and* naturopathic treatment. If the woman is in a downgraded health condition generally, then antibiotics may be needed as the body's vitality may be too low to respond rapidly enough to prevent damage.

For a patient with a chronic condition, especially one who has a history of previous antibiotic prescriptions, little can be lost from an extended application of naturopathic treatments. This is probably the patient's only hope, short of surgery, of removing her disorder. After a reasonable period of treatments, if little response is forthcoming, antibiotics may be tried in conjunction with therapy, in the hope of preventing surgery.

Diet

Depending on the patient and the condition, varying periods of vegetable juice fasting or fruit juice fasting are beneficial. With the catarrhal type of disorder short periods on the mucus-cleansing diet may also prove beneficial. These cleansing fasts may then be followed with periods on an all fruit or an all raw fruit and salads diet, followed by a good blood-building, primarily vegetarian protein, diet.

The following fast or simple elimination diets may be used:

Carrot juice: The high vitamin A content is useful to heal mucous membranes.

Carrot mono diet

Fruit juice diet

Apple mono diet

Raw fruit diet

Raw fruit and salads diet

Mucus-cleansing diet

These fasts will need to be continued until all symptoms are gone in an acute condition, or alternated with other less severe diets for the prolonged treatment necessary in the chronic condition. Acceptable interim diets are the anemia diet with only vegetarian proteins, or the asthma Stage 2, low-carbohydrate, mucus-cleansing, high fruit and vegetable diet. In general, all mucus-forming foods such as dairy products and concentrated starches are to be avoided, as well as all animal products or irritants such as coffee, alcohol, and any other negative health factor, until all symptoms have been removed.

With proper diet and supportive therapies an acute case should resolve in 5 to 10 days, but will require a further 2 to 3 weeks' therapy to prevent recurrence. The chronic case may take months of vigorous treatments, but once cure has been established, and providing the patient stays on a healthy regimen, the problem usually does not return.

Physiotherapy

• Sitz Baths

The use of alternating hot and cold contrast sitz baths is the most effective measure in removing pelvic congestion and inflammation.

Directions: Obtain two containers or utility tubs 12 to 14 in. or more deep. These should be big enough to allow immersion from midthigh to the umbilicus, including the entire pubic and pelvic regions. Fill one container with very hot water (as hot as comfortably bearable) and the other with ice-cold water. First sit in the hot tub and place your feet in the cold tub. After 3 minutes reverse so that your bottom is in the ice-cold tub and feet in the hot tub. In 3 minutes reverse again and repeat the cycle three times, beginning with bottom in the hot water and ending with bottom in the cold water. Then briskly dry off with a rough bath towel. Repeat two to three times or more per day, depending on the severity of the condition. The alternate hot and cold bath will pump blood vigorously through the pelvic region to remove congestion and speed nutrition to these areas to hasten healing.

• Alternate hot and cold compresses:

These are applied directly over the painful pelvic region, 2 to 3 minutes hot, 2 to 3 minutes ice-cold. Thick toweling folded in four thicknesses should be used to retain heat or cold. A hot water bottle wrapped in moist toweling will help prolong the hot application, and an ice bag wrapped in moist toweling will prolong the cold.

- Cold compresses:
  In the acute stage, repeated cold applications 20 minutes on, 5 to 10 minutes off, will be very beneficial (heat is often contraindicated with acute inflammation).

- Abdominal or full trunk packs:
  These should be applied nightly in acute and chronic conditions.

- Depletion pack (with doctor's supervision only):
  In a 1 lb capacity jar mix ½ lb anhydrous magnesium sulfate. Add glycerine (approximately 6 tbs) until soupy. To this add 4 to 6 oz tincture of *Hydrastis* and 1 to 2 oz Tea tree oil. Optionally, 1 to 2 oz tincture of thuja may be added. Finally, mix one bottle VM120 (see Appendix II) while constantly stirring. Apply to the upper third of a tampon and insert into vagina twice daily (morning and evening), retaining for 3 to 6 hours. This formula may be obtained premixed from Eclectic Institute (see Appendix II).

Therapeutic Agents

VITAMINS AND MINERALS

Vitamin A: 25,000 IU three or more times per day for 6 weeks (under supervision). *Use any dose of vitamin A over 50,000 IU per day with medical supervision only.* *

Vitamin C: 500 to 1000 IU four to eight times per day.*

Vitamin E: 400 IU two times per day (prevents scarring).*

Zinc: 15 to 45 mg one to two times per day (aids in healing).*

BOTANICALS

Bearberry (*Arctostaphylos uva-ursi*)

Black cohosh (*Cimicifuga racemosa*)

Black haw (*Viburnum*)

Coneflower (*Echinacea angustifolium*): 20 drops of tincture four to six times per day.*

Goldenseal (*Hydrastis canadensis*)

---

*Asterisks indicate the most frequently used therapeutic agents.

Saw palmetto (*Serenoa serrulata*)

Wild yam root (*Dioscorea villosa*)

SCHIZOPHRENIA

Definition and Symptoms

Mental illness characterized by abnormal or disturbed associations, a reduced range of emotional response, detachment from reality, and severely mixed feelings that can become incapacitating. Hallucinations and delusions are also present in some cases.

Etiologic Considerations

- Altered biochemistry in the brain
  Genetic enzyme deficiency
  Genetic excessive requirement of certain vitamins, minerals, essential fatty acids, or enzymes
- Toxicity
  Heavy metal poisoning
  Drugs
  Pesticides
  Chemicals
- Nutritional deficiency
  Excess need
  Deficient diet
  Excess of some minerals (copper)
  Deficiency of some minerals (zinc, manganese)
  Vitamin B deficiency (B_3, B_6), subclinical pellagra
- Hypoglycemia
- Gluten intolerance, dairy product intolerance
- Alcoholism
- Pep pills, prolonged weight reduction diets
- Excess use of recreational drugs (pot, cocaine, LSD)
- Cerebral food allergy (allergic reactions affecting behavior or perception)
- Stress, nervous exhaustion
- Traumatic event

- Glandular imbalance
  Pineal
  Pituitary
  Thyroid
  Adrenal
- Deficient brain circulation
- Spinal lesions
  Coccyx to occiput
  Incoordination of spinal centers
- Destructive, self-condemning thoughts

Discussion

Schizophrenia is a fairly common disorder affecting about 3 percent of the population at some time in their lives. Patients may show no previous symptoms until a severe trauma suddenly initiates symptoms (reactive schizophrenia) or the condition may be the end result of slow deterioration in an individual with a history of being shy and withdrawn.

The orthodox approach to schizophrenia is the use of various tranquilizers, all with severe side effects, electroconvulsive shock therapy, and psychotherapy. Within the past 20 to 30 years a great deal of research and clinical trials have led many in the psychological world toward diet and nutrition as a factor in the cause and cure of some cases of schizophrenia and other mental illnesses.* The main conclusion is that psychoanalysis alone, or combined with drug therapy, is of little or no use in the actual cure of mental disease in most cases, since the real cause involves an abnormal brain biochemistry due to a genetic or acquired condition involving one or many nutrients, or in some cases, toxins. In spite of the rather large body of evidence supporting these views, the average psychiatrist still denies that nutrition plays any part whatsoever in mental illness. This belief that nutrition has no bearing on mental disease, or any disease for that matter, is prevalent among many physicians.

It has long been known that severe deficiencies of some of the B complex vitamins cause psychological symptoms which in some cases are strikingly similar to schizophrenia. Severe vitamin B_{12} deficiency causes difficulty in concentration, poor memory, hallucinations, agitation, and manic or paranoid behavior. Biotin deficiency, another B complex member, will cause depression, lassitude, panic, and hallucinations. Severe vitamin B_3 (niacin) deficiency (pellagra), with its characteristic nervousness, loss of memory, confusion, paranoia, insomnia,

*Williams, Roger, A Physician's Handbook on Orthomolecular Medicine, Pergamon Press, New York, 1977, pp. 1–200.

depression, and hallucinations, so closely resembles schizophrenia that in 1966 Dr. Abram Hoffer suggested that schizophrenia may be a vitamin-dependency disease. * He cites several examples where experimental animals and prisoners of war were kept on diets deficient in vitamin B_3 for prolonged periods, only to find that when B_3 was again available in the diet, the body then required up to sixty times more B_3 than the average person to prevent pellagra. As in other typical vitamin-dependency diseases, these victims had developed an increased need for a particular substance, greater than could be derived on a diet containing ordinary amounts.

Dr. Hoffer also describes B_6-dependent pellagra and schizophrenia, although occurring less frequently. It was found that schizophrenics excrete a highly toxic pyrrole known as KP (kryptopyrrole), which reacts chemically with vitamin B_6, forming a complex which binds strongly with zinc, producing not only a severe vitamin B_6 deficiency, but also one of zinc. Supplemental B_6 and zinc in these pyroluric patients produces favorable results.

Dr. Carl Pfeiffer, of the Princeton Brain Bio Centre in New Jersey, is another pioneer in the brain biochemistry of schizophrenia, as well as in the nutritional implications of these findings. Dr. Pfeiffer has recognized two major subgroupings depending on their blood histamine levels. †

The low histamine (histapenic) group is characterized by symptoms including thought disorders, grandiosity, paranoia, overarousal, hallucinations, hypomania, and mania. Associated with this grouping are low zinc and folate levels, and a high serum copper. The elevated copper may cause depression or paranoia. Treatment for this group includes supplementation of folic acid, vitamin B_{12}, niacin, vitamin C, with zinc and manganese taken to reduce elevated copper levels.

The less frequent high histamine (histadelic) group Dr. Pfeiffer characterizes by "fast oxidation, little fat, long fingers and toes, severe depression, compulsion and phobias." He has found that folic acid aggravates these patients severely, turning mild depression into severe agitated depression. ‡

Other aspects of diet and nutrition are associated with schizophrenia. Hypoglycemia is a common concurrent finding. Although it is not entirely certain that low blood sugar precedes schizophrenia, it is well accepted that hypoglycemics experience many emotional and perceptual changes, similar to other mental diseases.

Dr. Cleave, in *The Saccharine Diseases*, made similar conclusions about the

---

*Hoffer, Abram, and Osmond, H. "Nicotinamide adenine dinucleotide as treatment for schizophrenia," *Journal of Psychopharmacology*, 1:79, 1966.

†Pfeiffer, Carl, *Mental and Elemental Nutrients*, Keats Publishing Co., New Canaan, Conn., 1975, pp. 396–421.

‡Ibid., p. 399.

effects of a refined diet, independently implicating refined carbohydrates in the cause of schizophrenia. Dr. Cleave found schizophrenia uncommon in tribal Africans living on a traditional unrefined diet, but found it a common psychosis among their urbanized brothers consuming refined carbohydrates. It is significant to note that consumption of carbohydrates is involved in the causation of both hypoglycemia and pellagra.

Cerebral allergies also may be a factor in schizophrenic behavior. Literally any food may be the cause of learning disabilities, manic depressive states, hyperactivity, confusion, lethargy, and other abnormal perceptual states such as are seen in schizophrenia. Gluten-containing grains are particularly suspect and contain neuroactive peptides.*

Other recent research has implicated faulty essential fatty acid metabolism or deficiency as a cause of some psychotic and neurotic mental disorders, schizophrenia included. Pioneering research by D. F. Horrobin† suggests a genetic biochemical defect in essential fatty acid metabolism. Whether or not there exists a genetic defect, the therapeutic value of linseed oil, a rich source of the essential fatty acid alpha-linolenic acid, with a variety of "mental" problems is being confirmed in clinical trials. In 1981 Donald O. Rudin, of the Department of Molecular Biology, Eastern Pennsylvania Psychiatric Institute, Philadelphia, Pa., reported very favorable response to 2 to 6 tbs per day of linseed oil in divided doses with cases of schizophrenia, manic depression, and agoraphobia. Other essential fatty acids such as oil of evening primrose, sunflower seed oil, and eicosapentaenoid acid (EPA) also may be of use (see Allergy for diagnosis and treatment).

Another major cause of schizophrenia-like symptoms is heavy metal poisoning. Although the physical and psychological symptoms of lead, mercury, or copper excess are well documented, it is very rare for a schizophrenic patient to be tested for elevated levels as a possible cause of this condition. I have one well-documented "schizophrenic" patient who had received the typical gamut of psychological therapy and drugs for over 2 years with no benefit. We discovered a severe lead poisoning due to his occupation as an auto body repairman. With detoxification and proper diet, his symptoms were gone completely within 3 months.

Treatment

Standard treatments for schizophrenia have an exceptionally low success rate, deplete many essential vitamins, and are highly toxic. If these facts alone were not enough for the average psychiatrist to try nutrition, specifically mega-niacin therapy, the evidence of the carefully conducted medical trials of niacin

*Pfeiffer, op. cit., pp. 415–419.

†Horrobin, D. F., *Clinical Uses of Essential Fatty Acids*, Eden Press, 1982, pp. 167–214.

should be. As early as 1939, nineteen schizophrenic psychiatric patients were treated successfully with niacin. In 1949 one study showed twenty-nine schizophrenic cases cured with niacin, none of which showed any physical signs of pellagra. Ten-year double-blind studies of niacin in 1962 showed a 75 percent success rate in schizophrenics with no rehospitalization as compared with 31 percent of the control group not receiving niacin therapy. These are just a few examples.*

Although niacin therapy has been found extremely useful, it is important to remember that in most cases the best results can only be obtained by first minimizing all negative health factors and optimizing the positive. Dr. Hoffer recognized this need and as a first course of action advises an optimum diet to lay the foundation for further therapies.

Diet

The best maintenance diet for schizophrenia is the hypoglycemia regimen outlined in Hypoglycemia. This helps keep the blood sugar level under control and minimizes symptoms while the rest of the nutritional therapy takes effect. Best results will be obtained, however, if this diet is modified to be gluten-free and dairy-free (refer to Celiac Disease for complete details of a gluten-free diet).

Some practitioners have obtained excellent results with prolonged fasting of 7 to 14 days in the treatment of schizophrenia. If done properly, a prolonged fast normalizes blood sugar levels and removes toxic substances from the body. In practice I have found that the major barrier to progress with nutrition for the average schizophrenic lies in the patient's family environment. It is absolutely impossible to enforce or suggest dietary changes unless the entire family is willing to modify their diets at the same time. Absolute consistency is required, to get the desired results. All persons in the family do not necessarily have to follow the details of the hypoglycemic regimen, but all must eat only the best of unrefined whole foods and these alone should be made available in the house for consumption. All sweets, pastries, refined foods, canned foods, soda drinks, and other devitalized products should be removed from the home. Hair analysis and allergy tests (RAST, cytotoxic) should be performed early in therapy and repeated at 6-to-12-month intervals.

Physiotherapy

- Spinal massage: Use peanut oil, olive oil, and lanolin.
- Spinal manipulation: Treat generally once a week.

*Hoffer, A., "Treatment of Schizophrenia," in A *Physician's Handbook on Orthomolecular Medicine*, Pergamon Press, Elmsford, N.Y., 1977, pp. 83–89.

- Meditation: Encourage meditation or relaxation exercises twice a day by example, and with guidance.
- Kindness and love: Give plenty of both daily.
- Home environment: Look internally to see the internal chaos you as parent, sibling, or partner represent.
- Sunshine, ocean, peace, and quiet: All will be helpful.

Therapeutic Agents

VITAMINS AND MINERALS

Vitamin A: With allergy, lung, or mucous membrane disorders, 25,000 IU one to two times per day. *Use any dose of vitamin A over 50,000 IU per day with medical supervision only.* *

Vitamin B complex: 50 mg three times per day.*

Vitamin B_3: 3 to 30 g per day. 3 to 6 g mixed niacin/niacinamide as initial dose.*

Vitamin B_1: With depression.

Vitamin B_2: With visual problems and cracked corners at the mouth.

Vitamin B_6: With flat glucose tolerance curve, allergies, hyperactivity, convulsions, or malabsorption, indicated in kryptopyrrhole (KP) syndrome schizophrenia, with B_3. Dose: 80 mg per day or 1 mg for each 15 mg of B_3 used. Higher doses may be needed.*

Pantothenic acid: With fatigue or allergy; 200 to 600 mg per day.

Vitamin B_{12}: 1 mg intramuscularly once per week or more in some cases.

Vitamin C: 6 to 40 g; low C in urine of schizophrenics.*

Vitamin D

Vitamin E: 800 to 1600 IU per day; reduces anxiety.*

Inositol: 200 to 1000 mg per day.

Vitamin B_6: 250 to 1000 mg per day with supervision.*

Folic acid: Especially needed where anticonvulsants have been used since these deplete folic acid stores. Also needed in histamine type schizophrenics (see C. Pfeiffer, *Mental and Elemental Nutrients*); up to 2 mg per day.

Biotin

Zinc: Especially with elevated copper levels. Reduces anxiety; particularly indicated with other skin rashes. 30 to 50 mg two to three times per day.

*Asterisks indicate the most frequently used therapeutic agents.

Magnesium

Manganese: Also helps restore raised copper levels and helps remove the Parkinson-like side effects resulting from long-term use of strong tranquilizers.

OTHERS

Atomodine (Cayce)*

Brewer's yeast (contains inositol and B complex): Dose: 4 to 6 tbs per day.*

Choline (as concentrated phosphatidylcholine lecithin): 6 to 12 g per day.*

EPA (eicosapentaenoic acid): 1 to 2 g three times per day.*

Glutamic acid (glutamine)*

Liver tablets, liver injections: Contain inositol plus B complex.

Oil of evening primrose: 3 to 6 g per day.*

Taurine

Tryptophan: 1 to 3 g per day.*

Tyrosine

BOTANICALS

Chamomile (*Anthemis nobilis*): Mild sedative.

Passion flower (*Passiflora incarnata*): Sedative.*

Therapeutic Suggestions

Obviously not all cases of schizophrenia are nutritionally related, and even when they are, many other variables do take part. It is, however, in the best interest of the patient to seriously try the nutritional approach prior to drug therapy being relied on completely.

SCIATICA (see Low Back Pain)

SENILE MEMORY LOSS

Definition and Symptoms

Loss of normal ability to think and remember present and past facts, events, names, places, etc.

*Asterisks indicate the most frequently used therapeutic agents.

Discussion

Senility is nearly synonymous in most people's minds with old age and yet we all know or have heard of someone 80, 90, 100, or older whose mind has remained sharp as can be. So ingrained is the idea of senility, however, that many businesses require those over 65 to retire on the assumption that they must be getting a little befuddled. Nothing could, or should, be further from the truth if the person has taken reasonable care of himself or herself.

Common causes of senility include poor circulation to the brain, cerebral arteriosclerosis, prolonged nutritional deficiency, heavy metal toxicity, prolonged drug use, and lack of exercise.

Treatment

Prevention of senility must begin early in life. The diet must be composed of plenty of uncooked foods. Daily exercise to the point of breathlessness is essential to maintain adequate circulation. Heavy metals must be avoided by refraining from using aluminum pans or canned foods. A diet similar to that found under Heart Disease is probably the best form of prevention and treatment.

Therapeutic Agents

VITAMINS AND MINERALS

In addition to the diet and exercise regimen and supplements recommended under Heart Disease, the following will be specifically useful:

Vitamin A: 25,000 to 50,000 IU per day. *Use any dose of vitamin A over 50,000 IU per day with medical supervision only.*

Vitamin B complex: 50 mg one to two times per day.

Vitamin C: Up to bowel tolerance.

Bioflavonoids: 300 to 1000 mg per day.

Lecithin (choline): 2 to 4 capsules three to four times daily.

Zinc: 25 to 50 mg one to two times per day.

Ice-cold head baths daily.

SINUSITIS

Definition

Inflammation of the accessory nasal sinuses.

Symptoms

Nasal congestion and postnasal discharge, headache, pain behind eye, tenderness, fever, loss of smell.

Etiologic Considerations

- Diet
  Excess milk and dairy products
  Milk allergy
  Excess carbohydrates
  Raw vegetable deficiency
  Acidity
- Allergy
  Food
  Inhalants
- Suppressive
  Treatment of previous colds
- Cervical spinal lesions
  Lower cervical, upper thoracic
  Vasoconstriction; poor circulation
  Poor lymph elimination
- Obstruction
  Enlarged turbinates
  Deviated septum
  Polyps
- Toxemia
  Bowel stasis
  Poor eliminations
- Liver congestion
  Toxemia
- Emotional
  Stress
- Irritants
  Adrenal exhaustion

Discussion

The typical patient with chronic sinusitis characteristically follows an acid-reacting diet, having an excess of starches and dairy products and lacking in sufficient raw green vegetables. It is well known by naturopaths that this type of diet causes an increase in the amount of mucus produced by the body and favors tissue congestion. One of the most common signs of this is sinus congestion and irritation. Mucus is not only produced in excessive amounts, but can contain irritating elements accumulated through an improper diet. This may be due simply to the overconsumption of foods that render the body fluids more acidic, or due to actual toxic eliminations from chemicals, pesticides, or other causes of toxemia, such as poor eliminations. These irritants set up inflammation and discharge in the mucous membranes of the sinuses. A secondary infection may then settle into the downgraded congested tissues, resulting in acutely painful sinus headaches.

Most of these patients also have a history of treating previous acute eliminations such as the common cold with suppressive or improper treatments. Often, similar causes such as those under Allergies will be found in these cases. Invariably, either cervical or thoracic spinal lesions will be found to aggravate these upper respiratory complaints.

Treatment

Acute sinusitis is extremely painful. Fortunately it is also fairly easy to relieve rapidly by natural methods. Even stubborn cases of the more chronic sinus conditions usually respond well. I remember one patient in particular who had received every orthodox treatment available for a period of 6 months with no relief. She came for naturopathic treatments out of desperation. She had already made plans to fly nearly 6000 miles to see a specialist she had heard of, if our treatments failed to give her relief within 1 week. She was free of pain within 3 days! I am constantly amazed at the effectiveness of the simple methods that follow.

Diet

It is always best to begin the dietary regimen with a 3-to-5-day mucus-cleansing diet as follows:

Stage 1

Breakfast	Citrus fruit (especially grapefruit)
Midmorning	Fresh vegetable juice (carrot)
Lunch	A large plate of boiled or steamed onions; a little vegetarian seasoning may be used to flavor, but no salt. An orange for dessert.
Midafternoon	Fresh vegetable juice (carrot)

Supper	Same as lunch
Evening	Potassium broth, or as midmorning
	Take 2 garlic capsules three times per day.

This diet may be followed with 1 to 2 days on fresh citrus fruit, or if desired you may go directly to a raw food diet for 3 to 7 days. Eat plenty of fresh fruit, fruit juice, fresh vegetable juice, and raw salads with onions. Follow this with the Stage 2 asthma diet (below) until all residual symptoms are cleared. In many cases repeated mucus-cleansing diets may be needed to correct the condition. It is absolutely essential to avoid all irritants in the diet during this process. This includes coffee, tea, alcohol, strong spices, salt, sugar, and cigarettes.

Stage 2

Breakfast	1. Any fresh fruit, raw or stewed, *or:*
	2. Stewed or baked apple with soaked or simmered raisins.
Lunch	1. A large, varied, raw salad composed of vegetables that grow mostly above ground, in the ratio 3 to 1 (e.g., lettuce, cabbage, celery) plus carrots and onions; (peppers, watercress, cucumber). Also have a large plate of boiled or steamed onions topped with vegetarian seasoning or miso. A few walnuts, almonds, or hazel nuts may be added to the salad.
	2. Tofu may be added to the meal.
Evening	1. Same as lunch, *or:*
	2. A vegetarian protein meal excluding eggs and cheese, plus steamed or baked vegetables. Fresh or stewed fruit as desired.
Later in regimen	
	3. Lean meat, fish, or poultry (not fried) with vegetables. Fresh or stewed fruit as dessert.
Drinks	When thirsty, choose from fruit juice, vegetable juice, potassium broth, or herb teas.

Take 2 garlic capsules with meals. Always include raw onions in the salad meals.

If allergy is the cause of repeat attacks, follow regimen for Allergy.

Physiotherapy

- Glycothymoline packs
  Soak three to four thicknesses of gauze or cotton cloth with glycothymoline
  (very warm). Apply to painful and congested sinuses for 15 to 20 minutes,
  renewing the compress as it cools, and repeat the application until passages
  clear. (*Note:* In some cases heat may cause more pain. Use ice-cold compresses while doing a very hot foot bath. Another alternative is heat to the
  back of the head and very cold to forehead.)

- Alternate hot and cold compresses

- Inhalations
  Hot water steam with oil of eucalyptus (or leaves), oil of pine (or pine
  needles), and thyme or cloves.

- Nasal irrigations:
  Beet root juice in ice-cold water
  Borax nasal douche
  Chlorophyll nasal douche
  Lemon and water douche plus nasal spray
  Thuja oil nasal spray

- Specific nasal technique (for congestive cases only)
  Performed by naturopathic and some chiropractic physicians.

- Neck exercises

- Spinal manipulation
  Cervical; cervical/thoracic; upper thoracic

- Daily vigorous exercise

- Epsom salts baths (see Appendix I) or compresses, locally

- Alternate hot and cold baths locally (in chronic condition, but not during
  acute stage. Will cause great pain if done in acute exacerbation).

- Olbas inhalation

Therapeutic Agents

Vitamins and Minerals

Vitamin A: 25,000 IU up to six times per day in acute cases; two to three
times per day in chronic cases. Anti-infection, mucous membrane nutrient. *Use any dose of vitamin A over 50,000 IU per day with medical
supervision only.* *

---

*Asterisks indicate the most frequently used therapeutic agents.

Vitamin B complex: 25 to 50 mg two to three times per day.*

Vitamin B_6: 100 mg twice a day.*

Vitamin C: 500 to 1000 mg hourly in acute cases. Anti-infection, anti-inflammatory.*

OTHERS

Cayce expectorant (Product 49): 1 tsp three to six times daily.

Cod-liver oil

Garlic: 2 capsules three times per day.*

Glycothymoline (internal antiseptic): 2 to 3 drops per day.

Horseradish

Horseradish plus lemon juice

Onion syrup: 1 tsp per hour in acute cases.*

Onions: Cooked and raw.

Raw adrenal

Raw thymus: 1 to 4 tablets per hour in acute cases.*

BOTANICALS

American elder (*Sambucus canadensis*)

Autumn crocus (*Colchicum autumnale*)

Barberry (*Berberis vulgaris*)

Beech leaf tea (*Fagus* spp.)

Black cohosh (*Cimicifuga racemosa*)

Cayenne (*Capsicum frutescens*)

Comfrey (*Symphytum officinale*)

Coneflower (*Echinacea angustifolium*)*

Dandelion (*Taraxacum officinale*)

Fenugreek (*Trigonella foenumgraecum*)

Juniper berries (*Juniperus communis*)

Mustard seeds (*Brassica juncea*)

Nettle (*Urtica dioica*)

Pokeroot (*Phytolacca* spp.) (highly toxic; see p. 62)

Queen of the meadow (*Eupatorium purpureum*)

*Asterisks indicate the most frequently used therapeutic agents.

Red eyebright (*Euphrasia officinalis*)

Sarsaparilla (*Smilax ornata*)

SMOKING

Definition

The addictive habit of smoking cigarettes for physical and psychological causes.

Symptoms

Pallor, premature aging, discolored teeth and skin, bad breath, coated tongue, frequent colds, bronchitis, emphysema, lung cancer, and many others.

Etiologic Considerations

- Emotional insecurity
- Stress
- Improper diet
- Hypoglycemia
- Peer group pressure
- Oral gratification
- Nicotine addiction
- Alcoholism

Discussion

The tobacco industry has to be given credit for the effectiveness of their advertising campaigns over the years. They spend more money than any other industry in advertising and have succeeded in creating the impression that when you smoke, sophistication, independence, and the macho look are yours, along with good times, beautiful companions, and success in your career.

Peer pressure has created most smokers, along with the industry's seductive advertising. The first cigarette is usually very unpleasant. Poisons are introduced into the body, which rebels with nausea and perhaps a headache. After a few attempts at smoking, however, the body slowly becomes accustomed to the poisons and the addictive effect of nicotine takes hold. Nicotine is most definitely a highly addictive drug, and once the addiction is implanted, the body continues to demand its "fix." The cigarette habit is then established. The usual physiological demand of the body is at least the nicotine content of ten ordinary cigarettes per day. Often it is much more.

As public awareness of the dangers of smoking grew, the industry produced low-tar, low-nicotine cigarettes. However, since the body has developed a need for a certain amount of nicotine daily, more of these low-tar cigarettes are usually smoked than regular ones. The low-nicotine cigarettes also produce more carbon monoxide than regular ones. In an effort to produce satisfactory taste for these low-tar, low-nicotine cigarettes, various additives are used, which in themselves may be carcinogenic. Recent research shows that nicotine metabolites in the blood are related to the number of cigarettes smoked, low-tar or not. Low-tar cigarettes do not lower the risk of heart disease or lung damage.

Besides the physical addiction, which is very real, smoking quickly becomes associated with positive actions, such as a good meal or conversation with a close friend. Persons attempting to stop smoking have great difficulty due to these associations, as well as not knowing what to do with their mouths and hands, which were busy in the process of smoking.

Each cigarette is estimated to take away 8 minutes of life. This means that for the one-pack-a-day smoker, every year he or she gives up 1 month of life. For the two-pack-a-day smoker, this totals up to 12 to 16 years less of life, and the much greater possibility that the quality of the shorter life will be severely diminished. Cigarettes contain over 4000 known toxic poisons, any one of which in sufficient quantity can kill. Only one drop of pure nicotine (which may be obtained from 145 cigarettes) is sufficient to kill a grown man.

Smoking is a causative factor in many diseases, reducing not only the length of life, but also the quality of life. Smokers have more colds, sinusitis, bronchitis, emphysema, heart attacks, strokes, and other upper respiratory and circulatory problems than nonsmokers. Smoking aggravates diabetes, ulcers, high blood pressure, Burger's disease, and glaucoma, and may help cause osteoporosis, smaller babies, miscarriages, stillbirths, and lung cancer.

Cigarettes affect the circulatory system in several ways. After only one cigarette the heartbeat is increased 20 to 25 beats per minute. This increases the load on the heart and increases the blood pressure. The heart itself requires more oxygen due to the increased work load; however, at the same time the carbon monoxide from the cigarette forces the oxygen from the bloodstream, depriving the heart of oxygen it needs.

Smoking also constricts the peripheral blood vessels, reducing blood flow to the hands and feet. After the last cigarette 6 hours must elapse before the circulatory system returns to normal. For the smoker who has the last puff just before going to bed, and the first puff on awakening, the circulatory system is normal for only a short 2 hours out of the entire 24-hour day.

The lungs and respiratory system are the most directly affected by smoking. The lung of a smoker is dark gray and less elastic than the pink, healthy lung of the nonsmoker. The natural cleaning mechanisms of the lung, the cilia and macrophages, are unable to do their necessary work due to the tar deposited within the lungs. This effect is even worse for smokers in cities with poor air quality. Lack of cilia action, which normally propels mucus and residues out of the lung in a wavelike action, and reduced functioning of the macrophage cells, which engulf irritants and unwanted material, lead to an increase in the cough reflex to expel this accumulated matter. Local irritations and a drying of the mucous membranes further stimulate the cough reflex. This smoker's cough may settle into chronic bronchitis, then emphysema. Shortness of breath is characteristic of most smokers.

Lung cancer is the end result of the local irritation and exposure to the carcinogenic components of cigarettes. Cigarette smoking also appears to have a deleterious effect upon the immune system. Circulating immunoglobulins and antibody responses to antigens are depressed. The immunosuppressive effects of smoking take 3 months to reverse once smoking has been stopped.

The effect of smoking on the skin is that of premature aging. The skin becomes very dry, has an unhealthy pallor, and wrinkles markedly. The irritation of cigarettes, pipes, or cigars on lips and tongue leads to an increase in cancer in these areas. Taste, smell, and even vision are affected by smoking. Most former smokers report an increased acuity of all senses once smoking has been discontinued. Smoking also produces an insulin reaction which creates low blood sugar, resulting in fatigue, irritability, and the desire for another cigarette, setting up a vicious cycle.

Osteoporosis, or loss of minerals from bone, with its consequent weakening, is either aggravated or caused by smoking.

Other diseases such as ulcers usually will not heal while the patient continues to smoke. Smoking in this case increases the acid secretions in the stomach.

Women smokers may suffer more severe menopausal symptoms as well as premature onset of menopause; male smokers suffer more problems with their prostate.

Smoking destroys the body's supply of vitamin C. Each cigarette will destroy up to 25 mg of vitamin C. At one pack a day, this far exceeds the normal intake of this vitamin, which is essential for so many psychological processes. This prolonged vitamin C deficiency may be a factor in the increase in cancer of heavy smokers.

In general, smokers are sick more often, are absent from work more often, and spend more money on drugs, doctor bills, and hospitals. Smoking workers usually are less efficient than nonsmokers, and get less work done in an average day.

Smoking while pregnant leads to smaller babies and more stillbirths. The babies suffer from drug withdrawal symptoms when born and for several days will cry more often than other babies. Nicotine passes through breast milk and affects the nursing infant by dosing it with nicotine. Children of smoking parents generally are sick more often and do less well in school. They are also more likely to become smokers at an early age.

Anyone in the same room with a smoker suffers damaging effects even though they are nonsmokers. The smoke causes tearing of the eyes, constriction of the mucous membranes of the nose, as well as constriction of the blood vessels. Nonsmokers are affected by the tar, nicotine, and carbon monoxide as well as many of the other poisons. For anyone suffering from a heart condition, emphysema, stroke, or any other weakened body condition, the results can be aggravated with possibly fatal results. Inhaling smoke in a confined area such as a closed car can be particularly dangerous. The smoke from a smoldering cigarette is the most dangerous type, producing three times the amount of tar and five times the amount of carbon monoxide.

Clearly, smoking is not a benign social habit. If the tobacco industry were not so strong an influence in politics, and if legislators themselves were not so addicted to its use, as is a good portion of the general population, tobacco would probably be a controlled drug. Certainly any drug or other substance that caused this many harmful effects would surely be made illegal.

Treatment

Many smokers have tried unsuccessfully to stop smoking many times. They have sometimes tried by cutting down, but this is almost impossible since the body makes its physical addiction demand of at least ten cigarettes as seen above. Each time the effort fails, the addiction becomes even more deeply entrenched. Frequently, depression and a lack of self-respect follow these failed attempts. A series of these unsuccessful attempts often leads the person to feel he or she will fail in other facets of life as well.

Many rationalizations are used by smokers to defend their smoking habit, which they know is very dangerous and yet which they are unable to control. "I like to smoke" is a frequent excuse. (What they really like is the "fix" or nicotine lift without which they would suffer the pains of nicotine withdrawal.) Or: "I think better with a cigarette!" (Actually, smoking constricts the blood flow and oxygen to the brain, making thinking less clear.) Or: "A cigarette calms me down." (After only one cigarette tremors in the fingers increase 39 percent. The insulin response with consequent irritability and fatigue causes adrenal exhaustion and nervousness, not calmness.)

The ingrained habits and associations in smoking are so deep that only a definite campaign to recognize and change these habits can have a chance to succeed. Only a fortunate 3 percent are able to stop smoking on their own. The remainder either continue smoking or seek help. No program will be effective, however, unless a person is properly motivated and each person has to provide that motivation himself or herself.

Programs to help people stop smoking are many and varied. The American Lung Association, the Cancer Society, and the Seventh Day Adventists sometimes provide lecture programs with films. Numerous hospitals provide similar programs. Hypnosis and even acupuncture are sometimes used. There is even a medical procedure involving a solution injected through the ear. Smokenders features a 13-week program which meets once weekly.

Some people are helped by these programs. A study made in 1977, however, showed that while long-term effectiveness of these programs varied, they were less than half as effective as those programs combining behavior modification and aversion therapy. The National Society of Stop Smoking Centers with individual Stop Smoking Centers in most major cities, and the Schick Centers, primarily on the West Coast, provide this combination therapy. They screen applicants and eliminate those who either do not have sufficient motivation, or who are unacceptable because of certain severe medical problems. Their programs are so effective in helping people that they offer a money-back guarantee which only rarely is required.

After a person stops smoking, however, he must realize that he can never have another cigarette or the habit is reinstated, and nicotine will once again latch its addictive hold on the individual.

Diet

The best diet for most smokers is found under Hypoglycemia. This diet helps maintain a constant blood sugar level and prevents many of the ups and downs that often stimulate the desire to smoke. Very high doses of vegetables, carrots, and citrus fruits are advisable for their detoxifying effects, and as a valuable source of vitamins and minerals. High fluid intakes help to detoxify nicotine in the early stages. When possible, dilute fruit and vegetable juice fasting may be tried. These help overcome the nicotine craving a little and of course detoxify the body rapidly. These fasts may be anywhere from 7 to 21 days, with supervision. This is a very effective way to stop smoking and get over the nicotine habit, if the patient is willing to follow it.

Habitual coffee drinking is frequently associated with excess smoking. Coffee consumption needs to be slowly reduced if great quantities have been taken, to avoid a toxic effect. The aim should be to reduce coffee from 6 to 10 cups every day to 1 to 1½ in the first 3 days of pre-therapy, and to stop altogether by the start of any behavior modification and aversion therapy, or any other therapy for that matter.

Physiotherapy

- Sweat baths, saunas: Daily in the detoxification regimen to get nicotine out of the system.

- Colonics: Two times per week for 1 to 3 weeks.

- Exercise: Increase all activity.

Therapeutic Agents

VITAMINS AND MINERALS

Vitamin A: 25,000 IU two to three times per day for 1 month. Beta carotene sources are best in this instance (necessary for proper health of mucous membranes). *Use any dose of vitamin A over 50,000 IU per day with medical supervision only.**

Vitamin B_1: 50 to 100 mg per day.

Vitamin B complex: 50 mg three times per day.*

Vitamin B_3 (niacin): 100 mg up to 1 or more g two to three times per day.

Vitamin C: 3000 to 10,000 mg per day, to detoxify nicotine. Up to 30 g intravenously to aid withdrawal.*

BOTANICALS

Lobelia (Indian tobacco) contains lobeline, which is very similar to nicotine. It helps wean the patient off nicotine but is nonaddictive so once the habit is broken, lobelia may then be discontinued. Smoke, or take 5 to 15 drops six times per day. Aversion therapy with lobelia may also be performed.

Procedure: No smoking is allowed except for a concentrated period of 1 hour per day when 15 drops of lobelia are taken internally ½ hour and then 15 minutes before the first cigarette is lit. With each 15-minute period, a further 15 drops diluted in water are taken while cigarettes are smoked end to end. The result will be nausea, which soon becomes associated with smoking. In 5 or 6 days the desire for cigarettes will probably have disappeared.

Calamus: Chew root, then smoke. Will also cause nausea as a negative feedback.

Chamomile: Take three to six times per day to relax.

*Asterisks indicate the most frequently used therapeutic agents.

SORE THROAT (see Colds)

SPASTIC COLITIS (see Colitis)

SPRAINS

Definition and Symptoms

Trauma to a joint (ankle, knee, back, wrist, etc.) with varying degrees of ligament injury or tearing, causing rapid swelling, pain, and discoloration.

Discussion

All sprained joints should be treated along the same lines. Most people think of ice application for a sprained ankle, but for some reason the average person feels at a loss when other joints are sprained. I am always surprised to see how many people will put heat and not ice on a sprained or severely strained back. A joint is a joint. Obviously, some joints cannot be easily treated with the standard RICE treatment (Rest, Ice, Compression, and Elevation), but ice and rest are the mainstays of such treatment and should always be employed.

Treatment

The general treatment for all sprains, where possible, is discussed below.

Rest

Do not use the affected joint from the first moment of injury for at least 2 days. If the ankle is involved, use no weight-bearing. Crutches are to be used when you must be upright, but avoid as much moving about as possible these first few days. Severe shoulder injuries require a sling to allow full rest. Severe back sprains require 24 to 48 hours of *complete* bed rest. Only after 24 to 48 hours, once pain and swelling has begun to subside, can you begin to mobilize the joint within the pain margin, taking care not to reinjure the joint.

Ice

Ice really should be the first item on the list, but ICRE is not so easily remembered. As soon as possible, hopefully within minutes, apply ice to the area. Swelling begins immediately, so it is essential to reduce this as rapidly as possible to minimize pain, reduce possibility of adhesions, and speed healing. Apply ice over one layer of toweling to prevent burning the skin or immerse joint in ice water. Keep ice on for 30 minutes. Ice is also used in the recovery period as long as there is any sign of inflammation.

Compression

To further prevent swelling, cover crushed ice with a plastic wrap and apply an adhesive bandage. Leave on 30 minutes, unwrap for 5 to 15 minutes, and rewrap. After the second ice compression wrap, apply a standard compression bandage which consists of a layer of cotton, a layer of elastic, another layer of cotton, and a final elastic wrap. Keep toes or extremities exposed to make sure of adequate circulation. If toes turn blue, unwrap and rewrap less tightly. This compression bandage may stay in place for a full 24 hours when the joint is checked, or it may be removed every 2 hours for an ice application.

Elevation

Elevate the injured joint to prevent effusion into joint and surrounding tissues. As healing progresses over the first 24 to 48 hours, and swelling and pain are reducing, the joint is now ready for mobilization. Place the joint in hot water, or use a hot compress. Slowly move the area in all its normal movements to the point of pain, but not beyond. Some joints may require passive mobilization where the joint is taken through its movements without the patient's muscular assistance. Ice should still be used periodically throughout the day to speed healing and prevent the joint from swelling. If for any reason the joint swells after an activity, apply ice.

Once the joint begins to feel less traumatized and can perform most of its normal movements without much pain, even if some restriction of range of motion remains, it is time for muscle-assisted exercise. First, use no weights, and then increase by 1 to 2 lb, depending on the joint involved. Do not reinjure. Bring back to normal levels of activity with care.

Therapeutic Agents

VITAMINS, MINERALS, AND OTHERS

Vitamin C: 4 to 5 g at time of injury; 1 g per hour for first 2 to 3 days.

Bromelain: 2 to 3 tablets three to four times per day.

Dimethyl sulfoxide (DMSO): Topical.

Arnica tincture (topical): Apply four to six times per day.

(*Note:* All severe sprains should be checked for fracture. If severe effusion into the joint has occurred, it may best be aspirated to prevent adhesions.)

STAPHYLOCOCCAL INFECTION: Impetigo

Definition

Staphylococcus: A small round bacteria growing in clusters. May infect any area of the body.

Impetigo: A highly contagious, superficial skin infection usually caused by staphylococci, or occasionally *Streptococcus.*

Symptoms

Staphylococcal infection: Pimples, furuncles, boils, carbuncles, abscesses, osteomyelitis, enterocolitic pneumonia, bacteremia, occasionally fatal.

Impetigo: Red swellings becoming pustules or large pus-filled bullae which rupture and form a yellow crust. May rapidly spread in infants with risk of fatal systemic infection, although this is rare. May complicate other skin lesions such as eczema, scabies of fungus infections, or other types of dermatitis.

Etiologic Considerations

- Poor hygiene
- Diet
   Toxic
   Low protein
   Excess sweets, fruit
   Excess acidity
   Green vegetable deficiency
   Milk or other allergy with staph infection secondary
- Allergy with staph infection secondary
- Polluted bathing water (especially ocean, swimming)
- Insect bites
- Cuts at site of entry, poor care
- Predisposition
   Staph sensitivity
   Newborns
   Nursing mothers
   Skin disorders
   Diabetes
   Lung conditions

- Post antibiotic staph infection
- Postsurgery staph infection

Discussion

Staphylococcus bacteria are found almost everywhere in our environment. They live quite happily on the nasal membranes and skin of most healthy people. Normally, however, they cause no problem and go unnoticed.

An interesting fact about staphylococcal infections (and most other infections for that matter) is that some people seem more susceptible than others. In studying the differences between those who are very susceptible and those practically immune to staph infection, we can find both the cause and the cure.

General poor hygiene is considered a major cause of staph infection. This may be the cause in a few extreme cases where gross neglect leads to infection, especially where there is an abrasion or cut present. In general, however, with the exception of lack of attention to superficial injuries and neglect of basic sanitation or cleanliness, hygiene is probably one of the least significant causes of staph infection in the average situation. Exceptionally clean and hygienic people do indeed get staph infections.

Diet and its effect on immunity and general vitality is a significant causative factor in staphylococcal infections. Contrary to the popular "new age" belief that all disease may be cured by fruit juice fasting, staph is a disease frequently found to be precipitated by excess fruit, or at least some form of sugar, along with a pronounced protein deficiency.

As with most other diseases, we do see many with staph infections on a refined, devitalized, and toxic diet, but a large number are "new age" fruitarians or fairly strict vegetarians. These people often eat excess fruits in the belief that fruit is health-giving, and very little protein in the belief that protein is dangerous to the health.

Both beliefs are right and wrong. Fruit and fruit juice are excellent purifiers and may be used medicinally to encourage eliminations. It is superb as a medicinal agent. As a luxury food or source of vitamin C and a few other vitamins and minerals, again, it is superb. As a staple food, however, it fails miserably. The taste of fruit, we all know, is delectable. Most succulent fruits, however, contain little more than sugar, water, a few vitamins and minerals, and little, if any, protein. Not only is fruit in excess not particularly good for you, it may even be quite bad. Too much quickly absorbed sugar as found in most fruits can seriously upset the glucose-regulating system in the body, adversely affecting both the pancreas and adrenal glands (see Hypoglycemia).

More to the point of the present discussion, excess sugar in any form favors staph growth and multiplication. Staph doesn't care if your sugar comes from cane sugar, alcohol, honey, grapes, or apples. To a *Staphylococcus*, if it is sweet, "how sweet it is."

Protein is another example of a misunderstood food. All the negative publicity concentrated proteins have received in the past 20 years has turned many toward protein avoidance. Certainly it has become obvious that excess animal proteins are hazardous to health. The link between saturated fats and heart disease is now fairly well accepted. It is now clear that a partial or even total vegetarian diet is more conducive to long life and a reduction of many health complaints. But many people have rejected nearly all proteins to live exclusively on fruits and vegetables, even to the exclusion of nuts or beans. While it is possible to live on this diet if extreme care is made to supply vegetable matter with high protein content, any severely restricted diet of this nature may become a health risk. Staph infection is one of those risks.

I think it fair to point out that some people do follow these strict regimens with good results. If proper care is taken the result may be a healthy and strong vitality. I am more concerned with those who obviously are not well suited to this regimen, proven by their lack of vitality. Staph infection is *not* a cleansing process. The boils are *not* removing toxins from within in most cases, but result from reduced vitality and are a *disease process*. The end result of ignoring a staph infection or treating it through extended fasting could lead to bacteremia and death. Others who commonly contract staph infections are on no specific diet regimen but habitually eat little protein and eat excessive amounts of fruits and fruit juices, other sweets, or refined carbohydrates.

Antibiotics, so often used with even minor infections, are both a blessing and a curse as far as staph infection is concerned. I am strongly against the habitual and routine use of antibiotics for any and almost all infections, colds, fevers, etc., as they are routinely prescribed by most physicians. Not only is the natural way quite effective in these minor to moderate problems, but the overuse of antibiotics is rapidly creating a world health crisis.* In the old days when antibiotics were first produced, they truly worked miracles. Patients that surely would have died were saved. Weeks of agony ending in death were often replaced by apparent health within days, if not hours.

As the years have passed, however, it has now become clear that the longer we use antibiotics regularly, the more resistant strains of bacteria emerge.† Many diseases that were all but wiped out are now re-emerging even stronger than ever and are almost impossible to kill off. Not only is an individual these days exposed to antibiotics as medicine from cradle to grave, but they are even found in milk and meat products, to name just two. My objection to this abuse in this particular case is threefold. The first is that antibiotics destroy not only the target patho-

---

*Buist, Robert, "Antibiotics—An Achilles Heel?" *International Clinical Nutrition Review*, S(2): 51–52, April 1985.
†Ibid.

logical bacteria, but also destroy the entire ecology of the body, which in many cases depends on friendly bacteria for our health and protection. Once these allies are destroyed, *Staphylococcus* may take a strong hold.

My second objection is that the use of antibiotics for minor staph infections tends to cause antibiotic-induced yeast infections that may be very difficult to treat, especially if there is systemic spread.

Lastly, antibiotics used even for the most trivial infection often cause a chronic case of allergic dermatitis which may in turn become infected with a secondary staph infection, complicating an otherwise simple problem. Infants seem particularly sensitive to antibiotics. One of the saddest and most difficult problems that confront most naturopaths is seeing an infant who, upon receiving antibiotics for one or two small skin infections or a mild case of impetigo, develops an antibiotic dermatitis which then settles into a chronic eczema, covering the entire body. This then commonly becomes infected with a secondary staph infection!

It may now seem strange, after all I have just written about the evils of antibiotics, for me to say how life-saving antibiotics can be in severe staph infections. If the infection is allowed to get out of control and enter the blood stream and the patient has swollen glands and fever, or other signs of systemic infection, the time has arrived for antibiotics. At this point the infection has established too strong a hold to be treated with natural therapy safely. The general vitality cannot defend the body's borders and needs help.

It is unfortunate that something so useful and lifesaving when used with discretion as antibiotics should become one of the major threats to world health because of indiscriminate use. Antibiotics should be reserved for the few times of true health crises that most people do encounter within their lifetimes. With proper diet, preventative care, and simple natural treatments, even these few crises may often be avoided.

Treatment

To treat staph infections and impetigo properly with natural therapies, the infection should be caught early and treated vigorously. Haphazard treatment will not be curative and only allows the infection to spread.

Diet

Susceptibility to staph infection may be due to excess sugar in one form or another. The best therapeutic regimen in these cases is one high in green vegetables and vegetarian protein, with absolutely no sugar, honey, refined carbohydrates, or alcohol. Fruit consumption is severely restricted or eliminated until the infection and rash are gone. Protein supplements are recommended two to three times daily. In the case of impetigo, the child is usually on a diet high in fruits, fruit juices, and carbohydrates with a deficiency of vegetables other than potatoes and other starches. For these children, the best diet is one of raw and cooked vegetables, especially green and yellow or orange foods, no fruit or fruit juice, and only unrefined carbohydrates, along with adequate protein.

Hygiene

The skin and mucous membranes normally function as a protective barrier for the body. Subtle qualities of pH, cilia hairs, bacteria flora, and quality of secretions help prevent infection. Once these barriers are breached by an abrasion or cut the internal immunological defenses act as secondary protective mechanisms. The integrity of the immunological system may be affected by diet, nutritional deficiency, glandular disorders, stress, and many other factors. Some people seem virtually immune to staph infections. They can receive deep gashes and give them little or no attention, even to the extent of leaving the wound dirty and unattended, and it will still heal quite happily without infection. Other people can get the slightest prick and will develop a staph infection almost overnight. It is obvious that individual resistance is very important and varies from individual to individual. Once again we see that it is not the germ that causes disease, but a favorable environment that allows ever-present germs to flourish.

Still, it is not wise to allow a wound to go untreated. Clean cuts need less attention than jagged ones. Any situation that causes the skin to lose its normal circulation is more likely to lead to infection. Deep, penetrating punctures or wounds that cause much tissue damage always need to be treated. Dirt and foreign matter must be removed and the area washed with soap and water and flushed with hydrogen peroxide. Although alcohol and iodine do kill bacteria, they also destroy healthy cells and should not be used. Tea tree ointment or oil is the best application for a cut or wound. It is much more effective than other antibiotics such as bacitracin and is also an antifungal agent.

Goldenseal or calendula tea may be used as a wash. Give the wound fresh air and sunlight, and avoid prolonged immersion in water. Avoid salt water contact as this delays healing and may encourage spread. Expose to strong sunlight if possible.

Local Treatments

Wash area with full-strength tincture of green soap. Crust should be removed for rapid healing. Apply warm goldenseal tea compresses to firmly adherent crust. Flush with hydrogen peroxide and then apply tea tree oil full strength. Repeat every 2 waking hours. Apply tea tree ointment at night. Ultraviolet exposure daily as an antibacterial agent is encouraged where possible. Another approach is to follow the same procedure as above, but instead of using a tea tree oil application, use castor oil, 3 parts; to eucalyptol, ½ part. This may be more useful in some cases of impetigo, where the skin is so raw that the tea tree oil causes severe pain or aggravation. Change pillow covers and sheets nightly. Take care to disinfect these along with any towels, washcloths, or clothes that may cause reinfection, or spread to other family members.

Therapeutic Agents

VITAMINS AND MINERALS

Vitamin A: Very high doses (for short term):*
10,000 to 20,000 IU daily (infant)
20,000 to 60,000 IU daily (child)
75,000 to 200,000 IU daily (adult)
Use any dose of vitamin A over 50,000 IU per day with medical supervision only.

Vitamin C: Very high doses:*
500 to 1000 mg daily (infant)
1000 to 3000 mg daily (child)
3000 to 20,000 mg daily (adult)
(Vitamins A and C are very low in infections.)

Zinc: Necessary for healing.*

Garlic: Antibiotic.*

Raw thymus: 2 tablets four to six times daily.*

Essential fatty acids

BOTANICALS

Comfrey (*Symphytum officinale*)

Coneflower (*Echinacea angustifolia*)*

Garlic (*Allium sativum*): Internal, external to lesion; external as foot compress (see Appendix I).*

Gentian violet (use with care; this will stain everything): Apply two times per day (1%).

Oil of bitter orange (*Citrus aurantium*): Antibiotic.

Tea tree oil: External; antifungal, antibiotic.*

Eucalyptus (*Eucalyptus globulus*)*

Goldenseal (*Hydrastis canadensis*)*

*Asterisks indicate the most frequently used therapeutic agents.

STRESS

Nearly every disease we know can be aggravated or even caused by stress or destructive emotions. We have discussed stress-related hypoglycemia, headaches, colitis, ulcers, enuresis, fatigue, high blood pressure, and a whole host of other conditions. No list of supplements will cure stress if the cause is primarily emotional, or due to external conditions. The following list of supplements will help deal with *results* of stress, and if taken in conjunction with efforts to deal with the cause of stress, will be instrumental in the overall therapy. Some cases of stress are solely due to nutritional deficiencies and these will be corrected by dietary changes and nutritional supplementation alone.

Treatment

Vitamins and Minerals

Vitamin A: 25,000 to 100,000 IU per day.

Vitamin B complex: 50 mg two to three times per day.

Pantothenic acid: 25 to 50 mg one to two times per day.

Vitamin C: To bowel tolerance.

Vitamin E: 400 to 800 IU per day.

Calcium: 800 to 1000 mg per day.

Magnesium: 600 to 1000 mg per day.

Zinc: 25 to 50 mg one to two times per day.

Others

Essential fatty acids
    Eicosapentaenoic acid

    Oil of evening primrose

    Flaxseed oil

    Gamma-linolenic acid (GLA)

Hypothalamus: 1 tablet two to three times per day.

Raw adrenal: 1 tablet two to three times per day.

Thymus: 1 to 3 tablets two to four times per day.

Note: Stop drinking coffee!

STROKE (see Heart Disease)

SUGAR DIABETES (see Diabetes)

SUNBURN (see Burns)

TEETH AND GUM DISEASE: Caries, Periodontal Disease (Gingivitis, Pyorrhea)

Definition

Caries: Gradual dissolution and destruction of tooth enamel and dentin, eventually involving the tooth pulp.

Periodontal disease:

Gingivitis: Inflammation of the gums surrounding the teeth.

Pyorrhea: Inflammatory enlargement and degeneration of the soft tissue and bone surrounding teeth, leading to recession of gums and loosened teeth.

Symptoms

Dental caries
> Frequent cavities
> Irregular enamel

Periodontal disease
> Bad breath; foul taste in mouth; red, swollen, bleeding gums
> Sensitivity to hot or cold
> Receding gums
> Loose teeth
> Loss of teeth

Etiologic Considerations

- Refined carbohydrates (foods stick to teeth)
- Vitamin deficiency
- Sugar
- Excess meat-based protein and/or processed foods

- Soft drinks
  Phosphoric acid in soft drinks dissolves enamel, and they contain up to 7 tsp sugar, as well
- Overcooked foods
- Vitamins A, C, D, calcium, magnesium, phosphorus, trace mineral, or protein deficiency
- Heredity (some families show poor tooth calcification)
- Excess hot or cold foods lower gum vitality
- Prolonged bottle feeds, especially at night (milk or fruit juice bottle syndrome)
- Poor hygiene
  Improper brushing
  Lack of flossing
- Poor diet of mother during pregnancy or lactation
- Severe infection in infancy leaves poorly developed layers of enamel
- Diabetes

Discussion

Both caries and periodontal disease are diseases of civilization related to abnormal dietary habits. Archeological findings show clearly that Stone Age peoples had remarkably little of either tooth or gum disease. Further findings show that the peasant classes of ancient Egypt who could afford only simple whole grains had far fewer cavities than the ruling class, who lived on more refined foods. Recent studies of rural populations eating unrefined foods showed very strong gums and teeth but once they are exposed to a more modern diet containing sucrose and refined cereal grains, a rapid deterioration takes place.

Healthy gums and teeth begin early in gestation and depend to a large extent on the diet of the mother. Strong teeth specifically require adequate supplies of vitamins A, C, D, calcium, magnesium, phosphorus, trace minerals, and protein. If the mother's diet was marginal in any of these nutrients prior to pregnancy, the deficiency would be magnified by the increased needs of the fetus. In most cases, nutrients needed by the growing infant will be leached from the mother to the extent they are available. This is the reason for the old adage, "a tooth lost for every child." Calcium and other minerals are extracted from the mother's bones and teeth to provide for the growing needs of the infant. This obviously sets the stage for dental problems in the mother, but evidence also suggests that nutrient-deficient mothers make babies with poor teeth.

Rats fed on a good diet give birth to baby rats with teeth strongly resistant to disease. Poorly fed nutrient-deficient rats, however, produced offspring with teeth highly subject to decay. Repeated pregnancies closely following each other is another factor in dental problems for the mother and infant. Studies show that later siblings have statistically more dental disease than the first-born child.

Although the mother's diet during pregnancy is very important in the subsequent development of strong teeth in her newborn, the baby's diet in early infancy and childhood is equally important. It is important to remember that teeth are made from within and require not only a few vitamins and minerals, but a generally good diet. A sound diet makes sound teeth and is a child's best guarantee that he or she will have little or no dental problems. No amount of external cleaning measures will be of much benefit if the diet produces weak teeth.

Once the teeth are formed and hopefully have an even, tough layer of hard, impervious enamel, proper diet once again is essential to prevent tooth decay and gum disease. The biggest enemy of healthy gums and teeth is plaque. Colonies of microorganisms form difficult-to-remove plaque, which then causes fermentation of carbohydrates, producing acids that dissolve away minerals in the tooth's enamel. The enamel becomes brittle and ultimately is breached, allowing destruction of the inner pulp.

Although carbohydrates are implicated in the process, it is the ultrarefined carbohydrate of sucrose (sugar), along with other refined grains such as white flour or white rice that are the main offenders. A gluelike substance called dextran is produced by a specific *Streptococcus* in the mouth, and is necessary to fix the plaque in place on the tooth margin. Dextran, however, can only be produced from sucrose. Other refined carbohydrates such as white bread are very sticky and become easily lodged between teeth and gum margins, providing ideal fuel for plaque to ferment. This leads to erosion of the enamel and irritation of the gums. The gums may develop pockets, which act as further reservoirs of impacted food materials, creating an ideal environment for bacterial proliferation. Eventually the gums become inflamed (gingivitis) and begin to recede (pyorrhea), leaving the tooth root exposed. Finally the tooth loosens and falls out or must be removed due to infection. Gum disease also creates a foci of infection which may have profound effects on the general health.

Another possible factor in tooth loss is periodontal disease where alveolar bone surrounding the tooth becomes weakened and less dense. According to present statistics, two-thirds of the population of the United States suffers some degree of periodontal disease. Recent research has implicated modern diet in both periodontal disease and osteoporosis, or a generalized bone loss. A diet high in phosphorus and low in calcium seems to be a major factor. The typical western diet high in red meat has a ratio of between 1 part calcium to 25 to 40 parts phosphorus. The normal ratio should be 0.7 calcium to 1 part phosphorus. Other foods high in phosphorus are refined foods and carbonated soda beverages. As the phosphorus level increases in relation to calcium, the parathyroid glands are stimulated to produce a hormone, parathormone, which acts to withdraw calcium from bones. This causes a weakening and shrinking of the alveolar bone surrounding teeth and allows bacteria to proliferate in these spaces, initiating gum disease and tooth loss.

Prevention and Treatment

Diet

Since a high-phosphorus and refined diet is the major cause of tooth and gum disease, the best prevention and treatment is a diet high in raw fruits, raw and conservatively cooked vegetables, nuts, fermented dairy products, and whole unrefined grains. Such foods are very rough and chewy, cleaning the teeth and massaging the gums as they are eaten. Excess meat, sugar, soda, candy, refined cereals, and overcooked foods are to be strictly avoided. In several studies where sweets were replaced after a meal with an apple, dental caries in subjects were reduced drastically. If this single dietary change could do so much to reduce dental problems, imagine how few cavities children would have if everyone avoided all the refined foods that make up such a large proportion of our diets today. Periods of restricted diet on all fruit or all raw foods will speed recovery in cases of established pyorrhea.

Local Hygiene

Proper brushing and flossing of the teeth helps prevent plaque buildup and removes food residues. The proper brushing technique now recommended is to use a soft, rounded-end nylon brush, and with the edge of the brush applied at a 45° angle at the gum-tooth junction, gently massage the gum in small, circular, vibrating movements. The object is to massage the gum-tooth margin and loosen plaque and food particles. Later, the typical tooth polishing and stroke/brushing from gum to tip of tooth is used. Follow with dental flossing.

Recently an old Edgar Cayce treatment for gum disease has become popularized by several prominent dentists. Several modifications of this are advised, but the original Cayce recommendations advise brushing one to two times per day with an equal combination of baking soda and salt. Some dentists recommend rinsing with hydrogen peroxide. I have never used this rinse with any of my patients and so cannot comment on its effectiveness. The baking soda brushing, however, is effective in removing plaque. In addition, I find the following procedure very effective if followed regularly:

• Daily dental flossing

• IPSAB massage

    After the baking soda and salt brushing, massage the gums vigorously with IPSAB (Cayce product) twice a day. IPSAB is anti-infective, astringent, a glandular tonic, and increases local circulation. It contains prickly ash bark, sea water, calcium chloride, sodium chloride, iodine trichloride and essence of peppermint. Apply IPSAB to loose teeth with cotton.

- Glycothymoline, myrrh, and *Hydrastis* rinse—follow IPSAB massage with mouth rinse from a mixture of:
    14 oz glycothymoline
    1 oz tincture of myrrh
    1 oz tincture of *Hydrastis*
- As instructed on every bottle of IPSAB, have at least one large salad each day!

    Other local therapies sometimes used are:

- Gum massage
    Eucalyptus oil: Massage once a day
    Witch hazel massage once a day
    Vitamin E massage
    1 oz *Hydrastis*, 1 oz myrrh, 1 pint water
    Infusion: Rinse three times per day
- Ipsident (Cayce product)

Therapeutic Agents

VITAMINS AND MINERALS

Vitamin A: 25,000 IU per day.

Vitamin B complex: 25 to 50 mg one to two times per day.

Vitamin B_3

Vitamin B_6

Folic acid: 800 mcg per day.

Vitamin B_{12}

Vitamin C plus bioflavonoids: 500 to 1000 mg three times per day.*

Vitamin D: 400 to 1000 IU per day.*

Vitamin E: 400 IU per day (chew); plus local application to gums.*

Zinc: 15 to 25 mg one to two times per day.

Calcium and magnesium in a ratio of 2:1. Usual dose is calcium, 800 mg per day, magnesium 400 mg.*

Trace minerals*

OTHERS

Cod-liver oil

Green vegetables, sea vegetables*

*Asterisks indicate the most frequently used therapeutic agents.

Hydrochloric acid, cider vinegar: Acid helps calcium absorption.

*Lactobacillus**

Spirulina

BOTANICALS

Cayenne (*Capsicum frutescens*)

Coneflower (*Echinacea angustifolia*)

Goldenseal (*Hydrastis canadensis*)

Myrrh (*Commiphora myrrha*)

THORACIC OUTLET SYNDROME AND BRACHIAL NEURALGIA

Definition

Compression of the lower cord of the brachial plexus of nerves as it passes between the first rib and clavicle, due to a lowering of the shoulder girdle, the presence of an abnormal seventh cervical rib, enlarged seventh cervical transverse process, or strong fibrous band.

Symptoms

Pins, needles, numbness, and pain in one or both hands, occurring 2 to 3 hours after falling asleep, which usually wakes the patient due to discomfort. Wasting of small muscles in hands may occur, as well as coldness or swelling.

Etiologic Considerations

• Lowering of the shoulder girdle
  Muscle weakness in middle age (weakness of shoulder elevator muscles, upper trapezius, and levator scapulae)
  General fatigue
  Carrying excess heavy weights
  Overuse of arms
  Poor posture

- Seventh cervical rib abnormality
- Enlarged seventh cervical transverse process
- Strong fibrous band

Discussion

Thoracic outlet syndrome is a fairly common problem, occurring due to compression of the lower branch of the brachial plexus of nerves which exit from the lower cervical vertebrae to pass underneath the clavicle and on into the arm. The lowest cord of the brachial plexus lies in close proximity to the first rib, where it is subject to compression between the first rib and the clavicle, if the muscles that help support the shoulder girdle in elevation become weakened. This is the common adult-onset syndrome which usually progresses gradually, causing pins and needles sensations and numbness and pain in one or both arms. The discomfort usually occurs in the middle of the night.

Other structures in the region, such as an abnormally developed transverse process, cervical rib, or a hard fibrous band, may compress the lower brachial nerves or in some cases restrict blood flow in the subclavian vessels and cause circulatory symptoms similar to Raynaud's disease with resultant coldness, pallor or redness, and some swelling.

Cervical rib syndrome or that of an enlarged transverse process usually differs from thoracic outlet syndrome of muscular weakness origin in that the former conditions are more frequent in younger persons and the pain or paresthesia occurs shortly after heavy lifting, wearing a heavy coat, or simply having the arms hang in a dependent position. Nocturnal pain is not usually present. X-rays will clearly show the abnormal bony development of the seventh cervical vertebra in most cases; however, even a strong fibrous band in this area may cause compression which will not be noticeable with a routine x-ray.

Typical adult-onset thoracic outlet syndrome is almost always caused by poor muscular tone. The average patient is middle-aged, with a lowered shoulder girdle due to the cumulative effect of weakness of the upper trapezius and levator scapulae muscles along with gradual reduction of disc space, normal with the aging process, and consequent changes in spinal curves. The patient complains that he or she is awakened by pronounced pins and needles sensations, numbness, and pain in one or both hands, 2 to 3 hours after having fallen asleep. Getting up into a sitting or standing position helps relieve the disagreeable symptoms. These symptoms may recur, leaving the hands literally numb on awakening. During the day few symptoms are present unless heavy lifting is performed. In some cases even a heavy overcoat will instigate symptoms of pins and needles. Over time the symptoms may include the lower arm, upper arm, and even the shoulder, and are usually worse on days where heavy lifting or exertion has been performed.

Nocturnal symptoms are usually the result of prolonged nerve compression occurring during the day and are a nerve recovery phenomenon. Only when the nerve compression caused in the shoulder weight-bearing position is relieved, in this case by lying down to sleep, can the nerve recover. This recovery takes time in the case of a prolonged compression, which is the reason it takes several hours before symptoms are sufficiently strong to wake the patient.

Treatment

The basis for therapy in the muscle weakness type of thoracic syndrome relies on muscular and postural reeducation. The following exercises must be repeated twice daily until the muscles gain strength. The number of repetitions may be increased as well as the weights used.

- *Shoulder shrugs:* Stand with arms at sides, with a 2-lb weight in each hand, shrug shoulders upward and forward. Hold 1 to 2 seconds and relax slowly. Repeat ten times. Shrug shoulders upward and backward. Hold 1 to 2 seconds and relax slowly. Repeat ten times. Shrug shoulders upward. Hold 1 to 2 seconds and slowly relax. Repeat ten times. Gradually increase weights as these exercises no longer cause fatigue. The weights used may be the standard barbell type or sandbags, cans, jars, etc., as long as the weight is known.

- *Corner press:* Stand facing the corner of a room with feet 2 to 3 ft from the wall, one hand on each wall at shoulder height and arms outstretched. Slowly allow the chest to press forward into the corner as you inhale, and press outward back to the original position while exhaling. Repeat ten or more times.

- *Arm lift:* Stand with arms held out at shoulder level, palms downward, holding 2-lb weights. Raise arms sideways over the head until back of hands meet, keeping arms straight at all times. Slowly lower arms to shoulder level. Repeat ten times. Increase weights to 5 to 15 lb as muscles become stronger.

- *Neck exercise:* Stand erect with shoulders very slightly shrugged. Slowly bend head to right, attempting to come as close to your shoulder with the ear as possible, without shrugging the shoulder. Repeat to the left.

- *Upper trunk raise:* Lie face down with a small pillow under the chest and hands clasped behind the back. Raise the head and chest as high as possible off the floor, pulling the shoulders backward while keeping the chin close to the chest. Inhale while going up. Hold 3 to 5 seconds, exhale as you return to the starting position. Repeat ten to twenty times.

Spinal Manipulation

Twice a week initially; later one to four times per month.

Others

- Swimming: Three times per week.
- Medicine ball throwing: Keep ball shoulder high or higher.
- Evening armchair sitting: Sit with elbows supported on an armchair and shoulder girdle elevated for 20 to 40 minutes each evening to allow for nerve recovery while awake. Continue session until usual nighttime symptoms of pins and needles appear and then cease. This will prevent nighttime symptoms from occurring.
- Avoid heavy lifting and heavy overcoats.
- Lifting advice: Shrug shoulders first prior to lifting and keep in partly shrugged position while lifting proceeds. This will prevent nerve compression.

Diet

The general diet regimen is suggested, with plenty of raw green vegetables. Some cases benefit from a diet regimen similar to that under Arthritis.

Therapeutic Agents

VITAMINS AND MINERALS

Multivitamins

Multiminerals

Vitamin C: 1000 mg three times per day

See Arthritis for additional supplements.

THRUSH (see Vaginitis)

THYROID DISORDERS: Simple Goiter, Hypothyroidism, Hyperthyroidism

Definition

Simple Goiter

An enlargement of the thyroid gland. This may be due to iodine deficiency in foods or due to natural goitrogens in foods such as cabbage or kale that block synthesis of thyroid hormone and therefore stimulate thyroid-stimulating hormone (TSH) production via the hypothalamus and pituitary centers.

Hypothyroidism

Myxedema: Low thyroid function due to atrophy of thyroid, following radioactive iodine therapy for hyperthyroidism or secondary to hypofunction of anterior pituitary.

Cretinism: Juvenile hypothyroidism due to a deficiency of thyroid hormone during fetal period or early development. Causes are inborn errors of iodine metabolism, abnormally developed thyroid, enzyme blocks in thyroid hormone production, and dietary deficiency. The thyroid may be absent, reduced in size, or greatly enlarged.

Hyperthyroidism

Thyrotoxicosis, Graves' Disease: Excessive production of thyroid hormone with growth or atrophy of thyroid gland, increased metabolic rate, and possible bulging of the eyes (exophthalmos).

Symptoms

Hypothyroidism

Cretinism: Physical and mental development is retarded. Tongue is enlarged, lips thickened, and mouth is held open and drooling. Umbilical lesion common with pot belly. Apathy, constipation, sallow skin.

Myxedema: Large tongue; slow; deep speech; thickened dry skin; puffiness of hands, face, and eyelids. Baldness of scalp and outer one-third of eyebrows. Mental apathy, sensitivity to cold, constipation, menstrual disorders, low blood pressure, weight gain, insomnia.

Mild hypothyroidism: A wide range of symptoms is associated with this most common thyroid condition. These include easy fatigability, headaches, chronic or recurrent infection, eczema, psoriasis, acne, menstrual disorders, painful menstruation, depression, cold sensitivity, psychological problems, and anemia.

Hyperthyroidism

Thyrotoxicosis, Graves' Disease: Insomnia, nervousness, weakness, sweating, overactivity, sensitivity to heat, weight loss, tremor, stare, and exophthalmos (eye bulge). The heart is overactive and enlarged, with systolic hypertension and possible heart failure. The thyroid is usually enlarged or nodular. Psychosis occurs in severe cases of "thyroid storm," when all symptoms are severely aggravated due to stress, infection, surgery, or other causes, which may have a fatal outcome.

Etiologic Considerations

Hypothyroidism

- Iodine deficiency
- Vitamin E deficiency
- Vitamin A deficiency
- Zinc deficiency
- Pituitary disorders
- Postradioactive iodine therapy
- Posthyperthyroid surgery
- Enzyme deficiency in thyroid hormone production
- Diet pills
- Emotions
- Spinal lesions
- Hereditary predisposition

Hyperthyroidism

- Vitamin A deficiency
- Vitamin E deficiency
- Vitamin B_6 deficiency
- Liver damage: Insufficient enzymes are produced to inactivate thyroid hormones
- Pituitary tumor (causing an increase in TSH)
- Emotions
- Spinal lesions
- Diet pills

Discussion

The thyroid gland plays a key role in controlling the body's metabolic rate. It is in turn controlled directly by secretions from the pituitary and hypothalamus in the brain. The hypothalamus is affected greatly by strong emotions. For these reasons the thyroid is especially susceptible to the emotional state. When the Eastern understanding of body centers is studied, we find the thyroid to be in the throat *chakram* or energy center. This center may be hindered by emotions such as fear or inability of self-expression, sexual excess or frustration, and general frustration. Spinal lesions from C3 to T1 or T2 may affect the thyroid gland as well, producing either hyper- or hypothyroidism.

Since the thyroid has a major effect on metabolism and the blood glucose level, it also has a strong effect on the mental state, causing mental depression, lethargy, fatigue, and psychosis. This may play a role in abnormal mental states in puberty, pregnancy, postpartum depression, and menopause.

Dietary causes of thyroid disorders may work hand in hand with their emotional counterparts, or independently. The most obvious is iodine deficiency. Iodine may be deficient in foods grown in certain localities, creating what is called endemic goiter. This is easily corrected by consuming iodine-containing foods. The incidence of endemic goiter is now reduced due to the addition of iodine to condiments. Unfortunately, the condiment is table salt, which is on its own a health hazard and avoided by those aware of its harmful effects or by those on a salt-restricted diet. Certain foods called goitrogens actually hinder iodine utilization. These include kale, cabbage, peanuts, soy flour, brussels sprouts, cauliflower, broccoli, kohlrabi, and turnips.

Vitamin E deficiency reduces iodine absorption by the thyroid by 95 percent, causing the thyroid to become overactive and enlarge to compensate. This may be part of the reason thyroid disorders are so common in pregnancy and menopause where vitamin E deficiency is common.

Of specific importance in the causation of thyroid disorders is long-term use of "diet" pills. Various forms of "speed" or Dexedrine are often used to increase the metabolic rate and reduce the appetite. Used frequently, these upset the normal control mechanisms of the entire hormonal system and may permanently alter thyroid function, predisposing either to hyper- or hypothyroidism.

Surgical or radioactive iodine treatments for *hyper*thyroidism often cause a permanent case of *hypo*thyroidism that requires lifelong use of the hormone prescription thyroxine. The best course of action when possible is to strengthen the weakened glands, remove the causative factors, and promote healing from within. The basal body temperature test (see end of chapter) can be used, not only for diagnosis but also as a gauge of treatment effectiveness. If the treatment is working properly, the basal temperature will return to normal.

Treatment

The general treatment for thyroid disorders is based on a gentle stimulation of the thyroid through proper diet, physiotherapy, food supplements, and herbs to raise the local and general vitality and allow the imbalanced hormones to reach a proper equilibrium.

Diet

Some thyroid patients benefit from foods especially high in iodine, vitamins E, A, C, and B complex. Raw foods are generally excellent for the glandular system. Foods of specific usefulness in some cases are:

Seaweed	Seafood
Kelp, dulse	Egg yolks
Garlic	Wheat germ
Radishes	Mushrooms
Watercress	Brewer's yeast

At all times the food eaten should be unrefined and as close to its natural state as possible. Two to 4 weeks or longer on a raw foods diet of raw green salads, seaweed, nuts, seeds, sprouted seeds, sprouted beans, and vegetable juices will have a strongly tonic effect.

All treatments, even dietary, for thyroid disorders should be undertaken with the assistance of a qualified nutritionally minded doctor in conjunction with an endocrinologist. Some of the therapeutic agents could become detrimental if taken in improper doses for a particular patient or thyroid condition.

Physiotherapy

• Sauna baths
• General exercise until vigorously sweating
• Sea bathing and sun baths
• Meditation
• Spinal manipulation: C3 to T1 or T2
• Yoga exercises specific to thyroid disorders:
  Shoulder stand
  Plough

Therapeutic Agents

VITAMINS AND MINERALS

Vitamin A (preformed): 10,000 to 25,000 IU, one to three times per day. Hypothyroid patients do not convert Beta-carotene to vitamin A efficiently.

Use any dose of vitamin A over 50,000 IU per day with medical supervision only. *

Vitamin B complex: 25 to 50 mg one to three times per day. Intramuscular injections may be useful. *

Vitamin B$_6$: 50 to 100 mg one to two times daily. *

Vitamin B$_2$ (increased need in hyperthyroidism): 50 to 100 mg once a day.

Vitamin C: 250 to 1000 mg two to three times daily. *

Vitamin E: Increases iodine uptake by thyroid and heals scars in gland. 400 to 1200 IU per day. *

Zinc: 25 mg two to three times per day.

Copper: 1 to 3 mg per day.

OTHERS

Atomodine (Cayce): All iodine-containing medications should be taken only with a doctor's prescription. They can be toxic if taken in excess. *

Brewer's yeast

Calcium fluoride

Calcium and magnesium

Garlic

Iodine

Kelp*

Raw adrenal tablets (with doctor's prescription): 1, one to three times per day. *

Raw hypothalamus tablets (with doctor's prescription): 1, one to three times per day. *

Raw pituitary tablets (with doctor's prescription): 1, one to three times per day. *

Raw thyroid tablets (with doctor's prescription): 1 to 2, one to three times per day. *

Desiccated thyroid (prescription)

Thyroid (homeopathic dilutions)

Tyrosine: Helps activate thyroid in hypothyroid cases.

Wheat germ oil

---

*Asterisks indicate the most frequently used therapeutic agents.

BOTANICALS
  Barberry (*Berberis vulgaris*)
  Blue flag (*Iris versicolor*)
  Bugle weed (*Lycopus virginica*)
  Irish moss (*Chrondus crispus*)
  Lettuce (*Lactuca sativa*)
  Oak (*Quercus*)
  Pokeroot (*Phytolacca decandra*) (highly toxic; see p. 62)
  Yellow dock (*Rumex crispus*)

For exophthalmos:

  American hellebore (*Veratrum viride*)
  Bugle weed (*Lycopus virginica*)
  Cactus (*Cactus grandiflorus*)
  Hawthorn (*Crataegus oxyacantha*)
  Pheasant's eye (*Adonis vernalis*)
  Strophanthus (*Strophanthus hispidus*)
  Thyroid 6×: Very useful in thyroid complaints.

Note: A useful home test for hypo- or hyperthyroidism is the basal body temperature test as first suggested by Dr. Broda Barnes.* Axillary temperature is taken for 10 minutes first thing in the morning. Average ranges are 97.8 to 98.2°F. Temperatures below this range suggest hypothyroidism, and those above hyperthyroidism. Women must take temperature on days 2 and 3 of the menstrual flow to get an accurate measurement.

TONSILLITIS AND ADENITIS

Definition

Inflammation and possible infection of tonsils and/or adenoids.

Symptoms

Acute
    Fever, chills
    Sore throat, swollen, red

*Barnes, Broda, *Hypothyroidism: The Unsuspected Illness*, Harper & Row, New York, 1976.

Difficulty swallowing
Tender swollen lymph nodes

Chronic
Mouth breathing, foul breath
Lassitude, frequent colds
Poor hearing
Eustachian tube blockage

Etiologic Considerations

• Toxins

• Diet
Excess starches
Milk allergy
Excess dairy products
Excess sugar
Green vegetable deficiency
Improper weaning

• Poor eliminations
Skin
Constipation
Deranged stomach

• Spinal
Impairment of local circulation
Accumulation of toxins

• Suppressive treatments to previous acute colds

Discussion

The tonsils and adenoids are lymphoid structures designed by nature to act as filtering agents for viruses, bacteria, and toxins. Not only do they protect us from external agents, but they also act as sensitive barometers of our inner health. When the blood or lymph fluids become overburdened with toxic waste or bacteria, these organs become inflamed and infected. These toxic overloads are usually due to an improper diet and poor stomach, bowel, skin, kidney, and liver function.

The typical child with recurrent tonsil infection and enlargement has been weaned to a diet high in milk and carbohydrates and very low in green vegetables. This causes a relative acidity and toxicity in the system. Excess mucus is produced by the imbalance of consumption of mucus-forming foods, such as milk, cheese, and bread, and an almost complete lack of the elimination and cleansing elements in the vegetable kingdom. Junk foods, sweets, and other highly processed or devitalized foods lower the body's vitality and congest the system so that elimination is required.

Food allergy may also cause tonsillitis. The two most commonly involved foods are milk and wheat. Thus, a child on even a small amount of these foods might suffer severe physical distress if an unsuspected allergy exists. The incidence of milk allergy is very common. True milk allergy, however, need not be the only process by which dairy product consumption may aggravate the system. Milk contains the sugar lactose which requires the enzyme lactase for complete digestion. This enzyme is commonly found in the digestive system of young children. However, in many cases, this ceases to be produced as a child becomes older. This causes the milk to be incompletely digested, causing gastric irritation and mucus production.

The incidence of milk intolerance due to digestive enzyme deficiency is somewhere around 15 to 25 percent in Caucasians and up to 85 percent in Orientals.

Wheat also may cause physical distress in ways other than strict allergy. The protein gluten found in wheat and other related grains can cause intestinal irritation and loss of the small villi, necessary for proper absorption, which line the intestinal walls. The result is a thinning of these areas, inefficient absorption, toxic reabsorption, and systemic irritation which may lead to tonsillitis among other disorders. These two allergies or digestive incompatibilities are so common that a diet restricting dairy products and gluten-containing grains is usually the first course of treatment in these cases.

Poor eliminations are another major cause of tonsillar enlargement and infection. The highly refined diet of white bread, white rice, overly cooked vegetables, refined sweets, and other fiber-deficient foods causes the body to lose its regular natural eliminative function. This can cause serious health problems and almost always is involved in cases of tonsillitis (see Constipation).

Spinal lesions in the neck may also reduce blood and lymph flow to these vital structures, causing reduced tissue vitality and congestion.

As with other diseases, tonsillitis is also usually the result of suppressive treatments to other acute diseases such as the common cold. These eliminative efforts by the body have been suppressed by improper diet and drugs, leading to a toxic buildup finally expressed by tonsillitis, asthma, and other more serious diseases.

The old medical approach to a case of tonsillitis was tonsillectomy. Its routine use has been abandoned ever since it was observed that the incidence of Hodgkin's disease was slightly increased in patients who have had a tonsillectomy. This procedure did nothing to remove the basic causes of the condition and only denied us the service of a faithful defender. It made no more sense to routinely remove tonsils than it would to remove the red oil-pressure warning lights in a car. Only on rare occasions, when the condition of the tonsils has become *chronically* enlarged, fibrotic, and pustular, may it be best to have them removed. In such an instance, the tonsillar infection can be very difficult to heal and continues to act as a reservoir of infection to pollute the entire body. With this in mind, it becomes increasingly obvious that proper attention should be given to the first acute attacks of colds, sore throats, or tonsillitis, to prevent a chronic condition from developing.

Treatment

Simple acute tonsillitis, although very uncomfortable and disturbing, is relatively easy to treat. Once a throat culture eliminates strep throat (for which antibiotics are required), the acute inflammation and infection is not difficult to remove within 3 to 10 days by natural methods. Chronically enlarged tonsils and adenoids, however, take much more time. Once the adenoids have enlarged to the extent they interfere with nasal breathing and cause the patient to breathe through his or her mouth, we have a serious problem. This can totally change the developing features of the face, leaving it permanently altered. It also may severely reduce the normal hearing range in the critical learning years. It therefore becomes extremely important that we reduce the size of these structures as much as possible, and as soon as possible. By the time the child is 9 or 10 these enlarged adenoids are usually much less of a problem anyway, but we cannot afford to wait for the body to slowly grow out of the problem. Vigorous treatment is required.

Diet

The simplest initial treatment for children to follow with either acute or chronic tonsillitis is the all fruit diet (see Appendix I) or fruit juice fast. Fasting may be very difficult for young children to handle, except when the throat is so sore and painful that no solid food is possible anyway. If fasting is possible, it should be continued at least as long as pain exists and then the all fruit diet may be instituted. This allows any fruit or fruit juice except banana. When fasting do an enema nightly or on days 1, 2, 3, 5 and 7.

An alternative approach, which is very effective, is the 3-to-5-day mucus-cleansing diet, as follows:

On Rising	Hot water, lemon, and honey
Breakfast	Citrus fruit
Midmorning	Carrot juice or citrus juice
Lunch	A large plate of boiled or steamed onions. Natural soy sauce may be used. Citrus as dessert if desired.

| Supper | Same as lunch |
| Evening | Same as midmorning |

In chronic cases short periods of fasting should be rotated with longer periods of the all fruit diet, mucus-cleansing diet, and Stage 2 of the asthma diet, which stresses nonallergic, non-mucus-forming foods with plenty of vegetables (see Asthma).

All these diets must also be accompanied by the internal and external treatments suggested below.

Physiotherapy

- Epsom salts baths (see Appendix I)

- Enemas

- Gargles
    Hydrastis (goldenseal), myrrh, and glycothymoline. Mix 1 oz of the two herbs (as alcohol tincture) with 16 oz of glycothymoline. Gargle daily four to six times.*
    Hot water, salt, and lemon: Gargle three times per day.*
    Lemon juice
    Hydrastis
    Myrrh
    Fenugreek tea
    Chlorophyll

- Throat sprays or swabs
    Hydrastis
    Myrrh

- Throat compress
    Three parts mullein, 1 part lobelia for pain relief. Alternate hot and cold.*

- Throat pack
    Soak a small towel in ice-cold water. Wrap around throat and pin. Leave on 1 to 3 hours. Repeat two times per day and at night.

- Endonasal technique (see Appendix I)

- Spinal manipulation
    Cervical and upper thoracic. Frequently in acute cases, weekly in chronic.

*Asterisks indicate the most frequently used therapeutic agents.

Therapeutic Agents

VITAMINS AND MINERALS

Vitamin A: High doses are required. 10,000 IU three times a day for child if acute; 25,000 IU three times a day in adult if acute. *Use any dose of vitamin A over 50,000 IU per day with medical supervision only.* *

Vitamin B complex: 25 to 50 mg three times daily.

Vitamin C: 250 to 500 mg chewable every hour in acute cases, or six times per day in chronic cases. *

OTHERS

Caldwell's syrup of pepsin (laxative)

Garlic: 2 capsules three times per day. *

Glycothymoline: 2 to 3 drops (internal antiseptic).

Herbal laxatives (gentle)

Lemon juice

Lymph glandular

Onion syrup: 1 tsp three to six times per day. *

Pineapple juice

Spleen glandular

Syrup of figs (laxative)

Thymus: 2 every hour. *

Vegetable juice*

Zinc: 15 to 30 mg three times per day. *

BOTANICALS

Coneflower (*Echinacea angustifolium*): Internal and topical.

Eucalyptus (*Eucalyptus globulus*)

Goldenseal (*Hydrastis canadensis*): Local swab and gargle. *

Myrrh (*Commiphora myrrha*): Local swab. *

Pleurisy root (*Asclepias tuberosa*)

Marigold flowers (*Calendula officinalis*): Use tincture as throat swab. *

*Asterisks indicate the most frequently used therapeutic agents.

Pokeroot (*Phytolacca decandra*) (highly toxic; see p. 62): For painful, hard, glandular enlargements. 25 drops in water four to six times per day in acute cases; three to four times per day in chronic cases.*

Red raspberry tea and sage tea (*Rubus strigosus* and *Salvia officinalis*)

St. John's wort (*Hypericum perforatum*)

ULCER (see Peptic Ulcer)

UNDERWEIGHT

Definition and Symptoms

Failure to maintain optimal weight for height.

Etiologic Considerations

- Digestive disorders
    Hydrochloric acid deficiency
    Pancreatic enzyme deficiency
    Malabsorption syndromes

- Hormonal imbalance
    Hyperthyroid

- Improper diet
    Low-energy foods
    Junk foods
    Restricted diets (i.e., fruitarianism)
    Protein deficiency

- Excess exercise or energy output

- Lack of appetite
    Zinc deficiency
    Cancer or other wasting disease

- Emotional
    Stress, anxiety
    Anorexia nervosa
    Bulimia

*Asterisks indicate the most frequently used therapeutic agents.

- Drug use
- Hypoglycemia, diabetes
- Allergy

Discussion

We all know someone who can eat and eat while still remaining extremely slim. Although this may make an overweight person envious, it does not necessarily equate with optimum health. Frequently, these individuals have a very inefficient digestive system and are absorbing very little of the food eaten. Digestive enzyme deficiency or failure of food absorption is very common. Malabsorption syndromes due to allergy or food insensitivity are also very common.

Endocrine imbalances involving the thyroid, pancreas, and adrenal glands can make weight gain impossible. Hypoglycemics and diabetics have a particularly difficult time maintaining proper weight.

Occasionally we will see very emaciated patients as a result of a specific dietary regimen. I once saw a 76-lb woman who had been living on fruit exclusively for 14 months. She had about 2 more months before she would have died on such a diet, had she not added protein to her regimen. Some strict vegetarians who have no knowledge of complete proteins can have plenty of calories per se but inadequate protein, causing their body's own protein to begin breaking down.

Zinc deficiency has been known to reduce the appetite as can some wasting diseases, such as cancer.

Stress or emotionally based weight loss may require psychological help.

Treatment

The actual cause must be diagnosed, if possible. I always suspect digestive enzyme deficiency and allergy or food sensitivity. The consistency of the bowel movement, and a check for undigested foods, can be a valuable diagnostic aid. The diet most useful for weight gain is similar to that found under Hypoglycemia or Diabetes. Adequate and complete proteins are essential: 70 to 100 g of dietary protein should be adequate, along with a diet of 60 or 70 percent unrefined carbohydrates and 50 to 60 g of dietary fat, most of which should be from unsaturated sources.

Therapeutic Agents

VITAMINS AND MINERALS

Vitamin A: 25,000 IU per day.

Vitamin B complex: 50 mg, one to two times per day.
Zinc: 25 to 50 mg, one to two times per day.

OTHERS
Hydrochloric acid and pepsin
Pancreatic enzymes

URETHRITIS (see Cystitis)

URINARY TRACT INFECTION (see Cystitis)

VAGINITIS (Thrush or Candidiasis, Trichomoniasis)

Definition

Vaginitis: Inflammation and irritation of the vagina.
Thrush: Infection caused by *Candida albicans* fungus. May affect the vagina, anus, mouth, skin, or nails.
Trichomoniasis: Protozoal infestation (by *Trichomonas vaginalis*) of the genitourinary tract, either in the male or female.

Symptoms

Vaginitis: Irritation, redness, intense itching, odor, discharge, painful sex.
Thrush: Vagina: Profuse, offensive, curdy discharge with inflammation, burning, itching, and painful sex.
   Nails: Painful red swellings leading to hardened, grooved nails.
   Mouth: Creamy white patches on inflamed mucosa.
   Skin: Inflamed, with red rash.
Trichomoniasis: Female: Frothy, thin, nonbloody vaginal discharge; rash; burning irritation; itching; and painful sex.
   Male: Usually symptomless carrier.

Etiologic Considerations

• Antibiotics (damaged ecology)
• *Candida albicans*, overgrowth
• Birth control pill (B_6 deficiency and pH changes)

- Pregnancy (vaginal pH changes, glycogen content increase)
- Diabetes
- Corticosteroids
- Tight-fitting synthetic underwear (poor ventilation; warm, moist environment)
- Diet (deficiency in vitamins B complex, B_6; excess sugar and refined carbohydrates)
- Poor hygiene
- Coitus transmission
- Raised vaginal pH (pregnancy, diabetes, menstrual period, after miscarriage, or abortion)
- IgA immune deficiency
- Stress
- Spinal
- Allergy
- Congestion
- Elderly: postmenopausal hormone changes causing dryness of vagina and lack of lubrication during sex
- Debilitation

Discussion

The normal vaginal ecology is a balance between many commensal organisms normally found in the vagina. These consist of a very large number of microorganisms, fungi, bacteria, and protozoa. Certain of these coexisting organisms are essential to normal vaginal health, such as Döderlein's bacillus, a species of *Lactobacillus*. This diversity of flora is controlled by several factors. The most important of these are the amount of glucose present in vaginal secretions, the acid/alkaline balance, and the hormonal state. Clinical infections such as candidiasis or trichomoniasis only occur when this natural balance is upset, allowing these fungi or protozoa to flourish and multiply in a more favorable environment.

Role of Sugar and pH

Normal vaginal secretions contain a large amount of glucose. This gives a high pH (basic or alkaline) quality to these discharges. The organisms that cause vaginal infections thrive on glucose. Fortunately, the Döderlein's bacteria, a normal inhabitant of the vagina in its mucous membrane, convert this glucose to lactic acid. This lowers the pH (making it more acid) just enough to keep other microorganisms from taking over.

Role of Menstrual Cycle, Pregnancy, and Birth Control Pill

During the normal menstrual cycle estrogen rises to a maximum at ovulation. This causes an increase in thin, sticky, alkaline mucus produced by the cervical glands. As this mucus passes down the vagina it gathers vaginal cells which break down and release their sugar content. This raises vaginal pH, making infection more probable. The actual menstrual flow further raises alkalinity. During pregnancy these alkaline changes are more sustained and encourage the common vaginal infections that often occur at this time. Use of the birth control pill, which simulates pregnancy, provides the ideal environment for vaginal infection.

Role of Antibiotics

Antibiotics kill disease-causing bacteria and friendly flora indiscriminately. These friendly bacteria exist all over the body, but their most important sites are the intestinal tract, where they help synthesize B vitamins, and the vagina, as described above. The widespread use of antibiotics has led also to a widespread epidemic of vaginal infections in all ages. Vaginal and systemic *Candida* infections are an increasing concern following antibiotic use. It has been frequently observed that the most common aftereffect of antibiotic use in women is a vaginal yeast infection. With repeated antibiotic use, the fungi that normally are present in the colon in controlled numbers may begin to proliferate and colonize the entire gastrointestinal tract. This can be a very serious problem, and has been associated not only with repeated vaginal infections, but also with panallergic conditions where the patient develops multiple allergies. The actual mechanism that causes these allergic-like symptoms is as yet not entirely clear. It is suspected that either the yeast produces a toxic substance that acts on remote tissues and organs, or, what seems to be more likely, that the fungus alters the structure and functions of the small intestine, causing a thinning of the wall, which allows larger allergenic protein molecules to pass into the bloodstream.*

Other Factors

- Stress: Stress upsets normal hormonal balance and reduces blood flow to parasympathetically innervated organs such as female organs.

- Spinal imbalances: L1 to 5—disturbs normal blood and nerve flow to pelvic organs.

*Truss Co., "Metabolic Abnormalities in Patients with Chronic Candidiasis—The Acetaldehyde Hypothesis," *J. Orthomolecular Psychiatry*, 13(2): 66–93, 1984.

- Congestion: Poor blood flow due to stress, spinal imbalances, lack of exercise, poor adrenal tone, diet deficiency, or any other reason will downgrade tissue health and encourage infection.

- Diet: Excess sugar, fruits, refined carbohydrates, or alcohol will lead to excess sugar in vaginal secretions. Strongly alkaline diets increase vaginal pH. Excess acid diet will favor simple vaginitis with rash and itching.

- Toilet: Frequent douching will upset vaginal ecology. Children should be educated to wipe front to back to prevent infecting vagina.

- Clothes: Tight-fitting synthetic underwear reduces ventilation and creates a warm, moist environment ideal for infection.

- Sex: Excess sex or intercourse without proper lubrication will irritate vaginal walls.

- Age: Senile changes in vaginal walls can lead to irritation and rash.

Treatment

Simple vaginitis and thrush respond quite readily to natural therapies. Trichomoniasis, however, can be very stubborn. Occasionally, orthodox treatments (flagyl) fail to eliminate the infection, leaving a deepseated problem very difficult to relieve by any means. In such a stubborn case I sometimes recommend following the treatments outlined below with one final series of metronidazole (flagyl) for both male and female partners. This will often succeed where the orthodox approach alone has repeatedly failed. Unfortunately I know of no other regimen that will be as effective and know of few naturopathic alternatives for the male partner. This does not necessarily mean that natural alternatives do not exist, but simply that I am at present unaware of them. Recent reports, however, show that trichomoniasis in males responds to high levels of zinc.* Certainly, for the female with simple vaginitis, thrush, or less-entrenched trichomoniasis, the simple therapies below are sufficient without drug medication.

Diet

During the 2 weeks of intense vaginal treatments aimed at establishing a normal internal ecology, the food eaten needs to be at least 80 percent raw, with an abundance of fresh vegetables. Salads are recommended for the main course for both lunch and supper. This is necessary to provide the proper healing influence on the mucous membranes; however, the urine needs to be artificially acidified by drinking 3 to 4 glasses of unsweetened cranberry juice each day. This is very important. Garlic and onions should be part of each meal. In

*"Zinc Treatment Suggested for Trichomonal Infection," *International Clinical Nutrition Review*, 4(1):29, January 1984.

general, the type of diet regimen found under Cystitis will be adequate. With thrush, one must stop taking both contraceptive pills and brewer's yeast and make sure that the vitamin B complex used is from a nonyeast source.

Therapeutic Agents

VITAMINS AND MINERALS

Vitamin A (high dose): 25,000 IU two to three times per day. *Use any dose of vitamin A over 50,000 IU per day with medical supervision only.* *

Vitamin B complex (high dose): 25 to 100 mg two to three times per day.*

Vitamin B$_6$: 50 to 100 mg two times per day.*

Vitamin C: 1000 to 6000 mg per day.*

Vitamin E: 400 to 800 IU per day.*

Zinc sulfate: 220 mg two times per day (trichomoniasis).*

Garlic: 2 capsules three times per day.*

Lactobacillus: 1 tsp three times per day.

Thymus tablets: 6 to 10 tablets per day.*

DOUCHES

Yoghurt, lactic acid, or acidophilus: 1 tbs added to 1 quart warm water, twice a day.*

Apple cider vinegar douche: 2 tbs to 1 quart warm water twice a day.*

Goldenseal: ½ to 1 tbs to 1 quart warm water twice a day.

Tea tree oil: 1 tbs to 1 quart warm water douche twice a day.

Bay leaf or barberry tea douche

Oxysulfate plus *Hydrastis* douche: 2% copper sulfate solution. 1 tsp to one pint of warm water.*

Glycothymoline douche: 1 to 2 tbs to 1 quart water. Alternate with:

Atomodine douche: 1 to 2 tbs to 1 quart water.

White oak bark *(Quercus alba)* douche: for leukorrhea.

Hemlock *(Abies canadensis)* douche: for leukorrhea.

Douche: Use just enough permanganate of potash to color warm water. Add 1 to 2 drops myrrh tincture.

Iodine: 1/1000 solution retention douche once a day (trichomoniasis).

Suppositories
    Lactic acid wafers*

*Asterisks indicate the most frequently used therapeutic agents.

Boric acid: 2 00 capsules inserted nightly for 2 days; 1 per night for 1 week, 1 weekly maintenance dose.*

Goldenseal and cocoa butter: 1 inserted nightly.

Gentian violet plus tampon

Cabasil garlic inserted nightly

Depletion pack (see Appendix II for source)

BATHS

Salt water bath: ½ cup to a tub of water. Allow to enter vagina.

Fume sitz baths: Add 5 drops of myrrh tincture and 10 grains of balsam of tolu to 1½ gallons of boiled hot water. Sit over basin and expose irritated membranes to the rising steam fumes.

Local applications

Calendula lotion: Apply to irritated vaginal walls full strength or 50/50 with water.

Calendula powder, calendula ointment

Goldenseal powder

Goldenseal and witch hazel tincture diluted: Applied locally.

Calendula, *Hydrastis* and *Berberis*

Thuja, tea tree oil, and calendula

Ultraviolet ray: Internal application.

Ichthyol, 20%: Local application.

0.5 to 1% Gentian violet: Painted inflamed mucosa.

B_6 vitamin salve

Goldthread *(Coptis trifolia)* and goldenseal

Witch hazel

Chickweed ointment

THRUSH

Oral: Acidophilus: ⅓ tsp three times per day by mouth.

Niacinamide: 100-mg tablet crushed and put on infant's tongue; plus 100 mg twice a day to breastfeeding mother.

Nails: Tea tree soaks (water-soluble tea tree): Dilute with hot water. Soak twice a day for 15 minutes, then apply tea tree oil or cream.

*Asterisks indicate the most frequently used therapeutic agents.

Therapeutic Suggestions

With the large number of possibly useful therapeutic agents, the following outline of a suggested procedure may be of benefit:

TRICHOMONIASIS

Days 1 to 3:
Atomodine or iodine douche, morning
Tea tree oil douche, afternoon
Depletion pack, evening (see Appendix II)
Calendula lotion applied locally to irritated membranes

Days 4 to 6:
Oxysulfate and *Hydrastis* douche (see Appendix II, Boericke & Tafel), morning
Atomodine or iodine douche, afternoon
Hydrastis and cocoa butter suppository, evening
Calendula lotion locally

Days 7 to 11:
Apple cider vinegar douche, morning
Yoghurt or acidophilus douche, afternoon
Boric acid suppository, evening

Days 11 to 18:
Boric acid suppository, evening

THRUSH

Days 1 to 3:
Tea tree oil douche, morning
Oxysulfate and *Hydrastis* douche, afternoon
Hydrastis and cocoa butter suppository, evening
Calendula lotion, locally

Days 4 to 6:
Oxysulfate and *Hydrastis* douche, morning
Apple cider vinegar douche, afternoon
Hydrastis suppositories, evening
Calendula lotion, locally

Days 7 to 9:
Apple cider vinegar douche, morning
Yoghurt or acidophilus douche, afternoon
Hydrastis suppository, evening

Another regimen that works well with vaginal yeast infections is as follows:

Days 1 and 2:
Tea tree oil douche, morning and afternoon
Boric acid crystals suppository, evening (1 00 capsule)

Days 3 and 4:
Tea tree oil douche, morning
Apple cider vinegar douche, afternoon
Boric acid suppository, evening

Days 5 to 7:
Apple cider vinegar douche, morning
Yoghurt or acidophilus douche, afternoon
Lactobacillus capsule suppository, evening

Days 8 to 14:
One 00 capsule mixed boric acid plus *Lactobacillus* suppository each evening. Some cases may require oral nystatin therapy for a period of up to 6 months if the *Candida* has overgrown throughout the entire intestinal tract. Also useful is oral superdophilus, or megadophilus, garlic, biotin, caprilic acid, and a yeast-free, refined carbohydrate-free diet.

VARICOSE VEINS AND VARICOSE ULCERS

Definition

Abnormally dilated, lengthened, and sacculated veins. May cause ulceration in later stages.

Symptoms

Muscle cramps, fatigue of leg muscles, sore calf muscles, ankle swelling, eczema, and ulcers.

Etiologic Considerations

- Diet
    Refined carbohydrates·
    Deficiency of vitamins E and C
- Constipation
- Obesity

- Posture, poor body mechanics
- Poor circulation
- Lack of exercise, sedentary occupation
- Spinal
    Lumbar
    Sacral
    Coccyx
- Acidity, improper eliminations
- Congenital valve insufficiency
- Leg crossing
- Prolonged sitting or standing
- Pregnancy
- Liver damage
- Abdominal tumors
- Blood clot

Discussion

The veins are equipped with a series of one-way valves that allow blood to enter in the direction toward the heart and away from gravity. This is a necessary function since veins, unlike arteries, do not have a positive pumping action exerted by the heart itself, nor any intrinsic muscular activity. Venous pumping is performed by the leg muscles massaging the veins during muscular activity. This action slowly pushes the blood uphill through the series of valves toward the heart. This muscular venous pumping action is aided by the diaphragmatic action sucking blood up against gravity. Once the valves have been severely damaged or destroyed, there is no cure. If circulation to the superficial skin becomes reduced, a gradual process of tissue starvation occurs, leading to difficult-to-heal varicose ulcers.

Surgery has been performed to replace the dilated, damaged veins with veins from other parts of the body. This does remove the unsightly dilated veins and improves local circulation, but does nothing to prevent a recurrence, which is common.

Here again we have an extremely common ailment which can be considered one of the "diseases of civilization." Varicose veins are found very rarely in undeveloped nations whose inhabitants still live on unrefined foods. The same dietary factors that lead to constipation and hemorrhoids (which in fact are a form of varicose veins) also cause varicose veins (see Constipation, also Hemorrhoids). Our diet in developed nations includes a very large proportion of devitalized, fiber-deficient, refined foods. These nutrient-deficient foods cause the tissues of the body to become weakened and low in vitality. A low-fiber diet also slows the bowel transit time of foods, leading to toxic reabsorption and hard, difficult-to-pass feces. Often this process becomes so extreme that actual pressure from a loaded bowel can restrict the venous return of blood from the legs, leading to varicosity. In these cases it is usually the left leg which is most affected, since the descending colon, splenic flexure, and lower rectum are the areas most likely to be overloaded. Obesity will have a similar action, but its effects are usually bilateral. Girdles and other restricting clothing may be a cause. Poor spinal mechanics and posture can affect venous return, especially with a severe lumbar lordosis leading to visceroptosis, or a drooping of the entire abdominal and pelvic contents that restricts venous return.

Prolonged standing has, in the past, been cited as the major cause of varicose veins. However, recent studies find little difference between those whose occupations require standing or sitting. The key factor seems to be lack of demanding exercise and a sedentary existence.

Spinal lesions are a common cause of reduced circulation and tissue malnutrition, and may lead to valve degeneration or favor constipation and act indirectly, as discussed.

In women, pregnancy is commonly the time when varicose veins are first a problem. The hormones present during the latter part of pregnancy cause all the involuntary muscles to become lax, favoring constipation and dilated varicose veins. In the final states of pregnancy, the pressure of the baby's head lower in the pelvis may also act as a mechanical barrier to proper venous return.

Treatment

Diet

The first objective is to establish proper bowel eliminations. These patients usually have a history of chronic constipation and a laxative habit. The best initial approach is either a 3-day fruit juice fast with enemas nightly (and no further laxatives or enemas taken in the future), or a 3-day apple mono diet where all that is eaten are apples and apple juice. On the evening of the third day, 1 to 2 tbs of olive oil are to be taken. Follow this with the full constipation diet (see Constipation). Cascara sagrada tincture is taken in tonic doses over a period of 4 to 6 weeks, beginning with 25 drops in water four times a day and gradually reducing to three times, two times, one time, and then stopping altogether as the bowels show renewed regularity. Cascara, when taken in this way, becomes a tonic rather than a laxative to the bowels.

Follow this diet with a high-fiber one based on the constipation diet, but more flexible in nature once regularity is established. A large amount of citrus fruit and salads is encouraged. 1 tbs raw bran with a glass of water is to be taken three times per day, both during the initial diets (except when fasting) and later as a bowel regulator on a permanent basis.

Physiotherapy

- Slant board abdominal exercises
- Upper leg and calf exercise
- Wet grass walking
- Salt water walks kneedeep in the ocean
- Walking, bicycling, swimming, etc.
- Headstands
- Elevate foot of bed 4 in.
- Keep affected leg elevated whenever possible
- Alternate hot and cold leg sprays
- Alternate hot and cold sitz baths
- Alternate hot and cold showers
- Spinal manipulation
- Friction brush massage (see Appendix I)
- Flex and extend ankles frequently
- Local massage upward (not over thinned veins) with warm olive oil and myrrh
- Massage feet in fluid from old coffee grounds; also apply over thinned vessels
- Mullein poultice
- Hot sage tea compress
- Witch hazel compress
- Slippery elm poultice to ulcers
- Vitamin E to ulcers
- Clay poultice to ulcers
- Comfrey poultice to ulcers
- Ultraviolet light to ulcers and varicose veins
- White oak bark tea compress
- Bayberry tea compress

- Stoneroot (*Collinsonia*) tea compress or ointment
- Pressure bandage

Therapeutic Agents

VITAMINS AND MINERALS

Vitamin A: 25,000 IU two to four times daily. *Use any dose of vitamin A over 50,000 IU per day with medical supervision only.**

Vitamin B: 25 to 50 mg two times daily.*

Folic acid

Vitamin C plus bioflavonoids: 1000 to 6000 mg per day.*

Vitamin E: 400 to 1200 IU per day.*

Essential fatty acids: GLA, EPA, and oil of evening primrose.

Calcium

OTHERS

Blackstrap molasses
Bran: 1 tbs with water three times per day.*
Chlorophyll*
Garlic: 2 capsules three times per day.
Lecithin
Rutin: 2 capsules two times per day.
Wheat germ
Zinc

BOTANICALS

Mullein tea (*Verbascum thapsus*)
Stone root (*Collinsonia canadensis*): 1 to 4 capsules per day.*

WARTS (Verrucae)

Definition

Benign epithelial tumors caused by a virus. They may affect the hands, arms, face, body, feet, and anal or genital region. The three most commonly seen types are common, venereal, and plantar warts.

*Asterisks indicate the most frequently used therapeutic agents.

Symptoms

Raised, irregular (common, venereal), or flat (plantar) growths on the skin. These may be symptomless or cause pain and discomfort, especially in areas of constant contact, such as the sole of the foot.

Etiologic Considerations

• Virus infection

• Lowered resistance

• Reduced immunological state

• Glandular development

• Trauma

• Vitamin A deficiency

• Psychogenic causes

Discussion

Warts are virus infections. Naturopathically, the causes of warts are no different from any other bacterial, viral, or parasitic infection or infestation of the body. These infections occur due to a lowered vitality and lack of resistance on the part of the host.

A key factor with warts in particular is a state of lowered immunological activity. This may be due to an improper diet of nutrient-deficient refined foods. Certainly, deficiencies of vitamin A, vitamin C, and zinc have all been related to an increased incidence of viral infections. These often lower the body's ability to fight off even everyday viruses such as those that cause warts.

Warts tend to appear at times when general glandular development is occurring. Thus they are fairly infrequent in the very young, but common in the puberty and teen years. Coincidentally, these are also the years that nutritional deficiencies of vitamins A and C, and zinc are most common. Warts are much less common in the aged when glandular systems are no longer functioning as actively.

Warts are most frequently found in areas exposed to trauma or repeated friction. They rarely cause anything more than a cosmetic problem, except with the case of plantar or venereal warts. Plantar warts can cause severe discomfort, making normal walking very painful. Genital warts can totally upset normal sexual relations, causing physical discomfort and severe psychological depression. Women with venereal warts should get a Pap smear and also be examined by a gynecologist. External condylomata are sometimes accompanied by internal warts (cervical human papilloma virus has been recently linked to an increased risk of subsequent cervical cancer with an estimated increase in the range of 200 times as likely).

Psychogenic factors are well recognized in relation to warts. They seem very susceptible to all types of suggestion, either in their creation or cure.

Treatment

The usual methods of removing warts by acids, surgery, burning, electro-therapy, and freezing carry a high percentage of recurrence over a much larger area than previously affected. The reason this occurs is that attention has not been placed on the major causative factors. Best results are obtained when internal, external, and psychological measures are taken simultaneously. Vigorous treatment is needed especially with venereal warts, which may be very contagious, and spread rapidly to cover the entire anogenital region.

Diet

The nutritional state has a great deal to do with general host resistance and a strong immunological system. Dietary changes, however, may take 6 months or longer to alleviate the condition. Foods high in vitamins A, B complex, C, and in zinc in particular should be stressed. The diet should have a large proportion of raw foods. The internal dietary and nutritional approach is especially necessary where warts are so widespread and numerous that topical therapy is practically impossible.

In these cases, along with the general upgrading of the nutritional status, it may be necessary to acidify the entire system artificially for a 2-week period by the use of 20 to 30 drops of orthophosphoric acid taken in water daily. This has a very strong effect on systemic warts. It may be repeated two or three times after a 2-week interval. High doses of vitamins A, B complex, C, and of zinc are used with all warts for 1-to-2-month periods, with care not to extend vitamin A therapy at too high a dose for too long, causing toxic results. Generally, 50,000 to 100,000 IU for up to 6 weeks is nontoxic for adults, especially if the emulsified form is used.

Psychotherapy

Hypnosis for warts is very effective.

External Applications

All the following local therapies have been used with success for some people. Several may need to be tried to get results.

Garlic: Apply thin section over wart as continuous poultice. Avoid healthy tissue.

Castor oil and baking soda poultice: Mix castor oil and baking soda into a paste and apply to wart; keep covered with Band-Aid each night. Do not pick at wart during the day, but let it slough off within 3 to 6 weeks. This may at times cause some pain. If so, stop the application and then apply again on the following evening.

Castor oil: Apply three times per day and at night. Cover with Band-Aid. May take 2 or more months to be successful.

Vitamin E: Apply 400 IU capsules three times per day and cover with Band-Aid. Takes approximately 2 months.

Vitamin A (micellized):   25,000 IU applied topically three times per day and night. Cover. Especially useful in plantar warts.

Podophyllum tincture (May-apple or American mandrake) (highly toxic; see p. 62):   Antimitotic, caustic: Simmer ordinary tincture until reduced to one-fourth. Apply 1 drop carefully to wart one time per day. Protect surrounding skin with Vaseline, paraffin, or sticky plaster to prevent tissue damage. Keep covered with adhesive tape. Repeat daily for 2 to 3 weeks. Care must be taken in treating multiple warts simultaneously with *Podophyllum* since it is toxic, even by absorption through the skin. Never use *Podophyllum* unless under medical supervision.

Podophyllum tincture 20% and compound tincture of benzoin 80%:   Apply to anogenital warts.

Thuja tincture: Especially useful in anal and genital warts. Thuja oil is also used topically.

Salicylic acid and thuja: Apply with care. Protect surrounding skin. Repeat application two to three times per day.

Other treatments suggested by some:

Powdered vitamin C: Topical as paste and covered with Band-Aid.
Black walnut tincture
Comfrey ointment, root poultice, or leaf poultice
Plantain poultice for plantar warts
Fresh dandelion juice: Apply locally and then cover.
Oil of sulfur
Chickweed juice or poultice
Sassafras oil
Tormentil oil
Oil of *Gaultheria*
Thymol
Fresh greater celandine juice
Green fig juice

Green papaya juice
Aloe vera
Onion and salt compress

Internal Botanicals and Dilutions

Castoreum 30×
Nitric acid 30×
Thuja tincture, thuja 30×

Therapeutic Agents

VITAMINS AND MINERALS

Vitamin A (emulsified): 50,000 to 100,000 IU per day for 6 weeks. *Use any dose of vitamin A over 50,000 IU per day with medical supervision only.**

Vitamin B complex: 25 to 50 mg two to three times per day.*

Vitamin B₆: 50 mg two times per day.*

Vitamin C: 1500 to 6000 mg per day.*

Vitamin E: 600 to 1200 IU per day.*

Zinc: 50 to 100 mg per day.*

OTHERS
Garlic: 2 capsules three times per day.

WHOOPING COUGH (see Childhood Diseases)

WORMS

Definition
Infestation with various types of worms, including pinworms, roundworms, hookworms, and tapeworms.

Symptoms

None, or local irritation of anus, weakness, fatigue, lack of vitality, grinding of teeth at night, loss of appetite, irritability, frequent colds, brittle and hard fingernails with ridged longitudinal lines, anemia, loss of weight.

*Asterisks indicate the most frequently used therapeutic agents.

Etiologic Considerations

- Poor diet
  Sugar
  Refined carbohydrates
  Excess dairy
  Excess acidity
  Raw green vegetable deficiency
  Excess meat
  Excess cooked foods

- Constipation

- Lowered resistance

- Poor hygiene

- Lack of exercise

- Upset internal ecology

Discussion

The human body supports many life forms, both externally and internally. Some of these do little or no harm, and in fact are usually never noticed. Others are actually beneficial as are the bacteria that normally inhabit the intestine and vagina. These actually help to protect the body from invasion of other more detrimental viruses, bacteria, or parasites.

Worms of various kinds can enter the body through several avenues and, if conditions are favorable for their development, may multiply. If this colony is not kept in check by the body's own defenses, the infestation soon becomes a burden on the body and health is downgraded.

Threadworms, Pinworms (Oxyuris or Enterobius vermicularis)

This is the most common of worm infestations. The infection rate among children is often close to 100 percent. Most people have, have had, or will have a pinworm infestation at one or more times in their lives. Many have pinworms right now but do not even know it.

Pinworms are spread by inhaling or ingesting their eggs, which are widespread in the environment, especially where children live or play. These eggs are extremely tiny. The female worm emerges from the anus at night to lay her eggs in the external anal folds. This causes irritation and itching. The area is then scratched and the eggs pass from the fingernails to others directly or via food. If left on the anal region they hatch, reenter the anus and mature. The eggs also gather on the bedclothes and enter the air as the sheet or blanket is shaken out, spreading throughout the room and infecting by ingestion or inhalation. The worms may be seen as tiny, threadlike, maggot-sized worms in the stool, or at the anus at night. They infest the large intestine and may cause appendix irritation, leading to false appendicitis. A single female may lay 10,000 eggs, which then mature in 2 weeks.

Parents seem to suffer most psychologically when their child gets pinworms. I have seen parents completely beside themselves with disgust when they discover such an infestation. I would like to reassure you that pinworms are not that bad. Certainly a large infestation can be a negative health factor as the worms do compete for the body's food supply, but much less so than with the other worms we will talk about later. The first infestation is usually the worst, and then the body slowly develops an immunity so that a low threshold infection is maintained without much detriment, even without treatment. Drug therapy for worms is very appealing to the parent, since it offers a quick solution to a distressing condition. One dose of Povan is usually very effective in killing the worms. The reinfection rate, however, is nearly 100 percent. The problem, of course, is that the real causes were never removed and reexposure for a typical child is practically certain no matter how many precautions the parent may take.

As with other infections, pinworms develop best if vitality is low. It is clear from studies of children in the same classroom that some develop a strong immunity to worms and get either light or no infections, while others never seem to develop immunity and harbor large infestations indefinitely. The most documented difference between these two groups is not general hygiene, as some might expect. It is diet. Those who are most susceptible generally eat more refined carbohydrates and sugar than their classmates, and have much less fiber in their diet.

Roundworms (Ascaris lumbricoides)

Ascarids have been humanity's constant companions probably since we began domesticating pigs. Where soil pollution, warmth, and moisture are common, so are roundworms. Ascarids are large nematode worms reaching 8 to 14 in. in length. They have a narrow tapered head and the females have a blunt tail. They normally inhabit the small intestine where they feed on undigested food and have also been known to bite the mucous membranes of the intestine and suck the host's blood.

A single female produces about 200,000 eggs each day. These eggs pass out of the body with the feces and develop or remain viable wherever moisture and oxygen exist. They are very resistant to chemicals and can even survive long exposure to seawater. Complete drying is lethal, but with moisture the eggs may remain alive for years. When the eggs are swallowed the larvae then hatch in the small intestine and penetrate their mucous membrane. From here they are carried by the blood to the liver, heart, and lungs, where they burrow out into the trachea, esophagus, or throat, to be swallowed. They then settle down and develop in the small intestine where they reach maturity in 2½ months.

They are commonly spread by hand-to-mouth contact. This emphasizes the importance of hygiene in restaurants and is one of the main reasons it is a state law for employees in the food-handling industry to wash their hands after a visit to the toilet. Contamination is also spread readily in areas where human manure is used for fertilizer. Vegetables or fruit grown on such soil then spread the infection. Young children may also spread them by defecating in yard areas where others may then easily be infected.

Infection with *Ascaris* is not nearly as benign as with pinworm, and a serious health risk occurs with heavy infestations. As the worms pass through the lungs, a severe and possibly fatal pneumonia may result. Abdominal symptoms include diarrhea, abdominal discomfort, or vomiting. The worms may become tangled, causing intestinal blockage requiring surgery, or may block various organs or ducts such as the gallbladder, or even the appendix. There is some evidence that these worms may produce toxic substances causing delirium, nervousness, convulsions, or coma. They may even cause poor digestion of proteins by interfering with the digestive enzyme trypsin, leading to malnutrition. The body reacts to these worm infestations with antibodies which may be responsible for a number of allergies.

Prevention depends mainly on proper nutrition, as with all infections, proper disposal of human feces, good hygiene, and proper washing of vegetables, especially where "night soil" is used.

Hookworms *(Ancylostoma duodenale* and *Necator americanus)*

These worms cause much injury to humans. Hookworm infestations, however, are rarely spectacular, but year after year insidiously drain the vitality and undermine the health. Many so-called worthless or lazy people are suffering from hookworms that stunt them mentally and physically.

Hookworms are rather fat and about ½ in. long. They possess powerful teeth that latch onto the bowel walls and allow the parasite to inflict severe damage to the intestine while sucking large amounts of blood. Each female produces 5000 to 10,000 eggs each day. The eggs pass out in the feces and develop into larvae in moist, warm soil. These free-living larvae then feed on bacteria and other small matter in the excreted feces until they either die from lack of moisture, or are stepped upon by a barefooted host. They then bore into the skin, pass into the lymph channels or blood vessels, making their way to the heart and lungs, where they burrow out into the air spaces and are passed upward toward the throat by the action of cilia hairs within the lungs themselves. Here they are either expectorated and then die in the sun or are swallowed, to pass into the intestine to mature and grow. Each worm lives anywhere from 5 to 15 years.

Hookworms are primarily tropical in origin. Cold and dryness will kill the larvae as will salt within the soil. Animals such as pigs, dogs, and cattle may eat the eggs and aid in the spread of infection by voiding these eggs unharmed in areas most likely to affect humans. Infestations are more common among agricultural workers, or those living in rural areas, especially where shoes are not often worn, or where human feces (night soil) are used as a fertilizer.

Diet has a profound effect on hookworm infestation and host resistance. Most of the injury done by these worms results from the consequent anemia and protein deficiency from the blood lost to the parasites. This lowers host resistance and reduces the body's capacity to produce antibodies. It is well proven that patients recover best from hookworms on a diet high in protein, iron, and other blood-building elements. This diet is also essential in the prevention of large infections. The severity of hookworm disease in a community is influenced more by the adequacy of the diet than to the incidence of exposure.

The main health problems hookworms cause are bronchitis and pneumonia when in the lung, and nausea, abdominal discomfort, and sometimes diarrhea, but the principal effects are those of anemia. The effects of hookworm during pregnancy are especially severe when the demand for protein and iron by the developing fetus puts an extra drain upon the mother's nutritional state. Hookworm is implicated in a vast number of stillbirths and is considered a more severe complication of pregnancy than eclampsia.

Tapeworms (Various Species)

Tapeworms consist of extremely long chains of nearly independent, sexually capable segments. These chains may be anywhere from 6 to 60 ft long. The tapeworm attaches to the intestinal wall and absorbs food from the host. The life cycles vary with each species. The most common are spread by the host's eating uncooked or incompletely cooked pork, beef, or fish. They cause symptoms similar to other worm infections—abdominal pain, loss of weight, weakness, and particularly a severe anemia, especially the fish tapeworm, which uses up all the available vitamin B_{12}, to cause pernicious anemia.

Treatment

Drug therapy is recommended. It is rapid and fairly sure. Dietary therapies for these conditions are much slower. The role of diet and nutritional factors, however, should then be helpful in preventing reinfection. The exception to this is mild pinworm infestations, which are fairly easy to take care of with natural remedies. Some interesting references to botanicals sometimes used for other intestinal parasites are included for general interest.

Diet

Studies of those with high resistance to worm infestation show a diet high in unrefined carbohydrates, raw green vegetables, and adequate protein; with little meat, pork, or uncooked fish, and no sugar. It is clear that appropriate diet has a great deal to do with preventing worm infections by increasing host immunity and preventing obvious infection through proper preparation and cooking of food. Once infection has occurred, various regimens are useful to lower or completely remove the population. A few useful diet regimens are found below:

Day 1 to 3   Green cabbage (or carrots) plus pumpkin seeds eaten three to four times per day. Nothing else except garlic or garlic capsules three times per day. Take prescribed worm medication morning and evening. (Wormwood plus other prescriptions, depending on type of infection.)

Day 4   In morning take purging dose of Epsom salts, senna, or other cathartic. In the evening take an enema with bitterwood (*Picraena excelsa* (1 oz to 1 pint of water). Same diet as above.

Day 5   Repeat Day 4

Another version:

Day 1 to 3   As above

Day 4   Take ½ tsp Fletcher's Castoria every ½ hour until half the bottle is used. Next, take strong worm remedy specific to infection. When bowel movement occurs, finish Castoria, plus half bottle more.

Another alternative is the all garlic and onion diet instead of cabbage and pumpkin seeds. Follow the same directions as above for the worm medication and purge. Garlic water enemas may also be used.

Follow-up diet to include:

No sweets or refined carbohydrates.
Increased raw greens, especially lettuce and cabbage.
No milk.
Plenty of onions and garlic.
¼ lb pumpkin seeds per day.
Coconut meat and milk, if available.
Figs.
Raw pineapple.

Pomegranate: 1 to 3 per day when available.

It is important to change the intestinal environment by these measures. Worms love sugar, acid conditions, and constipation. High-fiber alkaline diets are the best prevention of infestation, and cure.

Physiotherapy

* Garlic clove inserted rectally at night
* Garlic foot compresses at night
* Abdominal exercise
* Sit in bowl of warm milk after purge, for tapeworm

Therapeutic Agents

Garlic	Papaya
Onions	Horseradish
Pomegranate	Fig
Raw pancreas	Lemons
Pumpkin seeds	Carrots
Cabbage	Pineapple
Lettuce	Bromelain

BOTANICALS

Fresh papaya seeds: 1 tsp chewed on empty stomach.

Pumpkin seed tea: 1 oz to 1 pint water; 1 teacup to 1 pint per day.

Wormwood (*Artemisia absinthium*): For pinworms, roundworms:*

1 teacup infusion morning and evening.
10 to 30 grains powder morning and evening
5 to 30 drops tincture morning and evening, then purge.

Wormseed (*Artemisia cina*): Contains santonin. Useful with tapeworms. Use small doses frequently. ½ to 1½ grains.*

Male fern (*Dryopteris filixmas*):
½ to 1 tsp powder morning and evening, then purge (senna plus butternut purge).

*Asterisks indicate the most frequently used therapeutic agents.

30 drops oil morning and evening, then purge (for tapeworm).
1 to 1½ drams of tincture in morning, then purge.

American wormseed, Jerusalem oak (*Chenopodium anthelminticum*):*
Children: 20 to 30 grains powdered seeds or 3 to 10 drops oil.
Adults: 1 to 2 tsp powdered seeds or 10 to 20 drops oil (for roundworms, hookworms, tapeworms).

Tansy (*Tanacetum vulgare*):
½ to 1 cup infusion (especially seeds) morning and evening.
Fluid extract: Children: 1 tsp
                        Adults: 3 tsp
Take cathartic 1 hour later

Pomegranate (*Punica granatum*): For pinworms, roundworms, tapeworms.
Decoction of root bark used.*

Santonica/wormseed (*Artemisia santonica*): For pinworm, roundworm, tapeworm.*

Prickly pear (*Opuntia* spp.): For amoebic dysentery. Use strong infusion of flowers. Dose: 1 cup morning and evening.

Kousso (*Berayera anthelmenthica*): For tapeworm.

Chips tea enema: For pinworms.

Thymol (tapeworm, roundworm)*

Bitterwood: Enema or decoction. Use wood and bark:*
1 tbs to 1 cup water; boil 30 minutes
Dose: 1 tsp in 1 cup water one to two times per day.

Cascara (purge)

Senna (purge)

Epsom salts (purge)

Pinkroot (*Spigelia marilandica*) with wormwood for pinworms, 15 to 30 drops two times per day.*

Areca nut (Betel nut) for tapeworm.

Aloe (*Aloe vera*)

May-apple, or American mandrake (*Podophyllum peltatum*) (highly toxic; see p. 62)

Butternut (*Juglans cinerea*): Laxative.

*Asterisks indicate the most frequently used therapeutic agents.

PRESCRIPTIONS

Cina 6×
Santoninum 3 to 6×
Spigelia anthelmia 1×
Podophyllum: ¼ grain, two times per day with diet and purge.
Zymex II (Standard Process Labs)*
Calomel: ¼ grain
Senna: ½ grain
Santonin: ¼ grain
Pomegranate
Male fern
Wormwood
Sulfax (Boericke and Tafel)*

WOUNDS, MINOR CUTS, BRUISES

All injuries that cause tissue damage should be placed in ice-cold water immediately. This will stop bleeding, reduce the chance of inflammation, and dramatically speed recovery. Cuts should be thoroughly cleaned while in the cold water, and freed of any dirt or foreign object. Apply tea tree oil to prevent infection, and reapply every 2 to 3 hours. Vitamin E may be used topically to accelerate healing and reduce scarring. Arnica tincture applied topically—three to four times per day—is excellent for any bruise. Arnica in potency form should be taken internally at frequent intervals. Fresh *Aloe vera* juice and/or comfrey poultice will also accelerate healing of superficial wounds.

Treatment

Vitamins and Minerals

Vitamin A: 50,000 to 100,000 IU per day. *Use any dose of vitamin A over 50,000 IU per day with medical supervision only.*

Vitamin C: 5 to 10 g per day.

Bioflavonoids: 300 to 1000 mg per day.

Vitamin E: 400 to 800 IU per day.

Zinc: 25 mg two to three times per day.

*Asterisks indicate the most frequently used therapeutic agents.

YEAST INFECTION (Candida Albicans)

Definition
Local or systemic colonization of the skin or mucous membranes by the yeast *Candida albicans*, also referred to as *Monilia albicans*, or thrush.

Symptoms
These depend on severity of colonization, area affected, and tissue response. Common symptoms include the following:

Recurrent vaginal infections (see Vaginitis)
Fatigue
Depression
Inability to concentrate
Constipation or diarrhea
Gas
Bloating
Abdominal pain
Muscle or joint pain
Headaches
Allergies
Skin rashes (i.e., hives, eczema, psoriasis, rash under arms, in crotch, etc.)
Nail fungus
Menstrual problems (premenstrual syndrome)
Prostatitis
Hypoglycemia
Hyperactivity
Athlete's foot

Etiologic Considerations
- Repeated antibiotic use
- Birth control pill use
- Consumption of refined carbohydrates or excess fruit or fruit juice
- Improper hygiene
- Nutritional deficiency due to improper diet or malabsorption
- IgA (gamma-A globulin) or other immune deficiencies
- Allergies

- Chemical exposure
- Pregnancy
- Menstrual cycle
- Constipation

Discussion

Yeast infections have been recognized since the days of Hippocrates. Most women are aware of yeast problems since they are such a common cause of vaginitis. The yeast involved is *Candida albicans*, a common, usually nonpathogenic inhabitant of the skin and mucous membranes. Under normal circumstances, the body's defense barriers and immune system keep this fungus in check, allowing it only a limited existence. If, however, the body's defenses are weakened by improper diet, or if the general or local ecology of the body or tissues is severely altered, as it is by antibiotic use, *Candida* can begin to flourish. As the yeast takes hold, it produces local irritation and sends systemic toxins throughout the body, causing the wide range of symptoms listed above.

The problem with *Candida* infections is diagnosis. Since *Candida* is a normal inhabitant of the vagina and gastrointestinal tract, a culture is of no use. The only diagnosis can be one suggested by the case history followed by a successful trial treatment of an antifungal regimen.

Treatment

Diet

Yeast seems to thrive on sugars and refined carbohydrates. This may be the reason that a history of hypoglycemia and sweets craving is so common in patients with *Candida* infections. By starving *Candida* of its favorite foods, a better internal ecology is favored. A diet composed mostly of vegetarian (fish is an exception) nondairy protein (except for yoghurt), unrefined grains, and vegetables is best. Onions and garlic are particularly useful.

I prefer to avoid meat-based proteins, since these are associated with abnormal bowel flora development. Milk also can result in abnormal flora; however, fermented dairy products such as buttermilk, kefir, and yoghurt are beneficial. Yoghurt should be included in the diet once or twice daily, unless obvious dairy allergy exists. Although whole grains are suggested, yeasted grains should be avoided. Some question has arisen about yeast avoidance, since the type of yeast in bread and baked products is not the same as *Candida*. While this is true, it is a common clinical observation that these yeast definitely do aggravate these conditions and are best avoided. This also includes yeast-source multivitamins,

or yeast-source B vitamins, and any foods commonly known to contain yeast.
The following summary of acceptable foods may be of use:

Proteins	Yoghurt Kefir Buttermilk Seeds Nuts Eggs Tofu Beans Fish Chicken (less frequently) Meat (less frequently)

Vegetables	Unrestricted, except for the following carbohydrate-containing vegetables, which should be eaten less frequently:
	    Potatoes
	    Sweet potatoes
	    Beans
	    Squash
	    Corn

Fruit or Fruit Juice	Little or none except for avocado or papaya
Whole grains	All grains are allowed unless obvious allergy exists. The only restriction is the amount in the diet. Some patients respond best by reducing the proportion of grains dramatically, even excluding them altogether; others may handle unrestricted quantities and still reestablish good external ecology. While the whole grains are composed of significant carbohydrate, the fiber and protein components help reestablish proper bowel function, a major factor in the causation of altered bowel ecology in the first place.

Therapeutic Agents

VITAMINS AND MINERALS

Vitamin A: 25,000 to 50,000 IU one to two times per day.

Yeast-free vitamin B complex: 25 to 50 mg one to two times per day.

Vitamin B_6: 100 to 250 mg one to two times per day, especially with premenstrual syndrome.

Vitamin C: Up to bowel tolerance.

Vitamin E: 400 to 800 IU per day.

Biotin

Caprilic acid

OTHERS

Garlic: I prefer pure clove garlic, however unsociable, in cases of yeast infections. 1 medium clove two to three times per day, although difficult to take, is the best garlic preparation available. I question Kyolic in this instance and would prefer the products made by Arizona Natural Products if the clove garlic is not being used. Take garlic preparations at least three times per day.

Lactobacillus: Since this is one of the most important medications, it is essential that the preparation be *viable.* I use Superdophilus or Megadophilus powder, 1 tsp three to four times per day. Other brands may be as, or more, useful, but unfortunately (and maybe fortunately!), the health food industry is not presently regulated to demand validated testing of product consistency and potency. This applies to all nutritional products in health food stores. How often is an unreliable product the cause of prescription failure? We presently cannot know.

Nystatin: Once *Candida* is entrenched, it can be very difficult to eradicate. Many cases will not be treatable with general internal ecology improvement, and will require nystatin or other antifungal medication. Since this is a prescription item, it must be prescribed by your doctor. Usual doses range from 50,000 to 100,000 units three to four times per day. Side effects are minimal. Nystatin seems to be fairly nontoxic. Many of its side effects are in reality the result of massive *Candida* death, the body's sudden burden of its breakdown products, and the body's inflammatory response to these materials.

BOTANICALS

Taheebo inner bark tea (antifungal): 1 cup infusion four times per day.

Tea tree oil (local use): Useful in nail fungus. Add 1 tbs water-soluble tea tree (Melasol; Metabolic Products) to 1 cup hot water. Soak nail 20 to 30 minutes one to two times per day. Apply tea tree oil to nail and nail bed two to three times per day. Continue treatment for 30 to 60 days.

Aloe vera juice: 2 oz four times per day.

See Vaginitis for local vaginal treatments.

PART III

Appendixes

APPENDIX I

Remedies

DIETARY INSTRUCTION

Mucus-Cleansing Diet

This diet is extremely useful for all conditions of excess mucus such as asthma, bronchitis, catarrh, colds, pneumonia, salpingitis, ear infections, and many others.

Breakfast	Citrus fruit (especially grapefruit)
Midmorning	Fresh carrot juice
Lunch	A large plate of steamed onions with a little natural soy sauce for flavor. In some cases steamed carrots are also allowed (up to 25 percent of the meal), with the rest being onions.
Midafternoon	Potassium broth, or as midmorning
Supper	Same as lunch
Evening	As midafternoon

All Fruit Diet

Eat any unsprayed fruit or fruit juice other than banana. Banana is considered too starchy for an elimination regimen. Take only one type of fruit per meal. Alternate the juice and fruit every 1 to 2 hours.

Honey/Onion Syrup

Slice a large onion thinly, place in a bowl, and cover with 1 to 2 tbs honey. Cover container tightly and allow to sit for 8 hours. Mash, strain, and take in 1-tsp doses four to eight times per day. Excellent in mucous conditions.

Potassium Broth

Take ¼ in. of outer peelings of potatoes (including the skin), fresh parsley, unpeeled carrots, beet greens, onions, garlic, and any other organically grown green vegetables on hand. Prepare broth by washing and chopping the vegetables and then simmering in a large covered pot of water for 30 to 40 minutes. Strain and drink the essence, discarding the vegetables. Excess may be stored in glass containers in the refrigerator for up to 2 days.

PHYSIOTHERAPY INSTRUCTIONS

Endonasal Technique

This is a method where obstructions from the upper parts of the respiratory system are removed by manipulating small bones in and surrounding the nasal area. The usual method is the introduction inside the nose of small balloons which are then suddenly inflated. Most naturopaths use this technique as well as many chiropractors and osteopaths.

· Coffee Enemas

First thing in the morning prepare a pot of caffeinated coffee (not instant) using a glassware, enamelware, or stainless steel container. Use 2 to 4 tbs of coffee grinds to 1 quart of water. Take a preliminary warm water enema to cleanse the lower bowel. When coffee has cooled to body temperature, place in enema container 18 to 20 in. higher than the body. Attach a 24-to-32-in. colon tube (obtainable from most drug stores) to the end of the enema tip. Lubricate tube with K-Y jelly and slowly insert 18 to 20 in. into the colon, slowly rotating the tube to prevent kinking. Lie on the left side as you allow the coffee to enter the colon. If fluid does not flow easily, the colon tube may be kinked. If so, slowly remove 4 to 8 in. of the tube until the flow of fluid is felt and slowly reinsert the entire 18 to 20 in. Once all the coffee has entered the colon, remove the colon tube slowly and remain on the left side for 5 minutes. Roll onto the back for a further 5 minutes and finally on to the right side for 5 minutes. Finish by expelling the fluid into the toilet. The coffee enema removes toxins and opens the bile ducts.

Garlic Foot Compress

This is an extremely valuable method to reduce excess mucus and combat systemic infections. It is especially useful with infants who cannot take garlic or onions by mouth. Care must be taken to follow these instructions explicitly to prevent severe blistering of the soles. It is entirely safe if applied correctly. *Oil* the soles of the feet with olive oil. Mash garlic and apply ⅛ to ¼ in. thick between gauze. Apply to soles with suitable nonstick tape and cover with a sock to secure. Leave poultice on all night.

"Salt Glow"

Mix 1 lb of fine salt in enough water to make a slurry. Begin with a warm shower and then with water off rub the salt all over the body firmly. Finish with an ice-cold shower. Your skin will "glow" for hours.

Skin Brushing

Obtain a medium-to-firm-bristle body brush. Brush your entire body vigorously at least once daily, dry or in the shower.

Epsom Salts Baths

Put 1 to 1½ lb of Epsom salts into a hot tub and soak for 15 to 20 minutes. Immediately go to bed under plenty of covers to sweat. Remain in bed 3 hours to all night. Rinse off with tepid water after the sweat and finish with a colder application, either a sponge bath or shower.

Castor Oil Packs

Obtain undyed cotton or preferably wool flannel (see Cayce suppliers) of sufficient size so that it will cover an area approximately 8 in. by 12 in. when folded two to four thicknesses. Soak this flannel in a pan of unrefined cold pressed castor oil (see Cayce suppliers). Wring out so that the cloth is just wet but not dripping, and apply to area of body to be treated. Cover this with plastic and apply a heating pad as warm as is comfortably bearable. Leave pack on for 1 to 1½ hours. After the pack is completed, wash the oil off with warm water and baking soda (1 tsp to 1 pint warm water). Store flannel in covered pan for future use. After 20 or 30 uses thoroughly cleanse the flannel and reuse.

APPENDIX II

Sources of Health and Nutrition Products

Edgar Cayce Products: Throughout this book various products have been examined that were first suggested by Edgar Cayce during psychic readings for individuals seeking health service. Cayce's unique talent applied over a period of years gradually revealed detailed diagnoses and therapeutic suggestions for many disease states. It must be stressed that each of the readings was given for a particular individual and therefore not easily generalized, due to the very specific nature of these readings. Still, many useful suggestions were often repeated for separate individuals with similar disease states. This information has been compiled from thousands of psychic readings by the members of the ARE (Association for Research and Enlightenment). For further useful information contact:

> ARE
> Membership Services Director
> P.O. Box 595
> Virginia Beach, Va. 23451

These are three reliable sources of the Cayce products:

> PMS
> P.O. Box 3074
> Virginia Beach, Va. 23453
>
> Heritage Store
> Box 444
> Virginia Beach, Va. 23458
>
> Home Health Products, Inc.
> 383 S. Independence Blvd.
> Virginia Beach, Va. 23452

Source for Dr. Reckeweg homeopathic remedies:

Botanical Laboratories, Inc.
Sumas, Wa. 98295

Distributor for Naturopathic Formulations

Source for many excellent nutritional products. This is a young, very reliable company that is growing rapidly:

Naturopathic Formulations
3363 South East 20th
Portland, Oregon 97232

White Crane
9010 E.S. St. Helens St.
Clackamas, Oregon 97015

Source for first aid homeopathic kit and some very high quality botanical tinctures:

Equinox Botanicals
Rt.1 Box 71
Rutland, Ohio 45775

Source for the VM120 needed for the Depletion Pack:

Vita Minerals
1815 Flower
Glendale, Ca 91201

Seroyal Products is an extremely reliable brand of nutritional and health products, available through physicians only. The same company also produces NF products, available in most health food stores:

Seroyal Brands, Inc.	Seroyal
Box 6500	P.O. Box 5004
Concord, Ca 94524	Kent, Wa. 98031
	Tel: 1 (206) 226-5063
	1 (800) 426-0976

Source of gentle prenatal supplements, plus other useful supplements and botanical tinctures. Also source of valuable reprinted botanical texts from early 1900s. They now supply the depletion vaginal pack in ready prepared form:

Eclectic Institute Inc.
11231 S.E. Market St.
Portland, Oregon 97216
Tel: 1(503) 256-4330

Other reliable suppliers:

Nutridyn
14802 N.E. 31st Circle
Redmond, Wa. 98052

Professional Specialities, Inc.
1803 132nd Ave. N.E.
Bellevue, Wa. 98005

Standard Process Laboratories
Inc.
Milwaukee, Wisc. 53201

Anabolic Laboratories, Inc.
Box 3, 19508
Irvine, Calif. 92713

Standard Homeopathic Co.
Box 61067
Los Angeles, Calif. 90061

Weleda
Box 121
841 So. Main St.
Spring Valley, N.Y. 10977

Luyties
Box 8080
St. Louis, Mo. 63156

Health from the Sun
Dept. R.O., P. O. Box 477
Dover, Ma. 02030

Source of good deodorized garlic:

Arizona Natural Products
7750 E. Evans Rd., #3
Scottsdale, Ariz. 85260

An excellent botanical and homeopathic pharmaceutical supply source. Nearly all tinctures or dilutions may be obtained, or will be specially prepared on request:

Boericke & Tafel
1011 Arch St.
Philadelphia, Pa. 19107

Another fine source for botanicals and homeopathic dilutions:

Borneman
1208 Amosland Rd.
Norwood, Pa. 19074

Source for olbas products plus some other useful herbal products:

Penn Herbs
603 North 2nd St.
Philadelphia, Pa. 19123

Source for a liquid B complex (50 mg). Very useful when pills are poorly taken or digestion weak:

LaSante Products
5506 35th Ave., N.E.
Seattle, Wa. 98105

Source for tea tree products:

Metabolic Products Corp.
Cambridge, Mass. 02141

Source for orthophosphoric acid, plus many other nutritional products:

VM Nu-ri Inc.
Box 286
1012 Hort Dr.
Lake Geneva, Wisc. 53147

APPENDIX III

Associations

American Association of Naturopathic
  Physicians (AANP)
P.O. Box 5086
New Haven, Conn. 06525

Canadian Naturopathic Association
Suite No. 306
Mid Park Center
259 Mid Park Way S.E.
Calgary, Alberta
Canada T2X1M2
Tel: (403) 256-0272

British Naturopathic and Osteopathic
  Assn. (BCNOA)
Frazer House
6 Netherhall Gardens
London, NW 3 England 5RR

APPENDIX IV

Periodicals

The Journal of the John Bastyr College
of Naturopathic Medicine
1408 N.E. 45th St.
Seattle, Wa. 98105

An excellent periodical for the serious student or practitioner of Naturopathic Medicine:

Metabolic Update
15615 Bellevue-Redmond Rd., Suite E
Bellevue, Wa. 98008

An excellent monthly nutritional information series on cassette tape compiled from a review and consolidation of current research on every aspect of nutritional therapy. Dr. Jeffrey Bland began this series in 1982. The cost is $200 per year, and in my opinion, a bargain at nearly any price. Dr. Bland presents the newest information in a very concise form. Highly recommended to the health care practitioner. Dr. Bland also has done extensive nutritional seminars which are still available in tape form. For more information on these truly exceptional informational tapes, contact:

Dr. Jeffrey Bland
Laboratory for Nutritional Support
  Analysis
Linus Pauling Institute of Science Medicine
3180 Porter Dr.
Palo Alto, Ca. 94304

American Journal of Clinical Nutrition
9650 Rockville Pike
Bethesda, Maryland 20014

Holistic Health Review
Human Sciences Press
72 Fifth Ave.
New York, N.Y. 10011

Human Sciences Press
3 Henrietta St.
London, England WC2E 8LU

Journal of Holistic Medicine
Human Sciences Press
3 Henrietta St.
London, England WC2E 8LU

British Naturopathic Journal and Osteopathic Osteopathic Review
Frazier House
Netherhall Gardens
London, England NW3 599

Presents evidence of a therapeutic role for vitamins, minerals, and specific nutrients in modern medicine. Current research data relevant to clinical application of vitamins, minerals, trace elements, enzymes, amino acids, fatty acids, etc., is gathered from biochemistry, metabolism, clinical nutrition, neuroendocrinology, nutritional pharmacology, and clinical ecology.

International Clinical Nutrition Review
Dartech Technical Services
Mariner Medical Plaza
355 Placentia Avenue, Suite 305
Newport Beach, Ca. 92663

APPENDIX V

Clinics and Colleges

Tringham Naturopathic Clinic
Newport Pagnal
Bucks, England
Tel: Newport Pagnal 610450

An inpatient naturopathic clinic utilizing a full spectrum of natural therapies.

Enton Hall
Nr. Godalming
Surrey, England
Tel: Wormley (042 879) 2233

An inpatient naturopathic, osteopathic, and hydropathic health center.

Ontario College of Naturopathic Medi-
cine
Box 131 Kitchener
Ontario, Canada N26 3W9

Graduates are eligible for licensure in the Province of Ontario as doctor of naturopathic medicine.

National College of Naturopathic Medicine
11231 S.E. Market
Portland, Ore. 97216

The oldest accredited naturopathic medical school in the United States. Provides 4-year full-time training. Graduates are qualified to take state licensing examinations in seven states now fully licensing naturopathic physicians.

British College of Naturopathy and Osteopathy
6 Netherhall Gardens
London NW 3 England
Tel: 01 435 7830

Students are eligible for public grants. Training includes noninvasive osteopathy and naturopathy. Course curriculum meets or exceeds academic requirements for licensing of naturopathic physicians in the United States. Licensing
is subject to successfully passing state licensing examinations.

The John Bastyr College of Naturopathic Medicine
1408 N.E. 45th St.
Seattle, Wa. 98105

A newly established, highly respected 4-year naturopathic medical school.

Bibliography

A *Clinician's Guide to Toxic Metals* (Hayward, CA: Mineralab Inc., 1979).
A *Physician's Guide to Hair Analysis Interpretation* (Phoenix, AZ: Analytical Research Labs, Inc.).
A *Visual Encyclopedia of Unconventional Medicine* (New York: Crown Publishers, 1979).
Abehsera, Michel: *The Healing Clay* (New York: Swan House Publishing Co., n.d.).
Adams, Rex: *Miracle Medicine Foods* (New York: Parker Publishing Co., Inc., 1977).
Adams, Ruth, and Frank Murray: *Body, Mind and the B Vitamins* (New York: Larchmont Books, 1972).
Airola, Paavo: *The Miracle of Garlic* (Phoenix, AZ: Health Plus, 1978).
———: *Health Secrets from Europe* (New York: Arco Publishing Co., 1976).
———: *How to Get Well* (Phoenix, AZ: Health Plus, 1974).
———: *There Is a Cure for Arthritis* (West Nyack, NY: Parker Publishing Co., 1968).
———: *Hypoglycemia: A Better Approach* (Phoenix, AZ: Health Plus, 1977).
———: *How to Keep Slim, Healthy and Young with Juice Fasting* (Phoenix, AZ: Health Plus, 1971).
———: *Everywoman's Book* (Phoenix, AZ: Health Plus, 1979).
Aman: *Medicinal Secrets of Your Food* (Mysore, India: Secretary, Indo-American Hospital, 1969).
An Edgar Cayce Health Anthology (Virginia Beach, VA: A.R.E. Press, 1979).
An Edgar Cayce Home Medicine Guide (Virginia Beach, VA: Edgar Cayce Foundation, 1982).
Arthritis in the Edgar Cayce Readings (Virginia Beach, VA: Heritage Publications, 1976).
Aschner, Bernard: *Arthritis Can Be Cured* (New York: Arco Publishing Co., Inc., 1975).
Ashmore, Edythe F.: *Osteopathic Mechanics* (Mokelumne Hill, CA: Health Research, reprint 1964).
Atkins, Robert: *Dr. Atkins' Nutrition Breakthrough* (New York: William Morrow & Co., Inc., 1981).
Bach, Jean-François, ed.: *Immunology* (New York: John Wiley & Sons, Inc., 1976).
Bagnall, Victor H.: *Nutritional Therapy: A Clinical Presentation* (Wenatchee, WA: Nutritional Publications, 1977).
Bailey, Covert: *Fit or Fat?* (Boston, MA: Houghton Mifflin Co., 1977).
Ballentine, Rudolph: *Diet & Nutrition* (Honesdale, PA: The Himalayan International Institute, 1978).
Barrington, Greville G.: *How to Cure Insomnia* (London: Lutterworth's Ltd., n.d.).

Benjamin, Harry: *Your Diet in Health and Disease* (Wellingborough, Northamptonshire, England: Thorsons Publishers, Ltd., 1931).

———: *Everybody's Guide to Nature Cure* (Wellingborough, Northamptonshire, England: Thorsons Publishers Ltd., 1936).

Bennett, Sanford: *Old Age: Its Cause and Prevention* (New York: Dodd, Mead & Co., 1924).

Berland, Theodore, and Robert G. Addison: *Living with Your Bad Back* (New York: St. Martin's Press, Inc., 1971).

Bethel, May: *The Healing Power of Herbs* (North Hollywood, CA: Wilshire Book Co., 1972).

Bieler, Henry G.: *Food Is Your Best Medicine* (New York: Random House, 1973).

Bilz, F. E.: *The Natural Method of Healing* (Leipzig, London, Paris: F. E. Bilz, Part first, Part second, 1898).

Bircher-Benner, M.: *The Prevention of Incurable Disease* (Cambridge, England: James Clarke & Co., Ltd., 1969).

Bircher-Benner Nutrition Plan for Arthritis and Rheumatism: Staff of the Bircher-Benner Clinic (New York: Pyramid Publications, 1976).

Bland, Jeffrey: *Your Health under Siege: Using Nutrition to Fight Back* (Brattleboro, VT: The Stephen Greene Press, 1981).

———: *Diagnostic Usefulness of Trace Elements in Human Hair* (Bellevue, WA: Northwest Diagnostic Services, 1981).

———: *Trace Elements in Human Health and Disease* (Bellevue, WA: Northwest Diagnostic Services, 1979).

———, ed.: *Medical Applications of Clinical Nutrition* (New Canaan, CT: Keats Publishing, 1983).

Boerick, William: *Materia Medica with Repertory: Pocket Manual of Homeopathic Materia Medica* (New Delhi, India: Jain Publishers, 1927).

Bricklin, Mark: *The Practical Encyclopedia of Natural Healing* (Emmaus, PA: Rodale Press, 1976).

———: *Rodale's Encyclopedia of Natural Home Remedies* (Emmaus, PA: Rodale Press, 1982).

Brinker, Francis: *An Introduction to the Toxicology of Common Botanical Medicinal Substances* (Portland, OR: National College of Naturopathic Medicine, 1983).

British Herbal Pharmacopoeia, Part 1 (London: British Herbal Medicine Association, 1971).

Brodsky, Greg: *From Eden to Aquarius: The Book of Natural Healing* (New York: Bantam Books, Inc., 1974).

Buchman, Dian Dincin: *The Complete Book of Water Therapy* (New York: E. P. Dutton & Co., 1979).

———: *Herbal Medicine, The Natural Way to Get Well and Stay Well* (New York: Gramercy Publishing Co., 1979).

Budoff, Penny Wise: *No More Menstrual Cramps and Other Good News* (New York: Penguin Books, 1980).

Burroughs, Stanley: *Healing for the Age of Enlightenment* (Kalua, HI: Stanley Burroughs, 1976).

Carque, Otto: *Rational Diet* (Los Angeles, CA: Times Mirror Press, 1926).

Carrington, Hereward: *Vitality, Fasting and Nutrition* (New York: Rebman Co., 1908).

Carroll, David: *The Complete Book of Natural Medicines* (New York: Summit Books, 1980).

Carter, Mary Ellen, and Wm. A. McGarey: *Edgar Cayce on Healing* (Paperback Library, 1972).

Cayce, Edgar: *Hair Treatment: Crude Oil* (Virginia Beach, VA: Heritage Publications, 1978).

Charmine, Susan E.: *The Complete New Juice Therapy* (Wellingborough, Northamptonshire, England: Thorsons Publishers, Ltd., 1977).

Cheraskin, E., and W. M. Ringsdorf, Jr.: *New Hope for Incurable Diseases* (New York: Arco Publishing Co., Inc., 1971).

Chiropractic Reference Notebook (Virginia Beach, VA: A.R.E. Press, 1973).

Christopher, John R.: *Childhood Diseases* (Provo, UT: Christopher Publ., 1978).

Clark, Linda A.: *Know Your Nutrition* (New Canaan, CT: Keats Publ., Inc., 1973).

———: *Get Well Naturally* (New York: Arco Publ., Inc., 1978).

———: A Handbook of Natural Remedies for Common Ailments (New York: Pocket Books, Inc., 1976).

Cleave, T. L.: The Saccharine Disease (Bristol, England: John Wright & Sons, Ltd., 1974).

———: Peptic Ulcer (Bristol, England: John Wright & Sons, Ltd., 1968).

———: Fat Consumption & Coronary Disease (Bristol, England: John Wright & Sons, Ltd., Stoneridge Press, 1957).

Clement, Mark: Aluminum: A Menace to Health (London: True Health Publishing Co., 1949).

Clements, Harry: Self-Treatment for Colitis (London: Thorsons Publishers, Ltd., 1978).

———: Nature Cure for Constipation and Other Bowel Disorders (London: Thorsons Publishers, Ltd., 1968).

———: Self-Treatment for Skin Troubles (London: Thorsons Publishers, Ltd., 1951).

———: Headaches and Migraine (London: Thorsons Publishers, Ltd., 1957).

———: Prostate Troubles (London: Thorsons Publishers, Ltd., 1977).

———: Nature Cure for Shingles and Cold Sores (London: Thorsons Publishers, Ltd., 1977).

Clymer, Swinburne: Nature's Healing Agents (Quakerville, PA: Humanitarian Society, 1905).

Coca, Arthur A.: The Pulse Test (New York: Arco Publishing Co., Inc., 1967).

Coon, Nelson: Using Plants for Healing (Martha's Vineyard, MA: Hearthside Press, 1963).

Cotton, H. D.: Relax Your Way to Health (Surrey, England: Health for All Publishing Co., 1968).

Coulter, Harris L.: Homeopathic Medicine (Washington, DC: American Foundation of Homeopathy, 1972).

Culbreth, David M. R.: A Manual of Materia Medica and Pharmacology (Portland, OR: Eclectic Medical Publications reprinted in 1983 from early 1900).

Cyriax, James: Textbook of Orthopaedic Medicine, Volume One: Diagnosis of Soft Tissue Lesions (London: Cassell Ltd., 1978).

Davidson, Stanley, R. Passmore, J. F. Brock, and A. S. Truswell: Human Nutrition and Dietetics (London: Churchill Livingstone, 1975).

Davis, Adelle: Let's Get Well (New York: Jovanovich, Inc., 1965).

Deal, Sheldon C.: New Life through Nutrition (Tucson, AZ: New Life Publ., 1974).

de Bairacli Levy, Juliette: Nature's Children (New York: Schocken Books, 1971).

Dextreit, Raymond: Our Earth Our Cure (New York: Swan House Publishing Co., 1974).

Downing, Carter Harrison: Osteopathic Principles in Disease (Carter Harrison Downing, 1935).

Ehret, Arnold: Rational Fasting (New York: Lust Publ., Beneficial Book Edition, 1971).

———: Mucusless Diet Healing System (Beaumont, CA: Ehret Literature Publishing Co., 1953).

Ellingwood, Finley: American Materia Medica, Therapeutics and Pharmacognosy (Portland, OR: Eclectic Medical Publications, reprinted in 1983 from early 1900).

Felter, Harvey Wickes: The Eclectic Materia Medica, Pharmacology and Therapeutica (John K. Scudder, 1922. Portland, OR: Eclectic Medical Publications reprinted in 1983).

Finnerty, Gertrude Brentano, and Theodore Corbitt: Hydrotherapy (New York: Frederick Unger Publishing Co., 1960).

Fredericks, Carlton: Nutrition Guide for the Prevention and Cure of Common Ailments and Diseases (New York: Simon & Schuster, 1982).

———: Look Younger, Feel Healthier (New York: Grosset & Dunlap, 1977).

Fryette, Harrison H.: Principles of Osteopathic Technic (Carmel, CA: Academy of Applied Osteopathy, 1954).

Garten, M. O.: The Health Secrets of a Naturopathic Doctor (New York: Arco Publishing Co., Inc., 1967).

———: The Natural and Drugless Way for Better Health (New York: Arco Publishing Co., Inc., 1969).

Gerras, Charles, Joseph Golant, and E. John Hanna, eds.: The Complete Book of Vitamins (Emmaus, PA: Rodale Press, 1977).

Gerson, Max: A Cancer Therapy (Del Mar, CA: Totality Books, 1958).

Girdwood, R. H.: *Clinical Pharmacology* (Dilling) (London: Belliere Tindall, 1976).

Goldthwait, Joel: *Essentials of Body Mechanics* (Philadelphia: J. B. Lippincott Co., 1952).

Goodenough, Josephus: *Dr. Goodenough's Home Cures & Herbal Remedies* (Crown Publishers, Inc., 1982, previously published as *The Favorite Medical Receipt Book and Home Doctor*, 1904).

Goodhart, Robert W., and Maurice E. Shils: *Modern Nutrition in Health and Disease* (Philadelphia: Lea & Febinger, 1980).

Gordon, G. F.: *Lead Toxicity* (Beverly Hills, CA: American Academy of Medical Preventics).

Graedon, Joe: *The People's Pharmacy* (New York: Avon Books, 1977).

Graham, R. Lincoln: *Water in Disease and in Health* (Tyrone, PA: Bodley and Brooks, 1924).

Halcomb, Ruth: *Women's Bodies, Women's Lives* (Chatsworth CA: Books for Better Living, 1974).

Hall, George J.: *Overcoming Anaemia* (Surrey, England: Health for All Publishing Co., 1959).

————: *How to Overcome Anaemia* (Wellingborough, Northamptonshire, England: Thorsons Publishers, Ltd., 1959).

Hartmann, Franz: *Occult Science in Medicine* (London: Theosophical Publishing Society).

Hauser, Benjamin Gayelord: *The Eliminative Feeding System* (Chicago, IL: The New School Publishers, 1927).

Hayes, Brad M.: *Doctor's Guide to Patient Supplementation* (Tulsa, OK: Bran Printing, 1979).

Heinerman, John: *Science of Herbal Medicine* (Orem, UT: Bi-World Publishers, 1979).

Henshaw, George: *Years of Abuse of the Extensive Alimentary Canal and Its Appendages* (Mexico City: Delivered at XLII Annual Congress P.H.H.M.C., 1970).

Hill, Ray: *Propolis, The Natural Antibiotic* (England: Thorsons Publishers, Ltd., 1977).

Hills, Christopher: *The Secrets of Spirulina* (CA: University of the Trees Press in cooperation with the Journal of Nutritional Microbiology, 1980).

Hills, Hilda Cherry: *Good Food, Gluten Free* (England: The Henry Doubleday Research Assn., 1974).

Homola, Samuel: *Doctor Homola's Natural Health Remedies* (New York: Parker Publishing Co., Inc., 1973).

Hornibrook, F. A.: *The Culture of the Abdomen, The Cure of Obesity and Constipation* (London: William Heinemann Medical Books, Ltd., 1941).

Inglis, Brian: *The Case for Unorthodox Medicine* (New York: G. P. Putnam's Sons, 1965).

Irwin, M. Isabel: *Nutritional Requirements of Man: A Conspectus of Research* (New York: The Nutrition Foundation, Inc., 1980).

Jackson, Mildred, and Terri Teague: *The Handbook of Alternatives to Chemical Medicine* (Oakland, CA: Terri K. Teague and Mildred Jackson, 1975).

Janse, Joseph: *Chiropractic Principles & Technic* (National College of Chiropractic, Chicago: 1947).

Jarvis, D. C.: *Folk Medicine* (London: Pan Books, Ltd., 1961).

————: *Arthritis and Folk Medicine* (London: Pan Books, Ltd., 1962).

Jensen, Bernard: *Overcoming Arthritis & Rheumatism* (Solana Beach, CA: Bernard Jensen Publ. Div.).

————: *The Science and Practice of Iridology* (Escondido, CA: Bernard Jensen, 1952).

————: *You Can Master Disease* (Solana Beach, CA: Bernard Jensen Publ. Div.).

————: *Nature Has a Remedy (It Can Be Physical, Mental or Spiritual)* (Santa Cruz, CA: Unity Press, 1978).

————: *Tissue Cleansing through Bowel Management* (Escondido, CA: Bernard Jensen Publ. Div., co-authored with Sylvia Bell, 1981).

————: *How to Enjoy Better Health from Natural Remedies* (Solana, CA: Bernard Jensen Publ. Div.).

————: *Health Magic through Chlorophyll from Living Plant Life* (Provo, UT: BiWorld Publishing, Inc., 1973).

————: *Doctor-Patient Handbook* (Provo, UT: BiWorld Publ., Inc., 1976).

Kaye, Robert: Core Textbook of Pediatrics (Philadelphia: J. B. Lippincott, 1978).

Kellogg, J. H.: *Rational Hydrotherapy: A Manual of the Physiological and Therapeutic Effects of Hydriatic Procedures, and the Technique of Their Application in the Treatment of Disease* (Philadelphia: F. A. Davis Co., 1906).

Kent, James Tyler: *Lectures on Homeopathic Philosophy* (New Delhi, India: Jain Publ., 1979).

Kervan, Louis: *Biological Transmutations* (New York: Swan House Publishing Co., 1972).

Kirschmann, John D.: *Nutrition Almanac*, revised edition, Nutrition Search, Inc. (New York: McGraw-Hill Book Co., 1975).

Kloss, Jethro: *Back to Eden* (Coalmont, TE: Longview Publ., 1939).

Kneipp, Sebastian: *My Water Cure* (Bavaria: Jos. Koesel, 1886).

Kordel, Lelord: *Natural Folk Remedies* (New York: Manor Books, 1974).

————: *Health The Easy Way* (New York: Award Books, 1973).

Kraak, Anton: *Herbs and Phyto Therapy* (Ventura, CA: Silver Enterprises, 1971).

Krause, Marie, and L. Kathleen Mahan: *Food, Nutrition and Diet Therapy* (Philadelphia: W. B. Saunders Co., 1979).

Kunis, Richard A.: *Mega-Nutrition* (New York: McGraw-Hill, 1980).

Kuts-Cheraux, A.W.: *Naturae Medicina and Naturopathic Dispensatory* (Iowa: American Naturopathic Physicians & Surgeons Assn., 1953).

Lake, Thomas T.: *Treatment by Neuropathy and the Encyclopedia of Physical and Manipulative Therapeutics* (Mokelumne, CA: reprinted by Health Research, 1972).

Last, Walter: *Heal Yourself* (Whangarei, New Zealand: Healthprint, 1979).

Lectures of Dr. Jeffrey Bland (compiled and interpreted by Ron Schmidt, 1980).

Leek, Richard: Hair Analysis (1980).

LeHunte, Cooper, R. M.: *The Danger of Food Contamination by Aluminum* (London: John Bale, Sons & Danielsson Ltd., 1932).

Leung, Albert Y.: *Encyclopedia of Common Natural Ingredients* (New York: John Wiley & Sons, 1980).

Levine, Stephen A., and Jay Parker: *Selenium and Human Chemical Hypersensitivities: Preliminary Findings* (Tacoma, WA: Reprinted from The International Journal of Biosocial Research, 1982).

Levine, Stephen: *Allergy: An Expanded Concept* (Cassette: Allergy Research Group, 2336–C Stanwell Circle, Concord, CA, 1982).

Lewis, Walter: *Medical Botany Plants Affecting Man's Health* (New York: John Wiley & Sons, 1977).

Licht, Sidney, assisted by Herma Kamonetz: *Medical Hydrology* (New Haven, CT: Elisabeth Licht, 1963).

Linclahr, Henry: *Philosophy of Natural Therapeutics* (England: The Maidstone Osteopathic Clinic, edited and revised by Jocelyn C. P. Proby, 1975).

————: *Practice of Natural Therapeutics* (Chicago, IL: Lindlahr Publ., 1926).

Lucas, Richard: *Nature's Medicines* (CA: Wilshire Book Co., 1969).

————: *Common and Uncommon Uses of Herbs for Healthful Living* (New York: Parker Publishing Co., Inc., 1969).

Lust, John B.: *Raw Juice Therapy* (England: Thorsons Publishers, Ltd., 1959).

————: *The Herb Book* (Sun Valley, CA: Benedict Lust Publ., 1974).

Macdonald-Bayne, Murdo: *Heal Yourself* (London: L. N. Fowler & Co., Inc., Ltd., 1945).

Mackarness, Richard: *Not All in the Mind* (London: Pan Books, Ltd., 1976).

MacLeod, John: *Davidson's Principles and Practice of Medicine* (Edinburgh, London, New York: Churchill Livingstone, 1975).

Madaras, Lynda, and Jane Paterson: *A Gynecological Guide to Your Body* (New York: Avon Books).

Maigne, Robert: *Orthopedic Medicine, A New Approach to Vertebral Manipulation* (Springfield, IL: Charles C Thomas, 1972).

Markell, Edward, and Marietta Voge: *Medical Parasitology* (Philadelphia: W. B. Saunders Co., 1981).

McBean, E.: *Vaccinations Do Not Protect* (Yorktown, TX: Life Science, 1980).

———: *The Poisoned Needle* (Mokelumne, CA: Health Research, 1957).

McM. Mennell, John: *Back Pain, Diagnosis and Treatment Using Manipulative Techniques* (Boston: Little, Brown & Co., 1960).

Medical Group Theosophical Research Center: *The Mystery of Healing* (London: 1958).

Medicines for the New Age, from the Edgar Cayce Readings (Virginia Beach, VA: Heritage Publications, 1975, revised ed.).

Medicines for the New Age, from the Edgar Cayce Readings (Virginia Beach, VA: Heritage Publications, 1977, revised ed.).

Mellor, Constance: *Natural Remedies for Common Ailments* (Frogmore, St. Albans, Hert., England: Mayflower Books, Ltd., 1973).

Mendelsohn, Robert S.: *Confessions of a Medical Heretic* (New York: Warner Books, 1979).

Meséqué, Maurice: *Health Secrets of Plants and Herbs* (New York: William Morrow & Co., 1975).

Michele, Arthur A.: *You Don't Have to Ache (A Guide to Orthotherapy)* London: Pan Books, Ltd., 1974).

Miles, Eustace: *The Uric Acid Fetish (Exposure of a Popular Theory)* (London: Eustace Miles).

Mitchell, Ross G.: *Disease in Infancy and Childhood* (London: Churchill Livingstone, 1973).

Mitchell, W.: *Naturopathic Applications of the Botanical Remedies* (Seattle, WA: John Bastyr College of Naturopathic Medicine, 1982).

Moyle, Alan: *Self-Treatment for Insomnia* (London: Health for All Publ. Co., 1957).

———: *Self-Treatment for Digestive Troubles* (London: Health for All Publ. Co., 1951).

———: *Nature Cure for Asthma and Hay Fever* (London: Thorsons Publishers, Ltd., 1951).

Muramoto, Naboru: *Healing Ourselves* (New York: A Swan House Book published by Avon, 1973).

Murphy, Patrick: *Trace Minerals and Health* (Hayward, CA: D. J. Consultants, Inc., 1982).

Nittler, Alan H.: *New Breed—Digest of Metabolic Nutrition* (California: New Breed Enterprises Publication Division, 1977).

Nutrient Content of Foods (Hayward, CA: Mineralab, Inc., 1980).

Oliver, J. H.: *Common Ailments* (London: The C. W. Daniel Co., 1924).

Ott, John N.: *Health and Light* (New York: Pocket Books, 1976).

Passwater, Richard A.: *Super-Nutrition* (New York: Pocket Books, 1975).

Pfeiffer, Carl C.: *Zinc and Other Micro-Nutrients* (New Canaan, CT: Keats Publishing Co., 1978).

——— and the Publications Committee of the Brain Bio Center: *Mental and Elemental Nutrients* (New Canaan, CT: Keats Publishing Co., Inc., 1975).

Physician's Reference Notebook, Volume One (Virginia Beach, VA: A. R. E. Press, 1968).

Physicians' Desk Reference (Oradell, NJ: Medical Economics Co., 1980).

Potter's New Cyclopaedia of Medicinal Herbs and Preparations, R. C. Wren, reedited and enlarged by R. W. Wren (New York: Harper & Row, 1972).

Powell, Eric, F. W.: *The Natural Home Physician* (North Devon, England: Health Science Press, 1962).

Powell, Milton: *An Outline of Naturopathic Psychotherapy* (London: British College of Naturopathy and Osteopathy, 1967).

Quick, Clifford: *Nature Cure for Cystitis* (Wellingborough, Northamptonshire, England: Thorsons Publishers, Ltd., 1975).

Reference on the Significance of Hair Element Analysis (Hayward, CA: Mineralab, Inc., 1980).

Reilly, Harold J., and Ruth Hagy-Brod: *The Edgar Cayce Handbook for Health through Drugless Therapy* (New York: Macmillan, 1975).

Rodale, J. I., and staff: *The Complete Book of Minerals for Health* (Emmaus, PA: Rodale Books, 1977).

————: *Sugar the Curse of Civilization* (Emmaus, PA: Rodale Press, 1954).

Root, Leon, and Thomas Kiernan: *Oh, My Aching Back* (New York: New American Library, 1975).

Rosenberg, Harold, and A. N. Feldzamen: *The Book of Vitamin Therapy* (New York: Berkeley Publ. Corp., 1975).

Rudolph, Charles, Jr.: *Trace Element Patterning in Degenerative Disease* (Houston, TX: reprinted from the *Journal of the International Academy of Preventative Medicine*, 1977).

Saleeby, C. W.: *Sunlight and Health* (London: Nisbet & Co., 1923).

Samuels, Mike, and Nancy Samuels: *The Well Baby Book* (New York: Summit Books, 1979).

Saxon, Edgar J.: *Why Aluminum Pans Are Dangerous* (Essex, England: The C. W. Daniel Co., 1939).

School of Natural Healing (Provo, UT: BiWorld Publishers, 1976).

Scott, Cyril: *Health, Diet and Common Sense* (London: The Homeopathic Publishing Co., Ltd., 1944).

————: *Doctors, Disease and Health* (London: Methuen & Co., 1938).

Shelton, Herbert M.: *The Hygienic System, Volume II Orthotrophy* (San Antonio, TX: Dr. Shelton's Health School, 1935).

Sherman, John A., compiler: *The Complete Botanical Prescriber* (for the National College of Naturopathic Medicine; toxicology section by Bruce Canvasser, 1979).

Shook, Edward E.: *Advanced Treatise on Herbology* (Mokelumne Hill, CA: Health Research, 1974).

Smith, Lendon: *Feed Your Kids Right* (New York: McGraw-Hill, 1979; Delta Publ., 1979).

————: *Feed Yourself Right* (New York: McGraw-Hill, 1983).

Sneddon, J. Russell: *The Nature Cure Treatment of Varicose Veins and Ulcers* (Wellingborough, Northamptonshire, England: Thorsons Publishers, Ltd., 1950).

Some Unrecognized Factors in Medicine, 2d ed. (London: Theosophical Publishing House, Ltd., 1949).

Spoerke, David, Jr.: *Herbal Medications* (Santa Barbara, CA: Woodbridge Press Publishing Co., 1980).

Steiner, Rudolf, and Ita Wegman: *Fundamentals of Therapy* (London: Rudolph Steiner Press, 1925).

Stoddard, Alan: *Manual of Osteopathic Practice* (London: Hutchinson, 1969).

————: *Manual of Osteopathic Technique* (London: Hutchinson & Co., 1959).

Stone, Irwin: *The Healing Factor "Vitamin C" against Disease* (New York: Grosset & Dunlap, 1972).

Textbook of Medical Treatment (London: Churchill Livingstone, 1979).

The Atomidine Story (Virginia Beach, VA: Heritage Publications, 1978).

The Edgar Cayce Products, Ten Years of Research (Virginia Beach, VA: Heritage Publications).

The Encyclopedia of Common Diseases, by the staff of Prevention Magazine (Emmaus, PA: Rodale Press, 1976).

The Merck Manual of Diagnosis and Therapy (Rahway, NJ: Merck Sharp & Dohme Research Laboratories, 1982).

Thomas, Judith: *Fluoride and Its Effects on the Human Body* (London: Unpublished, 1982).

Tierra, Michael: *The Way of Herbs* (Mill Valley, CA: Unity Press, 1980).

Tilden, J. H.: *Impaired Health, Its Cause and Cure*, vol. 2 (Denver, CO).

Timms, Moira, and Zachariah Zar: *Natural Sources: Vitamin B–17/Laetril* (Celestial Arts, 1978).

Tissue Mineral Analysis (Phoenix, AZ: ARL Analytical Research Labs, Inc., 1977).

Tobe, John H.: *Milk: Friend or Fiend?* (Wichita Falls, TX: Foundation Publ., 1963).

————: *Cataract, Glaucoma and Other Eye Disorders: Prevention and Cure with Proven Natural Methods* (Ontario, Canada: John H. Tobe, 1973).

Tomlinson, H.: *Aluminum Utensils and Disease* (London: L. N. Fowler, 1967).

Turner, James S.: *The Chemical Feast* (New York: Grossman Publ., 1970).

Turner, R. Newman: *Self-Help for Gall-bladder Troubles* (Wellingborough, Northamptonshire, Thorsons Publ., Ltd., 1977).

Tyler, Varro, Lynn Brady, and James Robbers: *Pharmacognosy* (Philadelphia: Lea & Febinger, 1981).

Vithoulkas, George: *The Science of Homeopathy* (New York: Grove Press, 1980).

————: *Homeopathy: Medicine of the New Man* (New York: Avon Books, 1971).

Vogel, A.: *The Nature Doctor* (Teufen, Switzerland: Verlag A. Vogel, 1977).

Wagner, Frederick: *Popular Methods of Natural Healing* (Mexico City: "El Sobre Azul," 1940).

Waldbott, George: *Fluoridation: The Great Dilemma* (Lawrence, KS: Coronado Press, 1978).

Wale, J. O.: *Tidy's Massage and Remedial Exercises in Medical and Surgical Conditions* (Baltimore: The Williams & Wilkins Co., 1968).

Warmbrand, Max: *The Encyclopedia of Natural Health* (New York: Groton Press, 1962).

Weiner, Michael: *Weiner's Herbal* (New York: Stein and Day, 1980).

Weiner, Michael A.: *Earth Medicine-Earth Foods* (London: Collier-Macmillan, Ltd., 1974).

Whitehouse, Geoffrey T.: *Everywoman's Guide to Natural Health* (Wellingborough, Northamptonshire, England: Thorsons Publishers, Ltd., 1974).

Williams, Roger J.: *Nutrition against Disease* (New York: Bantam Books, 1973).

————, and Dwight K. Kalita, eds.: A Physician's Handbook on Orthomolecular Medicine (New York: Pergamon Press, 1977).

Useful Prescriptions, compiled by Cloyce Wilson (Cincinnati, OH: Lloyd Brothers Pharmacists, 1935).

Wilson, Frank: *Food for the Golden Age* (Essex, England: The C. W. Daniel Co., Ltd., 1954).

Wolfram, E.: *The Occult Causes of Disease* (London: Rider & Co., 1911).

Wright, Jonathan V.: *Dr. Wright's Book of Nutritional Therapy* (Emmaus, PA: Rodale Press, 1979).

Yudkin, John: *Pure White and Deadly* (Great Britain, 1972).

zur Linden, Wilhelm: *A Child Is Born* (London: Rudolf Steiner Press, 1973).

Index